Manual of Trauma and Emergency Surgery

Manual of Trauma and Emergency Surgery

David V. Shatz, M.D., F.A.C.S.
Associate Professor of Surgery
University of Miami School of Medicine
Miami, Florida

Orlando C. Kirton, M.D., F.A.C.S., F.C.C.M., F.C.C.P.
Associate Professor of Surgery
University of Connecticut School of Medicine
Farmington, Connecticut

Mark G. McKenney, M.D., F.A.C.S.
Associate Professor of Surgery
University of Miami School of Medicine
Miami, Florida

Joseph M. Civetta, M.D., F.A.C.S.
Professor and Chairman, Department of Surgery
University of Connecticut School of Medicine
Farmington, Connecticut

W.B. SAUNDERS COMPANY
A Division of Harcourt Brace & Company
Philadelphia   London   Sydney   Toronto

W.B. SAUNDERS COMPANY
A Division of Harcourt Brace & Company

The Curtis Center
Independence Square West
Philadelphia, Pennsylvania 19106

Library of Congress Cataloging-in-Publication Data

Manual of trauma and emergency surgery / David V. Shatz . . . [et al.].—1st ed.

p.   cm.

ISBN 0–7216–6437–7

1. Wounds and injuries—Surgery Handbooks, manuals, etc.   2. Surgical
   emergencies Handbooks, manuals, etc.   I. Shatz, David V.
   [DNLM: 1. Wounds and Injuries.   2. Emergencies.   3. Emergency
   Medicine.   4. Surgical Procedures, Operative.   WO 700 T7743 2000]

RD93.T673 2000   617.1—dc21

DNLM/DLC   99–22699

Manual of Trauma and Emergency Surgery   ISBN 0–7216–6437–7

Printed in the United States of America.

Last digit is the print number: 9   8   7   6   5   4   3   2   1

Contributors

John H. Armstrong, M.D.
Assistant Professor of Surgery,
 Walter Reed Army Medical Center,
 Uniformed Services University of
 the Health Sciences, Washington,
 D.C.
*Resuscitative and Emergent Diagnostic
 Procedures*
Resuscitation of the Burn Patient

Erik S. Barquist, M.D.
Assistant Professor of Surgery,
 University of Miami School of
 Medicine, Miami, Florida
Penetrating Trauma of the Extremity

Ivo C. Baux, M.D.
Attending Anesthesiologist, West
 Boca Medical Center, Boca Raton,
 Florida
Emergency Airway Management

Joseph M. Civetta, M.D., F.A.C.S.
Professor and Chairman,
 Department of Surgery, University
 of Connecticut School of Medicine,
 Farmington, Connecticut

Ray P. Compton, M.D.
Assistant Professor of Surgery, East
 Tennessee State University, James
 H. Quillen College of Medicine,
 Johnson City, Tennessee
Penetrating Neck Injuries

Matthew O. Dolich, M.D.
Assistant Professor of Surgery,
 University of Arizona College of
 Medicine, Arizona Health Sciences
 Center, Tucson, Arizona
Acute Gastrointestinal Hemorrhage

John J. Hong, M.D.
Assistant Professor of Surgery and
 Anesthesiology, St. Louis University
 School of Medicine, St. Louis,
 Missouri
Intestinal Obstruction

Dimiter B. Hristov, M.D.
Attending Trauma Surgeon, St.
 Mary's Hospital, West Palm Beach,
 Florida
Abdominal Vascular Emergencies

Omar F. Jimenez, M.D.
Senior Resident, Neurosurgery,
 University of Miami School of
 Medicine, Miami, Florida
Traumatic Brain Injury
Acute Injury to the Spinal Cord

**Orlando C. Kirton, M.D., F.A.C.S.,
F.C.C.M., F.C.C.P.**
Associate Professor of Surgery,
 University of Connecticut School
 of Medicine, Farmington,
 Connecticut
Blunt Thoracic Trauma
Blunt Abdominal Trauma
Blunt Genitourinary Trauma

Tammy R. Kopelman, M.D.
Associate Director of Trauma,
 Greenville Memorial Hospital,
 Greenville, South Carolina
Antibiotics

**Allan D. Levi, M.D., Ph.D.,
F.R.C.S.(C)**
Assistant Professor of Neurosurgery,
 University of Miami School of
 Medicine, Miami, Florida
Acute Injury to the Spinal Cord

Mark G. McKenney, M.D., F.A.C.S.
Associate Professor of Surgery, University of Miami School of Medicine, Miami, Florida
Penetrating Neck Injuries
Penetrating Trauma of the Extremity
Penetrating Chest Trauma

Nicholas Namias, M.D.
Assistant Professor of Surgery, University of Miami School of Medicine, Miami, Florida
Penetrating Injuries to the Precordium

J. Martin Perez, M.D.
Assistant Professor of Surgery, State University of New York at Stony Brook, Stony Brook, New York
Approach to the Acute Abdomen

Jon Christian Schauer, M.D.
Attending Anesthesiologist, Boca Raton Community Hospital, Boca Raton, Florida
Emergency Airway Management

Christopher K. Senkowski, M.D.
Attending Trauma Surgeon, Memorial Medical Center, Savannah, Georgia
Trauma Triage

David V. Shatz, M.D., F.A.C.S.
Associate Professor of Surgery, University of Miami School of Medicine, Miami, Florida
Crush Injuries
Organ Injury Scoring Systems
Pelvic Fractures
Penetrating Abdominal Trauma
Rib Fractures and Hypoxemia

Sydney J. Vail, M.D.
Assistant Director of Trauma, Carilion Roanoke Memorial Hospital, Roanoke, Virginia
Rectal Trauma

Philip A. Villanueva, M.D.
Associate Professor of Neurosurgery, University of Miami School of Medicine, Miami, Florida
Traumatic Brain Injury

Preface

Trauma accounts for more years of life lost in the United States than cancer and heart disease combined. The costs of long-term disability are astounding. To effect the best possible outcome, the severely injured patient requires aggressive and rapid intervention. This manual is designed to provide the practitioner with a rapid reference and an algorithmic approach to the initial therapy of specific injuries. It includes the acute therapy required beyond the initial resuscitation. Detailed text discussing the approach is provided for further reference.

Since patients are individuals, their care must be considered in this regard and in relation to their injuries. Treatment algorithms contribute to expedited care and help to minimize omission of details, but they are not absolute rules. Diagnostic and treatment options also vary among institutions and are often tailored based on local resources. Deviation from established protocols must be done with caution and well-reasoned justification. The treatment algorithms presented in this text should therefore be tailored to institutional resources, but close adherence to their recommendations is stressed.

Contents

Chapter 1

Trauma Triage

TRIAGE SCORING SYSTEMS

Triage is the separation or categorization of patients based on the need for medical attention and the possibility of survival given a specific and limited amount of medical resources. The term triage is of French origin and derives from the verb *trier*, meaning to sort, to pick, or to cull.[1]

The foundation of modern triage rests on the development and implementation of a reliable scoring system. In its simplest form, a trauma triage scoring system must satisfy the three R's: It must get the *right* patient to the *right* hospital at the *right* time. At face value this concept seems clear and basic. However, the creation of such a system contains many challenges. What follows is a discussion of the current trauma severity scoring systems, including their strengths, weaknesses, and applicability.

Glasgow Coma Scale

Developed in 1974 by Teasdale and Jennett[2] from the University of Glasgow, Scotland, the Glasgow Coma Scale (GCS) was the first attempt to quantify the severity of head injury. The scale includes assessment of three variables (Table 1–1). It is used as an initial assessment tool and also in continual reevaluation of head-injured patients. The strength of this system lies in the fact that it reliably predicts outcome for patients with both diffuse and focal lesions. Note that pupillary evaluation is not included in the score because it is not a measure of consciousness.

Trauma Score and Revised Trauma Score

In 1981, Champion and colleagues[3] published the trauma score (TS) as a system for field triage. It was found to predict survival outcome accurately in patients with both blunt and penetrating injuries.[4] Additionally, it was shown to have strong inter-rater reliability.[5] The TS includes five variables: GCS, respiratory rate, respiratory expansion, systolic blood pressure, and capillary refill. In 1989, the same authors reevaluated their system and created the revised trauma score (RTS).[6] In this system, capillary refill and respiratory expansion were dropped because these were often difficult to assess in the field (particularly at night) and had a wide margin of interpretation. There were also concerns that the TS underestimated the severity of head injury in certain instances. The RTS defines three variables: GCS, respiratory rate, and systolic blood pressure. A coded value ranging from 0 to 4 is assigned for each variable (Table 1–2). From these three coded values a score is generated. Heart rate is

Triage Algorithm

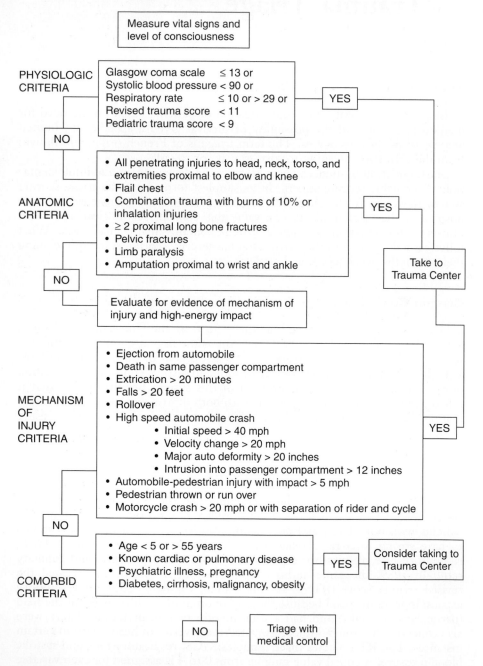

Measure vital signs and level of consciousness

PHYSIOLOGIC CRITERIA

Glasgow coma scale ≤ 13 or
Systolic blood pressure < 90 or
Respiratory rate ≤ 10 or > 29 or
Revised trauma score < 11
Pediatric trauma score < 9

YES

NO

ANATOMIC CRITERIA

- All penetrating injuries to head, neck, torso, and extremities proximal to elbow and knee
- Flail chest
- Combination trauma with burns of 10% or inhalation injuries
- ≥ 2 proximal long bone fractures
- Pelvic fractures
- Limb paralysis
- Amputation proximal to wrist and ankle

YES

NO

Take to Trauma Center

Evaluate for evidence of mechanism of injury and high-energy impact

MECHANISM OF INJURY CRITERIA

- Ejection from automobile
- Death in same passenger compartment
- Extrication > 20 minutes
- Falls > 20 feet
- Rollover
- High speed automobile crash
  - Initial speed > 40 mph
  - Velocity change > 20 mph
  - Major auto deformity > 20 inches
  - Intrusion into passenger compartment > 12 inches
- Automobile-pedestrian injury with impact > 5 mph
- Pedestrian thrown or run over
- Motorcycle crash > 20 mph or with separation of rider and cycle

YES

NO

COMORBID CRITERIA

- Age < 5 or > 55 years
- Known cardiac or pulmonary disease
- Psychiatric illness, pregnancy
- Diabetes, cirrhosis, malignancy, obesity

YES

Consider taking to Trauma Center

NO

Triage with medical control

Table 1–1. Glasgow Coma Scale

Best Motor Response	M Score	Best Verbal Response	V Score	Eye Opening	E Score
Moves limb to command	6	Oriented	5	Spontaneous	4
Localizes to painful stimulus	5	Confused	4	Open to speech	3
Withdraws from painful stimulus	4	Inappropriate words	3	Open to pain	2
Abnormal flexion response	3	Incomprehensible words	2	None	1
Abnormal extension response	2	No verbal response	1		
No motor response	1				

GCS = M score + V score + E score

Severe injury GCS less than 8
Moderate injury GCS 9 to 12
Minor injury GCS 13 to 15

not a predictive variable. An RTS score can range from 0 to 12 with the lower scores representing increasing severity.

The decision to transfer a patient to a trauma center based on an RTS of 11 or less provides a specificity of 82% while maintaining a sensitivity of 59%. Mortality related to RTS is presented in Table 1–3.

Injury Severity Scale

The injury severity scale (ISS)[7] was created to define the severity of injury for comparative purposes. It is not a field triage system. The ISS is most useful in providing researchers a method of controlling the variability of trauma severity in the evaluation of outcome. Before this system was developed it was exceedingly difficult for surgeons to judge the efficacy of treatment of trauma victims.

The strength of this system lies in the fact that it incorporates anatomic indices as well as severity indices. The authors began by grouping patients according to injury severity using the abbreviated injury scale (AIS).[8] The AIS

Table 1–2. Revised Trauma Score

Coded Value	Glasgow Coma Scale	Systolic Blood Pressure	Respiratory Rate
4	13–15	>89	10–29
3	9–12	76–89	>29
2	6–8	50–75	6–9
1	4–5	1–49	1–5
0	3		

Table 1–3. Predicting Mortality with Revised Trauma Score (RTS)

RTS	% Mortality
12	<1
10	12
8	33
6	37
4	66
2	70
0	>99

was developed in 1974 by the AMA committee on Medical Aspects of Automotive Safety. This committee defined nine categories of severity for several anatomic areas, of which five are applicable to ISS. The five categories are presented in (Table 1–4). Next, the levels of injury are described by anatomic area (general, head and neck, chest, abdomen, extremity). An example is provided in Table 1–5.

Baker and associates[7] evaluated 2128 victims of motor vehicle crashes during a 2-year period in Baltimore. For each patient the anatomic areas with the highest AIS scores were tabulated. In analyzing these data a nonlinear relationship became apparent, in that mortality was found to increase disproportionately with the AIS rating of the most severe grade. The best correlation was achieved by taking the sum of the squares of the three highest AIS scores. Thus, the ISS is calculated by using the AIS to determine the three anatomic sites of severest injury and then squaring the AIS score of each and taking the sum.

The ISS has become an excellent method of predicting injury severity and mortality.[9] Importantly, age has a significant effect on the ISS/mortality curve (Fig. 1–1). The strengths of the ISS are its ability to integrate the anatomic areas of injury in formulating a prediction of outcome. An ISS of 16 or more has been shown to be associated with a mortality of 10% in a review of 24,192 patients.[10] Therefore, any patient with an ISS of 16 or more should certainly be treated in a trauma center. However, the ISS is not a prehospital triage tool. Often the extent of injury, and thus the ISS, cannot be truly calculated until an operation or extensive diagnostic testing procedure has been performed. The strength of ISS becomes apparent in retrospective analysis of treatment quality, treatment effectiveness, and triage accuracy.[11]

Table 1–4. Abbreviated Injury Scale

AIS Value	Injury Severity
0	No injury
1	Minor
2	Moderate
3	Severe (not life-threatening)
4	Severe (life-threatening, survival probable)
5	Critical (survival uncertain)

Table 1–5. Abbreviated Injury Scale Classification for Abdominal Injury

AIS Value	Description	Examples
0	No injury	None
1	Mild	Muscle ache, seatbelt abrasion
2	Moderate	Major contusion of abdominal wall
3	Severe (not life-threatening)	Abdominal organ contusion, bladder rupture, ureter avulsion, lumbosacral spine fracture without neurologic signs
4	Severe (not life-threatening, survival probable)	Minor laceration of abdominal organ, ruptured spleen, spinal fracture with neurologic signs
5	Critical (survival unclear)	Rupture, avulsion, or laceration of abdominal organs or vessels except spleen, kidney, or ureter

Pediatric Trauma Score

The most frequent cause of death in the American pediatric population is trauma.[12] Most field triage tools are not applicable to pediatric trauma victims. For example, normal respiratory rate, heart rate, and systolic blood pressure vary considerably in infancy and childhood. Additionally, the verbal response as used in the GCS is obviously inaccurate for children. For these reasons, Tepas and colleagues created the pediatric trauma score (PTS).[13] Six variables are included in their scale (Table 1–6). Each variable is scored +2 for minimal or no injury, +1 for minor or potentially major injury, or −1 for major or life-threatening injury. The total score ranges from +12 for minimal or no injuries to −6 for very severe injuries.

TRISS

Combining the anatomic criteria of the ISS with the physiologic criteria of the RTS led to the "TRISS method" for analyzing trauma data.[14] Using logistic regression analysis, the TRISS method correlates the RTS with the ISS to create an S_{50} isobar on which a 50% survival rate is predicted.[15] Patients can

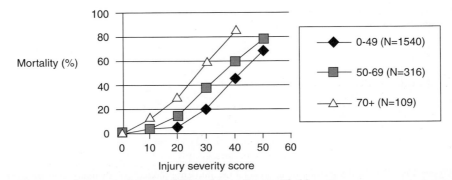

Figure 1–1. Injury severity score (ISS) and mortality stratified by age.

Table 1–6. Pediatric Trauma Score

Component	Category		
	+2	**+1**	**−1**
Size	≥ 20 kg	10–20 kg	< 10 kg
Airway	Normal	Maintainable	Unmaintainable
Systolic BP	≤ 90 mmHg	90–50 mmHg	< 50 mmHg
CNS	Awake	Obtunded, LOC	Coma or decerebrate state
Open wound	None	Minor	Major or penetrating
Skeletal	None	Closed fracture	Open/multiple fracture

Abbreviations: BP, blood pressure; CNS, central nervous system; LOC, loss of consciousness

then be plotted on the RTS vs. ISS graph (Fig. 1–2). With the isobar in place, survivors that fall above the isobar (unexpected survivors) and deaths that fall below the isobar (unexpected deaths) can be identified. It must be kept in mind that the 50% survivor cutoff rate is arbitrary and merely provides a method for isolating outlying cases in a particular series. These cases must then be analyzed on an individual basis. For example, a patient with a 55% chance of survival as predicted by TRISS who dies will appear as a preventable death when, in fact, that death may not have been preventable.

The TRISS methodology has been widely used in institutional internal quality assurance programs, for testing the efficacy of new protocols, and for evaluating outcome among different treatment centers.[16–18]

OVERTRIAGE AND UNDERTRIAGE

Overtriage is defined as the number of patients with minor injuries who are transported to a specialized trauma center. It can also be conceptualized as an

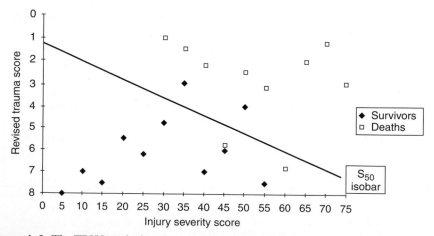

Figure 1–2. The TRISS method or the revised trauma score plotted against injury severity score (ISS) to predict mortality.

equation: overtriage = 1 − specificity. Undertriage is defined as the number of patients with severe injuries who are inappropriately sent to nontrauma centers. It can also be represented by the equation: Undertriage = 1 − sensitivity. There is general agreement that efforts to limit undertriage to less than 5% to 10% at the expense of increased overtriage is desirable.[19, 20] The American College of Surgeons (ACS) committee on trauma estimated that an overtriage rate of 50% would provide acceptable sensitivity and minimal undertriage.[21]

The adverse effects of undertriage are obvious: patients with severe injuries who do not arrive at designated trauma centers have increased morbidity and mortality. The adverse effects of overtriage include overburdening a specialized center with patients who do not need the resources, which is expensive and fatiguing for the hospital and staff.

The ACS algorithm shown at the beginning of this chapter provides a plan to direct the flow of trauma patients from the field so that undertriage rates are minimized and in-hospital systems can be constructed to lessen overtriage rates.

DISASTER MANAGEMENT

Disaster planning is hospital and region specific. The plan should be clear cut, and roles should be carefully defined and treatment areas known.[22] Mock disaster trials should be conducted regularly. When a real disaster arrives it brings chaos; there is no time to read a manual.

Triage should occur at three levels: (1) at the scene, (2) at the hospital, and (3) in treatment resuscitation areas. *At the scene* patients with the severest injuries and a chance for survival are transported first. Mental preparation is necessary for the physician to be able to leave those who are unlikely to survive for later transport. If possible, an experienced doctor should be dispatched to perform triage at the scene. *At the hospital* a senior physician again should be in charge of triage. *In treatment resuscitation areas* triage is fine-tuned in preparation for surgical intervention or intensive care unit admission.

The International Committee of the Red Cross recommends three levels of triage categories in disaster situations (Table 1–7).[23] Marking patients at the scene and at the hospital is essential in organizing the triage priorities in situations with mass casualties. One method of doing this is to mark the patients' foreheads with indelible ink.[23] This system is straightforward and clear but risks individual over- or undertriage and a reluctance to change a patient's category level once marked. For this reason, a single physician or small team should be in charge of all marking. Remember, triage is a continuous process and requires constant reevaluation. Patients who were initially

---

Table 1–7. International Committee of the Red Cross Triage Categories

I. Highest priority for surgery
II. Lowest priority because wounds are so severe patient will almost certainly die (only analgesics are given)
III. Safe to wait for surgery

categorized as Category III (need attention but can wait) may become much worse suddenly and change to Category I patients. Importantly, hopeless Category II patients sometimes survive beyond the expected time period and may then need reevaluation for treatment.

Plans for receiving victims at the treatment center must be prepared in advance. Without a plan chaos will be the inevitable result. A number of different types of victims can be expected to arrive at the hospital after a disaster.[24] In addition to severely injured patients arriving by medical transport, other vicitms with (both severe and minor injuries) arrive transported by friends or family. The "walking wounded" arrive later depending on the proximity of the hospital to the scene. A significant number of psychologically traumatized patients can be expected among this group. Finally, many community members arrive to volunteer help. While it is wrong to turn these people away, a plan must exist to identify this group of volunteers and distribute tasks to them while not distracting personnel from receiving the injured.

At the hospital receiving center different physical areas must be designated for the different needs of the disaster victims. An area designed for primary resuscitation (usually the emergency room [ER] proper) with ready access to operating room or intensive care unit should be located well away from the entrance. Ample basic supplies (intravenous fluids, dressings, and so on) should be available.[22] A separate area for the walking wounded should be created away from the path to the main resuscitation room. In this area, nurses and volunteer help can administer tetanus prophylaxis and dress minor wounds. Psychologically traumatized victims also belong in this group, and therefore it is advantageous to have appropriately trained staff available to treat these victims. Another area should be provided for the dead and for relatives of the dead to mourn.

SPECIAL SITUATIONS

Radiation Exposure

In a disaster in which significant ionizing radiation exposure has occurred, containment of contamination is added to the triage protocol.[24] Movements of patients and staff must be regulated clearly and in specific ways. Clothing must be collected and properly isolated. Radiation injuries to the central nervous system, gastrointestinal system, and hematologic system are difficult to judge in the initial triage process. The standard Advanced Trauma Life Support (ATLS) evaluation protocol for concomitant blunt or penetrating injuries should proceed expeditiously because those patients who require surgery are likely to do better with prompt intervention before the immunosuppressive effects of radiation emerge.

Hazardous Materials

Disasters involving hazardous materials can pose risks to caregivers if the material is not contained. The response to a hazardous material disaster is twofold: (1) to assess, triage, and attend to the victims, and (2) to deal with control of the hazardous material itself (i.e., stop the leak, control the spill, prevent explosions, and clean the site). Principles of management of such a disaster include removing all clothing and washing the victims. Thus decontamination stations with bags for clothes and showers at the treatment center are advised. Often medical cargivers do not know what the hazardous material is, and therefore they must take universal barrier precautions. The ABCs of trauma care are no different in these situations. Special attention, however, should be directed toward detecting inhalation injuries, chemical burn injuries, and possible toxic side effects such as depressed mental status or suppressed myocardial function.[25] The physiologic effects of chemical substances can easily fill a textbook. When the material is identified, its specific effects must be determined.

Biologic Disaster

With increasing terrorist threats worldwide, the possibility of biologic warfare exists. In these situations, decontamination centers with showers should be set up outside the treatment facility and all access to treatment must be routed through this area to the point of barricading all other doors. Protection of personnel and the treatment environment takes precedence over all else.[26]

References

1. Harper Collins French Dictionary. Harper Collins, 1990.
2. Teasdale G, Jennett B: Assessment of coma and impaired consciousness: A practical scale. Lancet 1974;2:81.
3. Champion HR, Sacco WJ, Carnazzo AJ, et al: The trauma score. Crit Care Med 1981;9:672.
4. Sacco WJ, Champion HR, Gainer P, et al: The trauma score as applied to penetrating trauma. Ann Emerg Med 1984;13:415.
5. Moreau M, Gainer PS, Champion HR, et al: Application of the trauma score in the prehospital setting. Ann Emerg Med 1981;14:1049.
6. Champion HR, Sacco WJ, Copes WS, et al: A revision of the trauma score. J Trauma 1989;29(5):623.
7. Baker SP, O'Neill B, Haddon W, et al: The injury severity score: A method for describing patients with multiple injuries and evaluating emergency care. J Trauma 1974;14(3):187.
8. American Medical Association, Committee on Medical Aspects of Automotive Safety: Rating the severity of tissue damage: The abbreviated scale. JAMA 1971;215(2):277.
9. Trunkey D: Panel: Current status of trauma severity indices. J Trauma 1983;23(3):185.
10. Champion HR, Frey CF: Report on the Major Trauma Outcome Study. Presented at the American College of Surgeons, Committee on Trauma. Chicago, American College of Surgeons, 1986.
11. Trunkey DD: Overview of trauma. Surg Clin North Am 1982;62(1):3.
12. Haller JR: Pediatric trauma: The number 1 killer of children. JAMA 1983;249:47.
13. Tepas JJ, Mollitt DL, Talbert JL, et al: The pediatric trauma score as a predictor of injury severity in the injured child. J Pediatr Surg 1987;22:14.
14. Champion HR, Sacco WJ, Hunt TK: Trauma severity scoring to predict mortality. World J Surg 1983;7:4.
15. Boyd CR, Tolson MA, Copes WS: Evaluating trauma care: The TRISS method. J Trauma 1987;27(4).
16. Cales RH: Injury severity determination: Requirements, approaches, and applications. Ann Emerg Med 1986;15(12):1427.
17. Hoyt DB, Hollingsworth-Fridlund P, Winchell RJ, et al: Analysis of recurrent process errors

leading to provider-related complications on an organized trauma service: Directions for care improvement. J Trauma 1994;36(3):377.

18. Bensard DD, McIntyre RC, Moore EE, et al: A critical analysis of acutely injured children managed in an adult level I trauma center. J Pediatric Surg 1994;29(1):11.
19. Knudson P, Frecceri CA, DeLateur SA: Improving the field triage of major trauma victims. J Trauma 1988;28(5):602.
20. Esposito TJ, Offner PJ, Jurkovich GJ, et al: Do prehospital trauma center triage criteria identify major trauma victims? Arch Surg 1995;130:171.
21. American College of Surgeons, Committee on Trauma: Resources for Optimal Care of the Injured Patient. Chicago, American College of Surgeons, 1993.
22. Coupland RM, Parker PJ, Gray RC: Triage of war wounded: The experience of the International Committee of the Red Cross. Injury 1992;23(8):507.
23. Gray R: Surgery of war and disaster. Tropical Doc 1991;21 (Suppl 1):56.
24. Yates DW: Major disasters: Surgical triage. Br J Hosp Med 1979;22(4):323.
25. Courbil LJ: Les agents vulnérants. Soins 1984;443/444:5.
26. Leonard RB: Hazardous materials accidents: Initial scene assessment and patient care. Aviat Space Environ Med 1993;64:546.

Chapter 2

Emergency Airway Management

Airway management is the first and perhaps the most important responsibility of the resuscitation team. During the initial assessment the team must quickly determine the patency of the airway, and this is done by asking the patient to speak. The ability to speak practically ensures a patent airway and also confirms the ability to breathe. If the patient is unresponsive but shows evidence of appropriate respiratory effort resulting in adequate ventilation and oxygenation (as confirmed by inspection, auscultation, and pulse oximetry), there is time to formulate a plan for airway management. If the patient is unconscious or not breathing, or if there is any question about the ability of the patient to protect the airway, endotracheal intubation should be performed emergently. Other indications for immediate intubation are included in Table 2–1.

Indications for intubation can be categorized as those showing either a need for mechanical ventilation (Table 2–1, numbers 1 to 5) or a need to protect airway patency (Table 2–1, numbers 6 to 8). Early intubation will prevent loss of the airway. Flail chest injuries are discussed further in Chapter 8.

EQUIPMENT NECESSARY FOR AIRWAY MANAGEMENT

The equipment that must be available for airway management is outlined in Table 2–2. All trauma patients are at increased risk of pulmonary aspiration of gastric contents. They are considered to have a full stomach due to presumed recent food, drug, or alcohol ingestion and also to the delayed gastric emptying that occurs in response to pain and catecholamine release. Recommended methods of securing the airway in these conditions include the following: awake intubation, rapid sequence induction with cricoid pressure, and surgical control of the airway.

The most common hypnotic agents used in trauma patients are sodium

---

Table 2–1. Indications for Intubation in the Trauma Victim

1. Shock or cardiac arrest
2. Respiratory failure (hypoxemia and/or hypercarbia)
3. Flail chest injury with respiratory compromise
4. Glasgow Coma Scale <9
5. Increased intracranial pressure (ICP)
6. Penetrating neck trauma with airway injury
7. Severe facial injuries
8. Airway or facial burns

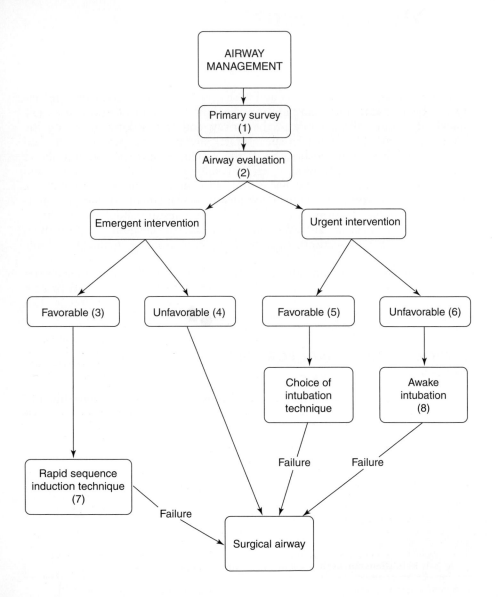

1. The urgency of airway intervention is determined during initial patient assessment.
2. The feasibility of intubation should be evaluated simultaneously. Favorable conditions include the ability to open the mouth more than three fingerbreadths, visualization of the uvula, absence of cervical spine injury, absence of facial or airway injury, and patient cooperation.[5] Unfavorable conditions include the absence of these conditions as well as morbid obesity and pregnancy.
3. In emergent situations, if the airway is considered favorable, rapid sequence induction is the method of choice. Failure of rapid sequence induction in experienced hands after two attempts indicates the need for an emergent cricothyroidotomy.
4. In emergent situations, if the airway is considered unfavorable and intubation is impossible, a cricothyroidotomy must be performed.
5. In nonemergent situations with a favorable airway, rapid sequence induction is the method of choice for intubation.
6. In nonemergent situations with an unfavorable airway or if the patient has suspected or proved cervical spine or airway injury, an awake intubation should be performed. Awake intubation using a flexible fiberoptic bronchoscope (FOB) and retrograde techniques are valuable adjuvants in these situations.
7. See Table 2-3 for pharmaceutical agents and doses. See Table 2-4 for rapid sequence induction technique.
8. Nasal or oral endotracheal intubation can be used. The fiberoptic bronchoscope may assist in placing the tube properly. Retrograde intubation can also be considered.

Table 2–2. Equipment Needed for Airway Management

1. Oxygen
2. Suction
3. Equipment for positive pressure ventilation (ambu bag)
4. Oral and nasopharyngeal airways, tongue depressor
5. Different sizes of endotracheal tubes and stylets
6. Laryngoscope with Miller and MacIntosh blades in various sizes
7. End-tidal CO_2 monitor and pulse oximetry
8. Medications: hypnotic agents and muscle relaxants
9. Alternative methods of ventilation (Combitube, laryngeal-mask airway, transtracheal jet ventilation)
10. Surgical airway kits (cricothyroidotomy and tracheostomy)

thiopental, etomidate, and ketamine. All share a rapid onset of action (arm-to-brain circulation time of about 30 seconds). Thiopental has vasodilatory and myocardial depressant effects. It should be avoided or administered in reduced doses in hypovolemic patients or those with compromised cardiac function. Thiopental and etomidate produce cerebral vasoconstriction, thus reducing cerebral blood volume and ultimately reducing intracranial pressure. They also increase the ratio of perfusion to metabolic rate by reducing the cerebral metabolic oxygen requirement. These properties make thiopental and etomidate particularly useful in the head trauma victim. The major benefit of etomidate is its cardiovascular stability. Although etomidate causes adrenocortical suppression (for up to 4 to 8 hours after an induction dose), this response has not proved to be clinically significant.

Ketamine is frequently used for induction of the trauma victim because of its catecholamine-releasing effects (which produce bronchodilation as well as elevations in blood pressure and heart rate). Side effects of ketamine include hypotension in the catecholamine-depleted patient and increases in intracranial pressure (ICP) due to its potent cerebral vasodilatory activity.

Succinylcholine is the muscle relaxant of choice for intubation of the trauma patient. It provides adequate muscle paralysis necessary for intubation within 60 seconds. Although patients with spinal cord, thermal, intracranial, or crush injuries are at increased risk for hyperkalemia and cardiac arrest after the administration of succinylcholine, this usually occurs 12 to 24 hours after injury and in general is not a concern in the acutely traumatized patient. Rocuronium is a nondepolarizing muscle relaxant that produces intubating conditions in 1 minute. It is a much longer acting drug than succinylcholine but is practically devoid of side effects. The doses for induction and muscle relaxant agents are given in Table 2–3.

TECHNIQUES FOR AIRWAY CONTROL

The most important factor in planning airway management in the trauma patient is determining the urgency of airway intervention. Other considerations include airway anatomy, potential for cervical spine injury, concomitant injuries, preexisting disease processes, patient cooperation, and physician expertise.

Table 2–3. Hypnotic and Muscle Relaxant Doses in Trauma Patients

Agents	Doses
Hypnotics	
Sodium thiopental	2–5 mg/kg
Ketamine	1–2 mg/kg
Etomidate	0.2–0.6 mg/kg
Muscle Relaxants	
Succinylcholine	1–2 mg/kg
Rocuronium	0.8–1.0 mg/kg

Rapid Sequence Induction Technique

Direct laryngoscopy with oral endotracheal intubation is the safest and most effective method of gaining immediate airway control in the trauma patient. It is usually performed after a rapid sequence induction in which a hypnotic and a muscle relaxant are given to facilitate intubation. Because trauma patients are considered to have full stomachs, cricoid pressure must be applied. This maneuver consists of temporarily occluding the upper esophagus by firmly applying pressure to compress the cricoid ring against the cervical vertebral bodies. When correctly performed, cricoid pressure seals the esophagus against intraesophageal pressures of up to 100 cm of water and is effective even in the presence of a nasogastric tube.[1] Failure of oral endotracheal intubation after induction of anesthesia requires an immediately available alternative method of ventilation. Administration of muscle relaxants for tracheal intubation should be done only by those skilled in bag-valve-mask ventilation of the lungs and in other methods of airway management. The appropriate technique for rapid sequence induction is depicted in Table 2–4.

Awake Intubation Techniques

Awake tracheal intubation reliably secures the airway but may be impractical when an emergent intubation is required in a combative patient. Awake techniques are indicated in any case when a difficult airway exists or a difficult intubation is anticipated (difficult anatomy, massive blood in the airway, full stomach, morbid obesity and so on). Some authors recommend awake intubation as the technique of choice in patients with cervical spine or airway injuries.[2]

Although they are controversial because of the risk of aspiration, airway

Table 2–4. Rapid Sequence Induction Technique

1. Equipment ready
2. Preoxygenation
3. Drugs given in rapid fashion
4. Cricoid pressure applied
5. In-line immobilization of cervical spine
6. Positive pressure ventilation avoided
7. Laryngoscopy and intubation
8. Confirmation of tracheal intubation
9. Removal of cricoid pressure

nerve blocks blunt the cough and gag reflexes when the endotracheal tube is advanced into the pharynx and larynx. These reflexes can be deleterious to a patient with increased intracranial pressure (ICP) or cervical spine fracture. Airway nerve blocks include blocks of the glossopharyngeal and superior and inferior laryngeal nerves. Aerosolized lidocaine provides topical anesthesia for the airway simply and effectively. A nebulizer and face mask is filled with 4 ml of 4% lidocaine. Ten minutes of oxygen given through this mask at 5 L/ minute provides superb topical anesthesia. Another way to provide topical anesthesia of the oral airway includes local application of spray or viscous lidocaine.

In awake nasal intubation an endotracheal tube (ETT) is inserted through the anesthetized nares, using the patient's breath sounds as a guide. Maximal breath sounds indicate close proximity of the ETT tip to the glottic opening. After expiratory breath sounds are heard, the ETT is advanced carefully through the vocal cords into the trachea. Continuous breath sounds during advancement of the ETT indicate endotracheal placement. The efficacy of this technique can be increased tremendously by using a flexible fiberoptic bronchoscope (FOB). The FOB is threaded through the endotracheal tube and guided into the trachea under direct visualization. The ETT is then advanced over the fiberoptic scope. Fiberoptic nasal intubation is particularly valuable in patients with trismus or cervical spine instability. Blind nasotracheal techniques are contraindicated in patients with possible basilar skull fracture because the ETT may traverse the fractured cribriform plate and damage brain tissue or increase the risk of meningitis in the presence of a cerebrospinal fluid leak.

Oral endotracheal intubation can also be accomplished in the awake patient by means of direct or fiberoptic laryngoscopy. A specially designed oral airway is available to assist in the performance of oral FOB intubation.

Another useful method of airway management in the trauma patient is the retrograde technique. After the cricothyroid membrane has been identified, a 16- or 18-gauge angiocatheter is inserted percutaneously. It is inserted cephalad at an angle of 45 degrees; the correct position is confirmed by aspirating air. Once this is accomplished, the catheter is advanced, and the needle is removed to decrease the risk of airway injury. A guidewire is passed through the catheter into the larynx and then advanced cephalad. The wire is visualized in the oropharynx, recovered with a clamp, and then used as a guide for the ETT tube or the FOB.

Surgical Options

Indications for taking surgical control of the airway are:

1. Inability to intubate and ventilate the patient.
2. Severe tracheal disruption.
3. Situations that make nasal or oral intubation impossible (e.g., massive facial fractures).

Surgical cricothyroidotomy is always preferred to tracheostomy in emergent situations, since the former is technically easier and quicker to perform. This surgical option must always be available even in the most routine intubation procedures (see Chapter 24).

SPECIFIC CLINICAL SITUATIONS

Cervical Spine Injury

Motor vehicle accidents cause 50% to 70% of cervical spine injuries. Ten percent of drivers in front-end collisions that occur at speeds greater than 35 mph suffer cervical spine injuries. At best, the sensitivity of plain x-ray films to rule out a cervical spine fracture is only 90%.[2] Important points are as follows:

1. If emergent intubation is required, rapid sequence induction with manual in-line immobilization of the cervical spine should be performed. In-line immobilization is applied by firmly holding the patient's head with both hands. Three points of contact should be maintained bilaterally: the second and third fingers on the zygomatic arch, the fourth and fifth fingers on the occiput, and the forearms on the chest. This allows the holder to be out of the way of the person placing the endotracheal tube. The thumbs can be used to facilitate opening the patient's mouth. This technique minimizes cervical spine movement during intubation.

2. A surgical airway is indicated if a difficult or impossible intubation is anticipated.

3. In nonemergent cases, awake fiberoptic intubation may be the method of choice to secure the airway.

Airway Injury

Airway injury can be the result of penetrating or blunt trauma to the neck. In one study, neither the zone nor the mechanism of injury correlated with the degree of difficulty of intubation.[3] There are three considerations in the airway-injured patient:

1. Intubation through a large open wound communicating with the airway can be lifesaving.

2. Blind awake intubation is discouraged because this can produce further airway damage or hematoma formation with subsequent loss of the airway.

3. It is wiser to secure the airway electively before edema compromises its patency and makes intubation impossible.

4. Direct visualization of the airway injury should be attempted to allow placement of the tip of the endotracheal tube distal to the injury.

Head Trauma

Specific considerations in the head trauma patient are:

1. Blind nasal intubation is contraindicated if a basilar skull fracture is suspected.

2. The primary concern should be to maintain adequate cerebral perfusion pressure and oxygenation.

3. During intubation, inadequate local or light general anesthesia can produce further increases in intracranial pressure.

Burns and Severe Facial Injury

Three points to keep in mind with these particular patients are:

1. In both groups, edema of the airway may become a major risk, justifying prophylactic intubation. Evidence of inhalation injury (history of closed-space fire, carbonaceous sputum, singed nasal and facial hairs) should prompt serious evaluation of the airway and early intubation.

2. In the burn patient, evidence of airway burns and possible carbon monoxide poisoning indicate a need for endotracheal intubation.

3. Succinylcholine should not be used for 24 hours in patients who have sustained a burn injury of more than 10% of the total body surface area.[4]

CONFIRMATION OF AIRWAY

After intubation of the trachea has been attempted, the correct position of the endotracheal tube is confirmed clinically by the auscultation of equal bilateral breath sounds. Detection of carbon dioxide using a disposable carbon dioxide detector can further confirm proper placement of the tube. It should be remembered that in cases of shock, little or no carbon dioxide will be exhaled. Pulse capnography can also be useful and is gaining widespread use in the prehospital setting. Ultimately, placement of every endotracheal tube should be confirmed by a chest x-ray.

References

1. Salem MR, Joseph NJ, Heyman HY, et al: Cricoid compression is effective in obliterating the esophageal lumen in the presence of a nasogastric tube. Anesthesiology 1985;63:443.
2. Hastings RH, Marks JD: Airway management for trauma patients with potential cervical spine injuries. Anesth Analg 1991;73:471.
3. Shearer VE, Giesecke AH: Airway management for patients with penetrating neck trauma: A retrospective study. Anesth Analg 1993;77:1135.
4. Furman W, Stiff J: Burn anesthesia. *In* Stene J, Grande C (eds): Trauma Anesthesia. Baltimore, Williams & Wilkins, 1991, p. 286.
5. Benumof J: Management of the difficult adult airway. Anesthesiology 1991;75:1087.

Chapter 3

Traumatic Brain Injury

EPIDEMIOLOGY

It is estimated that 1.9 million Americans suffer head injuries each year. Less than 25% of these require hospitalization. However, head injury has a significant impact on health care costs due to disability because more than half of disability days occur in patients with mild head injury. The reported rate of brain injury ranges from 132 per 100,000 to 367 per 100,000. The total estimate for 1990 included 499,265 fatal and nonhospitalized injury cases. Head injury takes a significant toll in younger people with peaks in patients in the mid to late teens and in the early to late twenties. These injuries are particularly common in large cities, where violence plays a significant role. The male-to-female ratio is 2:1. In addition, brain injury rates are inversely related to median income. Race does not appear to be a significant factor after income is considered. Traumatic brain injury can be classified as mild (61% to 84%), moderate (2% to 25%), and severe (3% to 9%).

The Glasgow Coma Scale (GCS) is a predictor of mortality. The mortality for patients with moderate head injury (GCS 8 to 12) is 12 times higher than that for mild head injury (GCS ≥13). Mortality is 100 times higher for patients with severe head injury (GCS <8).[1]

In the United States, the highest percentage of external head injury results from motor vehicle accidents (27% to 64%). Such accidents are the cause of injury in up to 70% of patients hospitalized with coma. Falls are the second most common cause, particularly in senior citizens (20% to 34%) and the very young. Gunshot wounds to the brain are more common causes of head injury in the inner city and in young adults (6% to 40%).[1]

ASSESSMENT AND THE GLASGOW COMA SCALE

The management of head injury, both penetrating and nonpenetrating, in a multitrauma patient is extremely challenging. The first priority is to follow the ABCs (airway, breathing, circulation) as outlined in the Advanced Trauma Life Support (ATLS) protocol. Early recongnition of head injury and aggressive management minimize morbidity and may be life-saving. In addition, because one must always assume the presence of a spinal fracture in a multitrauma patient, appropriate measures for immobilization should be taken. Nasotracheal intubation should be discouraged, particularly in patients with suspected basilar skull fractures, because of the possibility of penetrating the skull and the risk of meningitis. Patients with severe maxillofacial trauma may require a cricothyroidotomy; in patients younger than 12 years of age and in those with laryngeal separation, a cricothyroidotomy may be preferred instead.

Traumatic Brain Injury

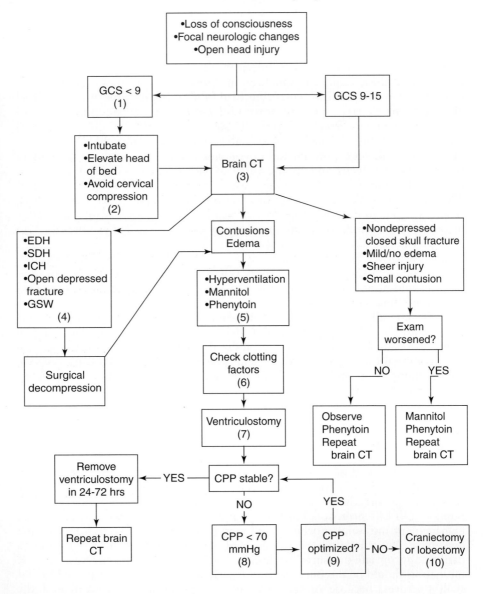

1. Neurologic assessment using the Glascow Coma Scale (GCS). In addition, proper evaluation of electrolytes and screens for alcohol and illicit drug use are essential. The patient should remain flat if the systolic blood pressure is less than 100 mmHg to optimize cerebral perfusion pressure.
2. Elevation of the head of the bed increases venous return and reduces intracranial pressure. Avoid tape or other devices that may compress the neck and decrease venous return.
3. Brain CT as well as bone windows are essential to rule out facial and skull fractures.
4. Epidural hematoma (EDH), subdural hematoma (SDH), or intracerebral hematoma (ICH) of greater than 1 cm with significant mass effect requires surgical decompression after full assessment of the patient's survivability. Depressed skull fractures of more than 1 cm or the thickness of the skull as well as open fractures and gunshot wounds require surgical decompression.
5. With signs of impending herniation, measures should be initiated to lower intracranial pressure. The quickest and easiest measure is hyperventilation, aiming for a $PaCO_2$ value of 30 to 34. Mannitol should be given at a rate of 1 g/kg over 30 minutes as an initial bolus, followed by a maintenance dose of 0.25 to 0.5 g/kg every 4 hours. Serum osmolarity must be followed and maintained between 300 and 315. Higher tonicity has no advantage and does carry a risk of renal dysfunction. Seizure prophylaxis is attained with phenytoin using a parenteral loading dose of 18 mg/kg in adults and 20 mg/kg in children. Adults should then receive a maintenance dose of 200 to 500 mg/day; this dose is 4 to 7 mg/kg in pediatric patients.
6. It is important to correct all clotting factor abnormalities to as near normal levels as possible before placing a ventriculostomy because of the potential risk of creating an intraparenchymal brain hematoma. Brain injury can also induce systemic coagulopathy through the release of tissue thromboplastin and plasminogen, both of which are abundant in brain tissue.
7. Alternatives to ventriculostomy include subdural and intraparenchymal monitors. The advantage of ventriculostomy is that cerebrospinal fluid (CSF) can be drained to lower intracranial pressures (ICP) as needed.
8. Prolonged high ICP and cerebral perfusion pressures (CPP) of less than 70 mmHg may signify severe edema and/or a space-occupying lesion (e.g., a hematoma). Brain CT should be repeated to rule out a developing surgically correctable lesion.
9. Lowering the intracranial pressure and maintaining an adequate systemic mean arterial pressure (MAP) will allow proper perfusion of the cerebral circulation ($CPP = MAP - ICP$). Methods of lowering the ICP include sedation, venting of CSF through the ventriculostomy, paralytic agents, and barbiturates. MAP may also be increased to raise CPP. Hypothermia may be considered, but this technique is considered experimental at this time.
10. Methods of increasing the space in which the brain is confined include craniectomy, which allows outward expansion, or lobectomy, which removes a less critical portion of the brain with the intent to save the more critical lobes. These procedures are very controversial and are rarely used.

Approximately 30% to 40% of patients with brain injury are hypoxic, a condition that may be difficult to identify in the acute setting.[2] It is important to obtain adequate oxygenation because hypoxia may lead to secondary brain injury. Patients who are verbalizing easily and appear to have a patent airway should not be intubated unless they show evidence of immediate compromise, either neurologic or systemic. Patients with severe head injuries who are unresponsive or agitated or have significant airway compromise, including facial trauma, require immediate intubation with in-line cervical traction.

Maintenance of adequate brain perfusion is essential to prevent secondary brain injury, particularly in the multitrauma patient who may have significant blood loss and hypovolemia. The goal of circulatory management is to maintain an adequate euvolemic state with the use of balanced or hypertonic saline, avoiding a hypo-osmolar state. A systolic blood pressure in the range of 100 to 160 mmHg is acceptable; while preventing hypertension, such a blood pressure stabilizes cerebral blood flow in a system in which cerebral autoregulation is disturbed. Vasopressor agents may be used to maintain an adequate blood pressure, and a pulmonary artery catheter may be used in patients who are hemodynamically compromised.

The first step in neurologic assessment is the evaluation of neurologic disabilty. The Glasgow Coma Scale is a means of assessing the severity of brain injury and functions as a uniform tool to reduce variability between observers. It is particularly valuable when neurologic assessment is performed prior to intubation or the use of sedative or paralytic drugs. It includes evaluation of the sensorium, eye opening, verbal response, and motor activity (Table 3–1). A GCS of 13 to 15 indicates a mild head injury, and such a patient may not require admission to the intensive care unit (ICU), although other neurologic findings and CT scans may dictate otherwise. A GCS of 9 to 12 indicates a moderate injury that has resulted from a significant insult. The possibility exists that a pathologic lesion may be present. A GCS of 8 or less signifies a severe head injury that warrants ICU admission and usually intracranial pressure (ICP) monitoring. With the addition of the brain stem examination, patient age, and mechanism of injury, the GCS can be used as a prognostic indicator for outcome.[3]

Other important aspects of assessment include differences in motor strength and right to left symmetry in the upper and lower extremities. Assessment of brain stem reflexes such as the oculovestibular, oculocephalic (once the cervical

Table 3–1. The Glasgow Coma Scale

Eye Opening	Verbal Response	Motor Response	Score
—	—	Obeys commands	6
—	Oriented	Localizes to pain	5
Spontaneous	Confused	Withdraws	4
To voice	Inappropriate words	Flexion to pain	3
To pain	Incomprehensible sounds	Extension to pain	2
None	None	None	1

A total score of 3 is the lowest score and represents the worst prognosis and highest mortality. A GCS of 8 indicates a severe head injury. A GCS of 9 to 12 indicates a moderate head injury, and a score of 13 to 15 indicates a mild head injury. The GCS is a prognostic indicator in neurologic outcome and survival.

spine has been assessed and cleared), and corneal reflexes, and respiratory patterns are important. Other important findings include a basilar skull fracture, as evidenced by a Battle's sign or raccoon's eyes, and evidence of a cerebrospinal fluid (CSF) leak.

Computed tomographic evaluation of the head is the current gold standard because of its speed and ability to delineate both intracranial and extracranial pathology. Skull x-rays, on the other hand, provide relatively little useful information about intracranial pathology, although the presence of a skull fracture, air fluid level in the sinus, pneumocephalus, or shifted calcified pineal body may suggest intracranial pathology warranting further evaluation. Skull x-rays are useful in searching for depressed skull fractures or penetrating injuries, but in general they are considered ancillary studies unless CT is not readily available. Magnetic resonance imaging (MRI) at present is not suitable for the initial assessment of head injury because of its uncertain availability and the variability of imaging techniques useful for the assessment of acute blood and bone windows.

INTRACRANIAL INJURIES

Neurologic damage following head injury is of two types: the primary injury is associated with the initial impact, and the secondary injury results from expansion of mass lesions, brain swelling, ischemia, hyperthermia, hypoxia, and hypotension. Acceleration and deceleration injuries may be seen in patients with blunt or penetrating brain trauma and may lead to coup and contracoup injuries. These result from the impact of the brain with the bony prominences and are more common in the frontal and middle fossae.

Cerebral concussions produce a brief loss of consciousness and retrograde amnesia in the absence of gross cerebral pathology and result from reticular activating and/or cortical electrophysiologic dysfunction. Intracranial hemorrhage occurs in half of head injury patients with prolonged unconsciousness.[4] Cerebral contusions consist of a mixture of damaged gray and white matter and interstitial hemorrhage appearing as a mixed-density mass lesion surrounded by a ring of low-density edema on CT scans. Acceleration and deceleration injuries can result in shearing of the subcortical white matter and can result in diffuse axonal injury, which is seen as white matter hemorrhages in the corpus collusum and cerebral peduncles.[5, 6] More violent impacts may produce brain laceration with secondary intracerebral hemorrhage. Delayed traumatic intracerebral hemorrhage occurs in up to 8% of patients who sustain significant head injury and may become manifest as late as 7 to 10 days after the injury, although the peak incidence occurs within the first 72 hours.[7, 8] Serial CT scans should therefore be considered in all patients who have significant intracranial pathology on admission, fail to improve neurologically, or exhibit neurologic deterioration.

Traumatic hemorrhage of the ventricles may result in obstructive hydrocephalus. Similarly, traumatic subarachnoid hemorrhage may cause diffuse meningeal irritation, nonfocal clouding of the sensorium, and late communicating hydrocephalus.

Subdural hematomas are the most frequently occurring type of extra-axial hemorrhage. They are termed acute, subacute, or chronic depending on the rate of progression of symptoms and the appearance of the hematoma after injury. Subdural bleeding usually results from tearing or avulsion of the bridging veins between the cortex and the dural venous sinus. Subdural hemorrhages with a significant mass effect of 1 cm or greater on the underlying cortex that show progressive neurologic deterioration should be considered surgical emergencies. Surgical decompression of these lesions within 4 hours is associated with a significant reduction in morbidity and mortality.[9]

Epidural (extradural) hematomas account for approximately 5% of intracranial hematomas and result from laceration of the middle or accessory meningeal arteries that lie within grooves of the calvaria. These vessels supply the dura and are ruptured in patients with linear skull fractures. Approximately 50% of patients with epidural hematomas give a history of a brief loss of consciousness (i.e., a concussion), followed by a lucid interval of several hours before the epidural hematoma expands sufficiently to cause deterioration in the level of consciousness. Early surgical evacuation may result in an excellent prognosis provided that irreversible brain stem compression has not occurred.[6] Extradural hematomas may also result from laceration of the dural venous sinuses. Because venous bleeding is involved, the rate of blood accumulation may be significantly slower, and symptoms may therefore appear up to 24 hours later.

PENETRATING INJURIES

The majority of penetrating injuries result from gunshot wounds and cause up to 35% of deaths from brain injuries in young adults.[10] Gunshot injuries are the most lethal type of injury because they result in tissue damage outside the actual tract of the bullet owing to kinetic energy dissipation, temporary cavitation, and shock waves in the viscoelastic neuroglial tissue.[11] Secondary injury results from shock waves of positive and negative energy oscillations that produce a conical cavitation, which is 30 to 50 times the volume of the missile. This generates a transient rise in intracranial pressure. The greater the velocity of the bullet, the worse the injury. The level of consciousness is very useful in assessing prognosis.[11] Approximately 95% of patients who are comatose on admission subsequently die. Other factors indicating a poor prognosis include a bullet trajectory that crosses the midline or passes through the center of the brain or the ventricles and evidence of a hematoma on CT.[12]

HERNIATION SYNDROMES

Because the cranial vault is only partly compartmentalized by the falx cerebri, tentorium, and foramen magnum, pressure gradients from expanding mass lesions result in anatomic compression and distortion of the brain and its supporting vasculature, leading to a herniation syndrome.[13] Delayed or progressive neurologic dysfunction may represent an ongoing dynamic process, such as an expanding hematoma or worsening cerebral edema, which heralds impending herniation. A hemispheric mass lesion, called a subfalcine herniation, may displace the medial cerebral cortex across the midline. If the distal anterior cerebral artery is trapped beneath the falx, contralateral monoplegia of the lower extremity results. A midconvexity or temporal mass lesion forces the medial temporal lobe through the tentorial incisura, resulting in an uncal herniation. This type of herniation leads to compression of the ipsilateral oculomotor nerve, resulting in pupillary dilatation and, most often, compression of the ipsilateral cerebral peduncle, causing contralateral hemiparesis. Occasionally, the entire brain stem is pushed across the tentorial incisura, pinning the opposite cerebral peduncle against its adjacent tentorial edge and resulting in ipsilateral hemiparesis (Kernohan's notch phenomenon).

Mass lesions cause progressive distortion of the upper brain stem and diencephalon, called a central herniation, which leads to progressive deterioration in neurovegetative functions. Significant distortions may cause avulsion of the brain stem vessels, resulting in catastrophic neurologic deterioration and Duret's hemorrhage of the brain stem. Mass lesions of the posterior fossa may produce cerebellar tonsillar herniation through the foramen magnum, causing signs of brain stem dysfunction such as skew deviation, respiratory and cardiovascular dysfunction, dysrhythmias, and terminal hypotension. Upward transtentorial herniation causes catastrophic strangulation of the superior cerebellar arteries, with fulminant brain stem dysfunction and bilateral pupillary dilatation resulting from compressed oculomotor nerves.[13]

SKULL FRACTURES

Skull fractures may be open or closed. They include linear, transverse, diastatic (involving a cranial suture), comminuted, and depressed. Basilar skull fractures can involve the anterior, middle, or posterior fossa. They may be associated with periorbital ecchymoses (raccoon's eyes) or mastoid ecchymoses (Battle's sign), CSF rhinorrhea, and otorrhea. Because of the risk of orbital, ethmoidal, or cribriform plate injury as well as the risk of CSF contamination, transnasal endotracheal and gastric tubes should be avoided if a basilar skull fracture is suspected. Most basilar skull fractures do not require treatment or prophylactic antibiotics. One exception is fractures through the nasal sinuses, which may be treated as an open fracture with broad-spectrum antibiotics. The criteria for surgical treatment of depressed fractures include the presence of depression of approximately 1 cm (the thickness of the skull), an associated underlying neurologic deficit, and the presence of an open fracture with evidence of a CSF leak. One exception, however, is a skull fracture overlying a dural sinus, where elevation may result in massive hemorrhage. Temporal bone fractures may be longitudinal (the most common type) and may result in hearing deficits. Transverse fractures are associated with facial and vestibulocochlear deficits.

SCALP LACERATIONS

Scalp lacerations occur very commonly in patients with head injuries and may result in significant blood loss due to the extensive supply of the scalp by five major branches from the external carotid artery. Copious irrigation and debridement of the wound followed by closure may prevent formation of a subgaleal abscess or osteomyelitis, particularly in patients with an underlying skull fracture.

INTRACRANIAL PRESSURE, VOLUME, AND BLOOD FLOW

The Monro-Kellie doctrine, proposed over 150 years ago, states that within the rigid cranial vault, the total volume of the intracranial contents remains constant. Because fluid is incompressible, mass lesions must displace blood, brain tissue, or CSF components if intracranial volume is to remain constant. Slowly growing intracranial lesions allow for volume compensation by means of decreased CSF production or displacement, atrophy of brain tissue, or decreased intravascular blood volume. Following an acute injury, however, the rapid development of space-occupying lesions and edema may outstrip the ability of the normal compensatory mechanisms to adjust, resulting in compression of brain tissue and a rise in ICP. Intracranial pressure represents the brain's resistance to cerebral perfusion pressure (CPP) and cerebral blood flow (CBF). These are related by the following equation:

$$CPP = MAP \text{ (mean arterial pressure)} - ICP$$

The ability of the brain to compensate for volume changes within the intracranial compartment is known as the pressure volume index (PVI). With progressive loss of compensatory reserves, small changes in intracranial volume can result in dramatic elevations of ICP, causing secondary derangements in CPP and CBF.

Normal ICP ranges between 10 and 15 mmHg in adults. An ICP of above 15 mmHg is considered abnormal, and intracranial hypertension is defined as a pressure above 20 mmHg.[14] Adequate cerebral perfusion pressure is critical and, in general, should be maintained at between 70 and 120 mmHg. Poor outcomes in patients with an elevated ICP reflect inadequate CPP, which results in cerebral ischemia.[15, 16]

Intracranial Pressure Monitoring

On admission to the ICU, the patient should be fully reevaluated. Assessment of the patient's vital signs, paying particular attention to signs of impending herniation or intracranial hypertension, such as an abnormal respiratory pattern (Cheyne-Stokes respirations, central neurogenic hyperventilation, ataxic apneustic respirations) or bradycardia with hypertension, should be carried out. Included in this evaluation is an assessment of the GCS score, the size and responsiveness of the pupils, and the movements of the upper and lower extremities and their comparative motor strengths. Adjunctive brain stem reflexes (eyelid, oculocephalic or oculovestibular, gag reflexes) may be assessed as the situation warrants once cervical spine stability has been assessed. Because brain edema and swelling reach their maximum levels 48 to 96 hours after injury, patients should receive at least 72 hours of neurologic monitoring. In patients with significant head trauma, follow-up CT studies should be performed 24 to 72 hours after the injury and again at 1 week post-injury, to detect the presence of occult delayed hemorrhages, particularly if hemorrhage is present on the initial CT scan.

Accepted indications for ICP monitoring include intracranial lesions that require surgical decompression postoperatively, a nonsurgical mass lesion that obstructs ventricular outflow or produces a significant mass effect on adjacent brain tissue, effacement of basal cisterns (in the presence of even a moderate head injury), a shift of the midline structures (particularly the pineal gland) of 7 mm or more, and GCS score of 8 or less. Head-injured patients requiring mechanical ventilation with elevated (>15 cm H_2O) positive end-expiratory pressures (PEEP) for treatment of pulmonary dysfunction may also require ICP monitoring. Similarly, patients who have been treated with pharamacologic paralysis for ventilatory support and a significant head injury can no longer be evaluated neurologically and may be considered for ICP monitoring, even if they have a relatively normal GCS.[17, 18]

Intracranial pressure should be monitored whenever the brain has sustained an injury that has a high likelihood of producing hemorrhage, edema, obstruction of CSF flow, or loss of cerebral autoregulation with vasodilatation, and a GCS of 8 or less on clinical examination. An intraventricular catheter connected to an external gauge remains the most accurate, cheapest, and most reliable means of monitoring ICP. It also permits CSF drainage to assist ICP control and allows assessment of brain compliance. Fluid-coupled systems that measure from the epidural, subdural, or subarachnoid space may allow CSF drainage, thus, decreasing ICP, but may not be as accurate as their intraventricular counterparts.[19] Parenchymal fiberoptic catheters are advantageous in patients with small ventricles and carry a low risk of intracranial hemorrhage. However, they are not easily recalibrated in vivo, and monitor drift may be a significant problem.[20] Daily aseptic sampling of the CSF allows it to be monitored for infection. If feasible, ICP monitors should be changed weekly (or more often if there is need for prolonged monitoring) to further decrease the risk of infection.

Increases in ICP may occur without any discernible change in GCS until a critical level is reached or brain stem distortion and dysfunction occur, when sudden, catastrophic decompensation may occur.[21] These insidious changes in ICP may occur particularly often in patients with a low GCS. ICP monitoring may detect such changes early and permit therapy to avoid further cerebral edema or neurologic deterioration.

TREATMENT OF INTRACRANIAL HYPERTENSION

Management of a patient with elevated intracranial pressure involves the use of increased jugular venous drainage, controlled hyperventilation, osmotic diuresis, CSF diversion, barbiturate administration, hypothermia, and surgical decompression. Elevation of the head increases jugular venous return and decreases intracranial pressure. Prevention of agitation, coughing, and hyperthermia and the use of anticonvulsant prophylaxis decrease cerebral metabolic demands, which aggravate ICP. The use of sedatives, analgesics, and muscle relaxants may be necessary to control muscle activity; agitation, coughing, straining, or anything that increases intra-abdominal or intrathoracic pressure may increase ICP.

Whereas intubation may prevent hypercapnia by protecting the airway, hyperventilation has an almost immediate effect in decreasing intracranial blood volume by inducing hypocarbia and cerebral vasoconstriction in those regions of the brain where autoregulation is preserved. Mild to moderate hyperventilation ($PaCO_2$ of 30 to 35 mmHg) is recommended.[22] Prolonged aggressive hyperventilation ($PaCO_2$ of 25 mmHg or less) causes severe vasoconstriction, which results in cerebral ischemia and a poor outcome.[23] However, this technique may be valuable in reducing ICP rapidly until other methods become effective.

If hyperventilation fails to decrease ICP to less than 20 mmHg, a mild diuretic can be given. Mannitol is the agent of choice. It is given in an initial bolus of 0.5 to 1.0 g/kg body weight, infused over 15 minutes, followed by 0.5 g/kg every 4 hours to maintain osmolarity at 10 to 25 mOsm above normal (300 to 315 mOsm). Osmotic diuresis helps reduce cerebral swelling by creating an osmotic gradient for interstitial brain water. The maximum effect occurs after approximately 20 minutes and lasts for 3.5 hours.[24] ICP monitoring can be used to assess the impact of therapy. Other osmotic diuretics available include 5% urea and oral glycerol. Mannitol, however, is preferred because it is associated with reduced rebound swelling. Loop diuretics may be effective in increasing osmolarity when they are administered after mannitol has been used, thus allowing a reduction in intravascular volume. It is important, however, to maintain an adequate hemodynamic state because hypotension may worsen CPP, resulting in greater secondary cerebral damage.

If the ICP remains over 20 mmHg, CSF can be vented if a ventricular catheter has been placed. Sufficient CSF is slowly removed to lower the ICP to 15 to 20 mmHg or to maintain CPP above 70 mmHg.

If the previous modalities, including sedation, use of muscle relaxants, and CSF drainage fail to reduce the ICP, and if no surgically accessible lesions are present, high-dose barbiturate therapy should be tried (barbiturate coma).[25, 26] Barbiturates reduce the cerebral metabolic rate, promote cerebral vasoconstriction, induce hypothermia, and depress cardiac output. All of these effects reduce ICP. Induction of barbiturate coma necessitates a commitment to careful monitoring because myocardial depression, hypotension, sepsis, and hypothermia may occur. ICP and arterial lines must be placed, and a pulmonary artery catheter should be used to monitor measured and calculated cardiac function. Cardiac inotropic support may be necessary in some instances. Because neurologic responses on examination may be lost at higher serum pentobarbital levels, alternative monitoring modalities must be employed; these may include serial CT scans, brain stem evoked potentials, and bedside transcranial Doppler flow studies. The electroencephalogram (EEG) is used to determine the degree of cerebral activity suppression that occurs with pentobarbital administration.

When used for control of ICP, pentobarbital is given as a loading dose of 10 mg/kg over 1 hour, followed by three doses of 5 mg/kg given over 30 minutes each. The maintenance dose is then given at 1 mg/kg/hour. The maintenance dose may be increased to 1.5 mg/kg/hour when a target serum level of 30 to 50 mg/L is obtained.[27] Occasionally, ICP may be controlled with lower doses. Once the desired serum level is obtained, further increases in dose to control ICP tend not to be effective. High-dose barbiturates have increased the number of patients with a useful recovery, but prophylactic use of the drug has not improved outcome.[28]

A successful response is defined as a reduction in ICP to 15 mmHg or less for 48 to 72 hours. Weaning from pentobarbital should be performed slowly, usually by half of the daily dose every 24 hours for 3 to 4 days, to prevent rebound intracranial hypertension. Therapeutic failure is evident by continual intracranial hypertension in the presence of maximum barbiturate therapy or the development of refractory cardiac dysfunction.

OTHER TREATMENTS

Glucocorticoids are not used in head trauma patients. Their effect has not been proved, and the resulting complications, such as hyperglycemia, immune suppression, and gastrointestinal bleeding, outweigh any potential benefit.[29–31]

Other modalities under investigation include medications such as N-methyl-D-aspartate (NMDA) antagonists and antioxidants. NMDA antagonists block the action of excitatory neurotransmitters such as aspartate and glutamate. These transmitters are released in patients with brain injury and lead to a massive influx of calcium, resulting in cell death. Antioxidants help to chelate free-radicals and other products of peroxidation that are involved in the pathophysiologic mechanisms of brain tissue destruction that take place during trauma.[32, 33]

The role of systemic moderate hypothermia (32°C) in the treatment of severe head injury is under investigation. Many laboratory and clinical investigations suggest that hypothermia results in neuroprotection, improved neurologic outcome, and reduced mortality.[34–37]

Fluid, Electrolyte, and Coagulation Abnormalities

Hyperglycemia may result from central nervous system stress responses that lead to release of growth hormone, catecholamines, and adrenal glucocorticosteriods and result in a hyperosmolar state. This state may be aggravated by the use of mannitol, which may lead to renal impairment. Hyperglycemia of greater than 150 mg/dl may lead to an increase in intracerebral lactate levels, thereby worsening the prognosis. The use of dextrose-containing fluids and hyperglycemia may increase cerebral ischemic damage in areas of brain injury.[38] Glycosuria may also cause severe hyperosmolar states, especially in association with mannitol or diabetes insipidus. Management of hyperglycemia requires frequent blood glucose checks and appropriate coverage with insulin.

Diabetes insipidus (DI) may result from injury to the pituitary stalk or hypothalamus and, in the comatose patient, may indicate a particularly poor prognosis. Decreased antidiuretic hormone (ADH) secretion results in polyuria, progressive dehydration, and a hyperosmolar state. DI may be self-limiting in patients with milder injuries. However, the persistent state is treated with desmopressin acetate, titrating the dosage against serum osmolarity, sodium levels, and urine output. Desmopressin acetate can be administered intranasally at a dose of 0.1 to 0.4 ml daily. Too rapid a correction may lead to rebound cerebral edema and elevated ICP. A safe rule is to correct 50% of the deficit over 24 hours and the remainder within 48 hours (a good method of correcting the deficit is to calculate the free water deficit [free water deficit = $0.6 \times$ usual body weight (kg) − total body water $(TBW)_{current}$]).

ADH secretion is a normal part of the body's response to stress (particularly in children). The syndrome of inappropriate secretion of ADH (SIADH) occurs frequently in patients with brain trauma and should be suspected if hyponatremia and low serum osmolarity are associated with high urine osmolarity and a high urinary sodium concentration. Because head-injured patients usually receive all their fluids intravenously, clinically significant SIADH is usually the result of excessive administration of free water to patients who cannot excrete free water because of excess ADH. In addition, atrial natriuretic peptide (ANP), which is secreted by the heart in response to stress, may mimic SIADH because it can cause urinary sodium loss with hyponatremia even in the absence of dilutional hypervolemia. Hypertonic saline solutions are required to treat a severe hyponatremic state (Na^+ <125 mEq/L). Correction of this hyponatremic state should be done cautiously by not administering a sodium dose of more than 1.3 ± 0.2 mEq/L/hour. Overzealous correction may lead to central pontine myelinolysis. This condition results in cerebral and pontine myelin loss (CPML). CPML leads to flaccid quadriplegia, mental status changes, and cranial nerve abnormalities as well as pseudobulbar palsy.

Disseminated intravascular coagulation or fibrinolysis may be seen in patients with severe brain injury. The brain has the richest supply of tissue thromboplastin, with plasminogen activity found in the dura, choroid plexus, and CSF. In patients with severe brain injury, tissue thromboplastin enters the systemic circulation, leading to a hypocoagulable state. Hypothermia may compound the effect, leading to vascular fragility, inactivation of tissue thromboxane, and poor platelet function. Treatment involves replacement of the depleted clotting factors using fresh frozen plasma (FFP). Close hematologic monitoring is warranted because of the risk of aggravating intracerebral hemorrhage or systemic bleeding complications.[39]

Seizure Prophylaxis

Antiepileptic drugs are used for seizure prophylaxis in patients with traumatic brain injury. Post-traumatic seizures can be categorized as acute or early (<24 hours), subacute (<1 week), and late onset (>1 week). Acute seizures resulting in loss of consciousness occur in 2.6% of children with traumatic brain injuries. This incidence increases to 30% in those suffering a severe traumatic brain injury (GCS of less than or equal to 8, loss of consciousness for more than 24 hours, intracerebral hemorrhage, or violation of the dura with brain laceration).[40] The incidence of late-onset epilepsy 2 years after injury is 10 to 13%.[41]

In the general population, the risk of post-traumatic epilepsy is 7.1% in the first year after a severe head injury and 11.5% at 5 years.[40] The majority of acute or early seizures occur within 24 hours, particularly in the pediatric population. Late-onset seizures are more common in adults than in children.

Many controlled studies on the effectiveness of seizure control have shown inconclusive results. However, the present recommendations are based on a randomized double-blind study of phenytoin given for prevention of post-traumatic seizures in 404 patients with serious traumatic brain injury (n = 208 for the phenytoin group and 196 for the placebo group). Patients were followed for 2 years, and their phenytoin levels were maintained in the high therapeutic range. At 7 days, 3.6% of patients treated with phenytoin had seizures, versus 14% of those given placebo. Between day 8 and 1 year, 21.5% of the phenytoin group had seizures versus 15.7 for the placebo group. At the end of 2 years, the incidence of seizures was 21.5% in the placebo group and 27.5 in the phenytoin group.[42] We therefore recommend seizure prophylaxis for the first week after a traumatic brain injury unless the injury is of the severe type as described previously. In that case, therapy may be continued for 3 to 6 months after the trauma event.

Management of late post-traumatic seizures, if they do develop, is the same as that for treatment of patients with epilepsy. Most data support a short-term course of prophylaxis; however, long-term treatment, with the attendant risks of medical and behavioral complications, has not been fully analyzed. At present we recommend follow-up with neurologic examination to optimize the treatment strategy.[43] In adults the parenteral loading dose of phenytoin is 18 mg/kg, and in children it is 20 mg/kg; the intravenous dose must be given slowly to prevent hypotension and arrhythmias (in adults <50 mg/minute, and in children <1 to 3 mg/minute). For maintenance, adults should receive 200 to 500 mg/day, and pediatric patients receive 4 to 7 mg/kg/day. Optimum serum levels range from 10 to 20 µg/ml. Fosphenytoin (Cerebryx), a pro-drug of phenytoin, has recently become available; it is reported to reduce the risk of hypotension and arrhythmias compared to phenytoin. It can be given parenterally or intramuscularly (75 mg/ml of Cerebryx = 50 mg/ml of pheny-toin). The loading dose is 15 to 20 mg phenytoin equivalents (PE)/kg at 100 to 150 mg PE/minute. The maintenance dose is 4 to 6 mgPE/kg/day.

CONCLUSION

The management of traumatic brain injury requires a multidisciplinary approach. The basic ABCs of the Advanced Trauma Life Support (ATLS) system are crucial in preventing secondary brain injury. Identifying which patients are at greatest risk of severe brain injury and maintaining a high index of suspicion for patients with associated spinal cord injury allow deliberate triage as well as aggressive management and treatment in an already compro-mised nervous system. Every minute is crucial because the prognosis of severe brain injury depends on aggressive control of intracranial pressure and decom-pression of large parenchymal, subdural, or epidural hemorrhages before herni-ation or disseminated intravascular coagulopathy dominates the clinical course. Other modalities for the treatment of secondary brain injury, including antioxidant medications and NMDA antagonists against "toxic amino acids," are under investigation. Moderate systemic hypothermia is also undergoing clinical investigation and appears to be a promising modality for providing neuroprotection and improving the neurologic outcome.

References

1. Vernberg D, Nedd K: Epidemiology of brain injury. *In* Greenberg J (ed): Handbook of Head and Spine Trauma. New York, Marcel Decker, 1993, pp. 3–13.
2. Popp AJ, Gottlieb ME, Paloski WH, et al: Cardiopulmonary hemodynamics in patients with severe head injury. J Surg Res 1982;32:416.
3. Jennett B, Teasdale G, Braakman R, Minderhound J, Heiden J, Kurze T: Prognosis of patients with severe head injury. Neurosurgery 1979;4:283.
4. Roberts JR: Pathophysiology, diagnosis and treatment of head trauma. Top Emerg Med 1979;1:41.
5. Peerless SJ, Rewcastle NB: Shear injuries to the brain. CMAJ 1967;98:577.
6. Geisler FH, Greenberg J: Management of the acute injury patient. *In* Salcman M (ed): Neurologic Emergency, 2nd ed. New York, Raven Press, 1990, p. 135.
7. Diaz GF, Yock DH, Larson D, Rockswold GL: Early diagnosis of delayed traumatic intracerebral hematoma. J Neurosurg 1979;50:217.
8. Kaufman HH, Moake JL, Olson JD, et al: Delayed and recurrent intracranial hematomas related to disseminated intravascular clotting and fibrinolysis in head injury. Neurosurgery 1980;7:445.
9. Geisler FH, Greenberg J: Management of the acute head-injury patient. *In* Salcman M (ed): Neurologic Emergency, 2nd ed. New York, Raven Press, 1990, p. 135.
10. Kaufman HH: Civilian gunshot wounds to the head. Neurosurgery 1993;32:962–964.
11. Villanueva PA: Cranial gunshot wounds. *In* Ordog G (ed): Management of Gunshot Wounds. New York, Elsevier, 1988, p. 257.
12. Greenberg M: Gunshot wounds to the head. *In* Greenberg M (ed): Handbook of Neurosurgery, 3rd ed. Orlando, Florida, Greenberg Graphics, 1994, pp. 559–562.
13. Plum F, Posner JB: The Diagnosis of Stupor and Coma, 3rd ed. Philadelphia, FA Davis, 1980.
14. Miller JD, Becker DP, Ward JD, Sullivan HG, Adams WE, Rosner MJ: Significance of intracranial hypertension in severe head injury. J Neurosurg 1977;47:501.
15. Jennett B, Teasdale G, Braakman R, Minderhound J, Knill-Jones R: Predicting outcome in individual patients after severe head injury. Lancet 1976;1:1031.
16. Rosner JM, Rosner SD, Johnson AH: Cerebral perfusion pressure: Management protocol and clinical results. J Neurosurg 1995;83:949–962.
17. Ropper AH: Lateral displacement of the brain and level of consciousness in patients with acute hemispheric mass. N Engl J Med 1986;314:953.
18. Frost EAM: Effects of positive end-expiratory pressure on intracranial pressure and compliance in brain-injured patients. J Neurosurg 1977;47:195.
19. North B, Reilly P: Comparison among three methods of intracranial pressure recording. Neurosurgery 1986;18:730–763.
20. Schickner DJ, Young RF: Intracranial pressure monitoring: Fiberoptic monitor compared with the ventricular catheter. Surg Neurol 1992;7(4):251–254.
21. Andrews BT, Chiles BW, Olsen WL, Pitts LH: The effect of intracerebral hematoma location on the risk of brainstem compression and on clinical outcome. J Neurosurg 1988;69:518.
22. Cruz J: An additional therapeutic effect of adequate hyperventilation in severe acute brain trauma: Normalization of cerebral glucose uptake. J Neurosurg 1995;82:379.
23. Muizelear JP, Marmarou A, Ward JD, et al: Adverse effects of prolonged hyperventilation in patients with severe head injury: A randomized clinical trail. J Neurosurg 1991;75:731.
24. Marshall LF, Smith RW, Rauscher LA, Shapino HM: Mannitol dose requirements in brain injured patients. J Neurosurg 1978;48:169.
25. Marshall LF, Marshall SB: Medical management of intracranial pressure. *In* Cooper PR (ed): Head Injury, 2nd ed. Baltimore, Williams & Wilkins, 1987, p. 177.
26. Ward JD, Becker DP, Miller JD, et al: Failure of prophylactic barbiturate coma in the treatment of severe head injury. J Neurosurg 1985;62:383.

27. Eisenberg HM, Frankowski RF, Constant C, et al: High dose barbiturate control of elevated intracranial pressure in patients with severe head injury. J Neurosurg 1988;69:15.
28. Rockoff MA, Marshall LF, Shapiro HM: High dose barbiturate therapy in humans: A clinical review of 60 patients. Ann Neurol 1979;6:194.
29. Braakman R, Schouten HJA, Blaauw-van Dishoeck M, Minderhound JM: Megadose steroids in severe head injury: Results of a prospective double blind clinical trial. J Neurosurg 1983;58:326.
30. Gudeman SK, Miller JD, Becker DP: Failure of high dose steroid therapy to influence intracranial pressure in patients with severe head injury. J Neurosurg 1979;51:301.
31. Marshall LF, King J, Langfitt TW: The complications of high dose corticosteroid therapy in neurosurgical patients: A prospective sutdy. Ann Neurol 1977;1:201.
32. Meldrum B, Millan MH, Obrenovitch TP: Excitatory aminoacid release induced by injury. In Globus NY-T, Dietrich WD (eds): The Role of Neurotransmitters in Brain Injury. New York, Plenum Press, 1992.
33. Stuart L, Bullock R, Jones M: The cerebral hemodynamic and metabolic effects of the competitive NMDA antagonist CGS19755 in humans with severe head injury. In Proceedings of the Second International Neurotrauma Symposium, Glasgow, 1993.
34. Clifton GL, Allen S, Barrodale P, et al: A phase II study of moderate hypothermia in severe head injury. J Neurotrauma 1993;10(3):263–271, 273.
35. Shiozaki T, Sugimoto H, Taneda M, Yoshida H, Iwai A, Yoshioka T: Effect of mild hypothermia on uncontrollable intracranial hypertension after severe head injury. J Neurosurg 1993;79(3):363.
36. Marion DW, Obrist WD, Carlier PM, Penrod LE, Darby JM: The use of moderate therapeutic hypothermia for patients with severe head injuries: A preliminary report. J Neurosurg 1993;79(3):354–362.
37. Metz C, Holzschuh M, Bein T, et al: Moderate hypothermia in patients with severe head injury: Cerebral and extracerebral effects. J Neurosurg 1996;85(4):533–541.
38. Lanier WL, Stangland KJ, Scheithauer BW: Effects of intravenous dextrose infusion and head position on neurologic outcome after complete cerebral ischemia (abstract). Anesthesiology 1985;63:A110.
39. Teasdale GP, Jennett B: Assessment of coma and impaired consciousness. Lancet 1974;2:81.
40. Annegers JF, Grabow JD, Groover RV, Laws ER Jr, Elveback LR, Kurland LT: Seizures after head trauma: A population study. Neurology 1980;20:683.
41. Young B, Rapp RP, Norton JA, Haack D, Walsh JW: Failure of prophylactically administered phenytoin to prevent post-traumatic seizures in children. Childs Brain 1983;10:185.
42. Temkin NR, Dikmen SS, Wilensky AJ, Keihm J, Chabal S, Winn HR: A randomized, double blind study of phenytoin for the prevention of post-traumatic seizures. N Engl J Med 1990;323:497.
43. Temkin NR, Dikmen SS, Winn HR: Management of posttraumatic seizures. Neurosurg Clin North Am 1991;2:425.

Chapter 4

Penetrating Neck Injuries

The diagnosis and treatment of penetrating neck injuries remain controversial. There is a wealth of literature showing contradictory results, with diagnostic measures ranging from simple observation to mandatory exploration.

Early operative management for neck wounds was advocated by Bailey in 1944 based on his experience in World War II.[1] Fogelman and Stewart in 1956 reviewed the results from Parkland Memorial Hospital and found a lower mortality rate in patients who were operated upon immediately compared to those who received nonoperative treatment or delayed exploration.[2] Early operative intervention became common practice for patients with penetrating neck wounds. Negative explorations were reported in up to 60% of patients, but these were accepted to keep the overall mortality low. Mortality rates from penetrating neck wounds range from 0 to 11% in the civilian population.[3-10] With advancements in invasive radiology, the concept of mandatory exploration was challenged. The surgical literature now abounds with articles advocating either mandatory operation or selective management. Those favoring mandatory exploration report a low morbidity and no mortality from a negative neck exploration with less than 1% missed injuries. Those who favor selective management report a lower rate of negative neck exploration, with the missed injuries often being inconsequential. Depending on the work-up and costs at a given institution, the mandatory operative approach or the selective approach may be more cost effective.

A working knowledge of the anatomy of the neck is required to implement an effective diagnostic workup for the vascular system (carotid and vertebral arteries, jugular vein, and subclavian vessels), the respiratory system (trachea and larynx), and the digestive system (esophagus and pharynx). The anatomy of the neck is complex and diverse. It is a crossroads for five different organ systems: respiratory, cardiovascular, nervous, digestive, and endocrine systems. Saletta and colleagues divided the neck into three regions, referred to as zones.[9] The problems encountered and the surgical approaches used vary with each zone. Zone I is the area extending from the clavicle to the cricoid cartilage; Zone II extends from the cricoid cartilage to the angle of the mandible, and Zone III encompasses the area from the angle of the mandible to the base of the skull.

Zones I and III are difficult to expose surgically. Exposure in Zone I is difficult because of the overlying clavicle and manubrium, whereas the mandible and vertebral column make exposure in Zone III a complex process. For these reasons, selective management is implemented in Zones I and III in patients who are stable and without massive hemorrhage. Zone II is controversial because the anatomy is familiar to most surgeons and exposure is simple relative to the other zones.

ANATOMY OF THE NECK

The platysma is a superficial subcutaneous muscle, which originates from the fascia of the deltoid and pectoralis major muscles and inserts onto the mandible. Below the platysma, the neck can be divided into five fascial compartments:

1. Superficial layer of the cervical fascia.
2. Prevertebral layer of the cervical fascia.
3. Infrahyoid fascia.
4. Cervical visceral fascia.
5. Carotid sheath.

The superficial layer of the cervical fascia encompasses the entire neck. Inferiorly, the fascia originates from the manubrium, clavicle, acromion, and spine of the scapula. Superiorly, it invests the masseter muscle and extends cephalad as the parotid fascia. Posteriorly, the superficial fascia is attached to the external occipital protuberance, the ligamentum nuchae, and the seventh spinous process. It divides to surround the sternocleidomastoid and the trapezius muscles.

The prevertebral layer of the cervical fascia is an extension of the superficial fascia. Posteriorly, it attaches to the same points as the superficial layer of the cervical fascia (external occipital protuberance, nuchal line, and the seventh spinous process). It then attaches to the cervical transverse processes and proceeds around the scalene muscles, the levator scapulae, the deep cervicals, the splenius, and the cervical sympathetic trunk. The prevertebral layer forms the floor of the posterior triangle. The prevertebral layer also becomes Sibson's fascia and embraces the brachial plexus as the axillary sheath.

The fascia of the infrahyoid muscles is composed of anterior and posterior layers. The anterior layer covers the omohyoid and sternohyoid muscles. Behind the sternocleidomastoid muscle, the infrahyoid fascia fuses with the superficial fascia. The posterior layer covers the sternothyroid and thyrohyoid muscles. In the anterior midline, the fascia of the infrahyoid and the superficial fascia blend with the pretracheal component of the cervical visceral fascia. Posteriorly, the infrahyoid fascia blends with the carotid sheath.

The cervical visceral fascia is composed of the pretracheal and buccopharyngeal fasciae. The pretracheal fascia is attached to the thyroid cartilage and is continuous with the pericardium. It is attached to the stylohyoid laterally and to the hyoid superiorly. The pretracheal component of the cervical visceral fascia encompasses four structures: the larynx, trachea, thyroid gland, and parathyroid glands. The buccopharyngeal fascia is attached to the pharyngeal tubercle superiorly, and inferiorly it blends with the pretracheal fascia at the posteromedial aspect of the thyroid. The buccopharyngeal fascia encompasses the esophagus and the buccinator muscle.

The last fascial compartment, the carotid sheath, covers the carotid artery, internal jugular vein, and vagus nerve. The carotid sheath may contain the superior ramus of the ansa cervicalis, or the nerve may run anterior to the sheath. The hypoglossal nerve and the first and second cervical nerves form the loop of the superior ramus that joins the inferior ramus (from the second and third cervical nerves) to form the ansa cervicalis.

The respiratory, vascular, nervous, digestive, and endocrine systems must be considered when evaluating a patient with a neck wound. The trachea originates from the larynx and extends down the midline of the neck, disappearing behind the sternum. A myriad of vessels and nerves pass through the neck. The anterior jugular vein is a confluence of small veins from the submental and submandibular triangles. The jugular venous arch often connects both sides. The external jugular vein is composed of the retromandibular and posterior auricular veins; it crosses the sternocleidomastoid muscle and pierces the superficial cervical fascia 2 cm above the clavicle to join the subclavian vein.

The common carotid artery originates from the aorta on the left and from the brachiocephalic artery on the right and divides into the internal and external carotid arteries. The internal carotid has no extracranial branches and enters the skull through the carotid canal. The external carotid artery has eight branches; these are, in order, the superior thyroid artery, lingual artery, facial artery, ascending pharyngeal artery, occipital artery, posterior auricular artery, superficial temporal artery, and maxillary artery.

Four structures cross the carotid artery: the hypoglossal nerve, the facial vein, the lingual vein, and the superior thyroid vein (inconsistent). The internal jugular vein is a continuation of the sigmoid sinus of the dura mater and descends in the carotid sheath. It combines with the subclavian vein to form the innominate vein. The internal jugular vein has seven tributaries: the inferior petrosal vein, lingual vein, pharyngeal vein, facial vein, superior thyroid vein, middle thyroid vein, and occipital vein (inconsistent).

The vagus nerve leaves the cranium through the jugular foramen with the glossopharyngeal and accessory nerves. It traverses the neck in the carotid sheath. The right vagus nerve passes between the subclavian artery and the brachiocephalic vein. The right recurrent laryngeal nerve loops around the subclavian artery and proceeds back into the neck. The left vagus nerve passes between the left subclavian artery and the left brachiocephalic vein, with the recurrent laryngeal nerve on this side looping around the arch of the aorta. The vagus nerve gives rise to the superior laryngeal nerve, which has an internal branch and an external branch. The internal branch travels through the thyrohyoid membrane with the laryngeal branch of the superior thyroid artery. It provides sensory innervation to the mucous membranes and parasympathetic innervation to the epiglottis, larynx, and tongue. The external branch travels medial and posterior to the superior thyroid artery and terminates in the cricothyroid muscle, supplying the inferior constrictor muscle of the pharynx. The recurrent laryngeal nerve passes back into the neck in the groove between the trachea and the esophagus. It supplies motor innervation for all intrinsic muscles of the larynx except the cricothyroideus muscle. The thoracic sympathetic trunk ascends into the cervical region and lies behind the carotid sheath. In the cervical region, the sympathetic trunk has three ganglia—inferior, middle, and superior.

The thoracic duct ascends through the aortic hiatus and is located to the left of the midline in the upper thorax. As it emerges into the neck between the esophagus and the left pleura, it then arches behind the carotid sheath and enters the vascular system at the junction of the left internal jugular and subclavian vein.

The subclavian artery arises from the aorta on the left and from the brachio-cephalic artery on the right. The subclavian artery is divided into three parts before it passes over the first rib and becomes the axillary artery. The first part is medial to the anterior scalene muscle, the second part is behind the anterior scalene muscle, and the third part is lateral. The first part is crossed by the vertebral vein, the internal jugular vein, and the ansa subclavia. The thoracic duct crosses the first part of the subclavian artery on the left, and the recurrent laryngeal crosses it on the right. The second part of the subclavian artery runs between the anterior and middle scalene muscles, and the third part of the subclavian artery is located in the omoclavicular triangle and lies against the inferior trunk of the brachial plexus. During its course, the subclavian artery gives off five branches: (1) the vertebral artery, which enters the costotransverse foramen of C6, (2) the thyrocervical trunk, which divides into the inferior thyroid, suprascapular, and transverse cervical arteries, (3) the internal thoracic artery, which run's inferiorly along the anterior chest, (4) the costocervical trunk, which divides into the highest intercostal and the deep cervical arteries, and (5) the dorsal scapular artery, which passes through the brachial plexus.

The subclavian vein passes in front of the anterior scalene muscle and the phrenic nerve. It has three tributaries: the external jugular, the dorsal scapular, and the thoracoacromial veins. In addition, the thoracic duct enters the junction of the internal jugular and subclavian vein on the left.

DIAGNOSTIC WORK-UP AND INITIAL EVALUATION

As in all trauma patients, the initial work-up should include evaluation of the airway, breathing, and circulation (ABCs) according to the Advanced Trauma Life Support (ATLS) protocol. If stridor, difficulty in breathing, or neck swelling is present, early intubation is warranted because the airway may be irrevocably lost if bleeding or swelling continues. In the presence of penetrating trauma to the larynx or trachea, a surgical airway may be required. The airway may become compromised or may collapse from bleeding into the pretracheal compartment, which encircles the larynx and the trachea. The fascial compartments of the neck can tamponade bleeding, but increased pressure in the compartment may also collapse the airway. A cricothyroidotomy is the fastest and easiest surgical access route to a compromised airway, since this membrane is superficial and usually has no overlying veins. If the injury to the airway is below the cricothyroid membrane, an emergency tracheostomy must be performed.

After the airway has been evaluated, breathing is assessed. Injuries to the subclavian vessels in Zone I may cause a hemothorax, or the penetrating injury may extend into the chest, resulting in a pneumothorax. A needle thoracostomy or chest tube should be placed in the patient with physical signs or symptoms of a pneumothorax or hemothorax. Decompression by needle thoracostomy should be used when there is evidence of tension pneumothorax or when a chest tube cannot otherwise be placed rapidly.

When airway patency and adequate breathing have been established, circulation is evaluated. All patients with penetrating wounds should have two large-bore (18-gauge or larger) peripheral intravenous lines placed. This rule should not be forgotten in stable patients who are not actively hemorrhaging because a soft clot that is temporarily occluding a major vessel injury could become dislodged, leading to unexpected massive bleeding.

Patients with unstable vital signs who have a penetrating wound of the neck should be taken directly to the operating theater. This decision evokes no controversy. The radiology suite or observation area are inappropriate locations for patients who have lost sufficient blood to alter their vital signs. The appropriate incisions and operations for specific presentations and injuries are discussed later in the section, Surgical Approach and Treatment of Specific Injuries. In addition to patients who are unstable, those with obvious vascular, tracheal, or esophageal injuries require surgical intervention without unnecessary delay for diagnostic evaluation.

After the primary survey and resuscitation, the secondary survey follows. The physical examination should include palpation of the neck and upper extremities for pulses and pulsatile masses, auscultation for bruits, and thorough investigation of all areas of bleeding or swelling. A neurologic examination must be completed with attention directed to major deficits such as hemiplegia or aphasia. It is important to identify any focal deficits. For instance, deviation of the tongue may indicate an injury to the hypoglossal nerve (cranial nerve XII). A hoarse voice may indicate an injury to the recurrent laryngeal nerve or the vagus nerve (cranial nerve X). Facial drooping indicates an injury to the facial nerve (cranial nerve VII). An examination should also be performed to identify brachial plexus injuries.

ZONE I INJURY

Initial Steps

The algorithm for penetrating injuriesin Zone I of the neck is complex. If the patient's vital signs are not stable or if massive hemorrhage is present, the cause must be quickly determined. These patients should undergo a rapid initial assessment and resuscitation following the ABCs of ATLS and should be taken rapidly to the operating theater.

The patient may have lost the airway owing to tracheal injury, compressive hematoma, or altered mental status secondary to hypoxia or exsanguinating hemorrhage. If the airway must be secured and there is no tracheal injury, oral intubation using in-line cervical traction or nasotracheal intubation should be done. If the airway is lost because of a tracheal injury, a difficult situation exists. Because the superior border of Zone I is below the cricoid cartilage, a cricothyroidotomy will not be helpful in these patients. This is one of the rare situations in which an emergency tracheostomy is necessary; it must be performed below the site of injury.

These wounds are in close proximity to the thorax and are frequently associated with thoracic injuries. In unstable patients, breathing is evaluated by physical examination; if breath sounds are decreased, a needle thoracostomy or chest tube is inserted prior to obtaining a chest radiograph. It is better to err on the side of occasionally placing a needle thoracostomy or chest tube in a patient who does not need it than to allow a tension pneumothorax or hemothorax to go untreated while wasting precious minutes obtaining a radiograph.

Zone I injuries can result in injury to the carotid, subclavian, or vertebral vessels. In addition, the wound may pass through Zone I and into other areas such as the mediastinum or thorax. If there is obvious external bleeding, direct pressure is applied to control hemorrhage while arrangements are made for emergency surgery. Massive hemorrhage can occur into the thorax without producing evidence of external bleeding. Once again, in the unstable patient, physical examination is necessary to quickly determine if there is a hemothorax. Chest tube placement prior to obtaining a chest radiograph can save precious time in the unstable patient.

Evaluation for Occult Injuries

If the initial assessment confirms the presence of a patent airway and adequate oxygenation, ventilation, and no signs or symptoms of circulatory collapse, the work-up for occult injuries is begun. A chest radiograph is obtained to determine whether intrathoracic penetration with subsequent hemothorax or pneumothorax has occurred. If necessary, a chest tube is placed to reexpand the lung and determine how much blood has been lost. Massive hemothorax (>1500 ml of blood over 30 minutes) requires immediate operative intervention. Persistent bleeding (>200 ml of blood per hour for 3 hours) is also an indication for operative intervention. If the patient continues to have a large air leak, a tracheal or major bronchial injury must be considered and surgical repair performed.

Evaluation for Vascular Injuries

After the thorax has been evaluated, the vascular system is assessed. Four-vessel arteriography (bilateral carotid and vertebral arteries) is performed, and the venous phase completes the study. In addition to making the diagnosis, radiologic intervention can also be used for therapy. The vertebral arteries are difficult to access surgically because of their protected location in the costotransverse foramina. If a vertebral artery injury is identified on arteriography, the artery can be embolized.[11] This is discussed later in the section, Surgical Approach and Treatment of Specific Injuries. The vascular system can be evaluated by an arteriogram of the vessels in proximity to the wound. Along with the carotid and vertebral arteries, the subclavian artery may also require evaluation.

Evaluation for Digestive Tract Injuries

If the tract of the bullet is in close proximity to the esophagus or the pharynx, the digestive tract must be investigated. An esophagogram is easily

Zone I Algorithm

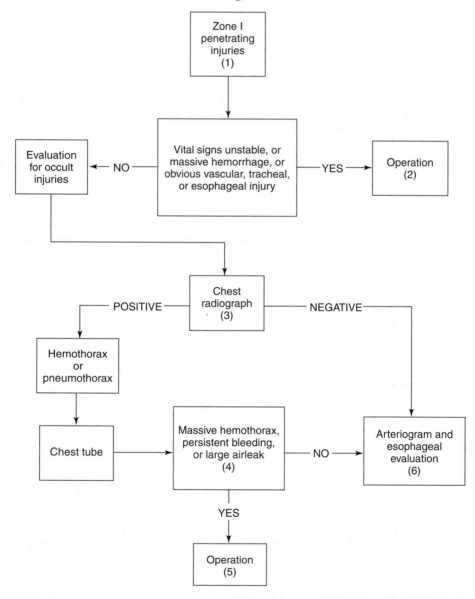

1. Zone I extends from the clavicle to the cricoid cartilage. Structures subject to injury include the carotid, subclavian, and vertebral vessels, trachea, esophagus, and thoracic duct. Additionally, the wound may pass through zone I and continue into the thorax and/or mediastinum.
2. Emergent operation is guided mainly by the physical examination findings. Exploration is directed at the main cause of the hemodynamic instability, which is usually a vascular or airway injury. After control of the injury has been achieved, exploration should continue and should include the esophagus, carotid and jugular vessels, thoracic duct, neural structures, and airway.
3. Chest radiograph should be reviewed not only for the common finding of a hemothorax or pneumothorax but also for more subtle findings such as a widened mediastinum, pleural capping, or mediastinal air.
4. Hemothorax is considered massive if it consists of greater than 1500 ml of blood over 30 minutes. Persistent bleeding is defined as greater than 200 ml/hour for 3 hours.
5. Operative control of a massive or persistent hemothorax or a suspected tracheal or major bronchial injury is determined by the site of the wound. For a vascular injury, a median sternotomy with supraclavicular extension gives the best exposure. For a tracheal or right mainstem bronchus injury, a right thoracotomy yields the best exposure. For a left bronchial injury, a left thoracotomy is preferable.
6. Arteriography must include all four cervicocranial vessels. Esophageal evaluation should include at least a contrast esophagram. Esophagoscopy can be reserved for situations in which the esophagram is equivocal or when a high index of suspicion remains even with a negative esophagram. Rigid esophagoscopy has been advocated in such situation, but the familiarity or skill level of most surgeons may make flexible esophagoscopy a more viable alternative.

obtained but has a sensitivity of less than 80%.[6, 12] Weigelt and colleagues found that no injuries were missed when they combined esophagography with rigid esophagoscopy, but there are several drawbacks to rigid esophagoscopy.[12] Today, many surgeons have little or no experience with the rigid esophagoscope because flexible endoscopes have been utilized almost exclusively for the past two decades. In addition, the patient must be sedated in order to undergo rigid esophagoscopy. The risk of iatrogenic injury, which existed even in experienced hands in prior years, is probably higher now because of the lack of familiarity with the technique. Weigelt and colleagues concluded that patients should be initially evaluated with esophagography. If the esophagram is positive, neck exploration should follow. If the esophagram is negative, observation is justi-fied. If the esophagram is equivocal, rigid esophagoscopy can be used to reduce the chances of a negative exploration. Many surgeons prefer to proceed with flexible esophagoscopy, which may or may not be as accurate in the diagnosis of cervical esophageal injuries. Many utilize only esophagography to evaluate the esophagus and pharynx, but with this technique an occasional injury will be missed. Adding endoscopy to the work-up will decrease the number of missed injuries.

ZONE II INJURY

Initial Steps

The major area of controversy concerns the management of penetrating injuries in Zone II of the neck in stable patients. Most practitioners would begin with local exploration in the emergency department or resuscitation unit. If the platysma muscle has not been penetrated, the wound is superficial, and only observation is required. Local exploration of the platysma should not be done by blind probing; a vascular injury with an overlying clot may be disturbed by such probing, leading to uncontrolled bleeding, and an opportu-nity for an easy operation can thus be lost. Instead, using good lighting and local anesthesia, the surgeon should explore the wound, extending it when necessary to examine the underlying platysma. There are two schools of thought about injuries that penetrate the platysma: one argues for mandatory operation, while the other argues equally forcefully for selective operation.

Evaluation for Vascular Injuries

If selective operation is chosen, nonoperative work-up is started to exclude a vascular injury. Arteriography can be performed as outlined in the Zone I algorithm for evaluation of a vascular injury; again, this approach can be both diagnostic and therapeutic.

Another approach is to use Doppler ultrasonography as a screening test for arteriography. In a prospective study of 55 patients, Doppler ultrasound was performed, followed by arteriography. Doppler ultrasound showed a sensitivity of 100% and a specificity of 85%.[13] If Doppler ultrasound is negative, no further work-up is required to evaluate the vessels. However, if the study is positive or inadequate, an arteriogram is obtained. The arteriogram is performed because Doppler ultrasound examination is known to produce some false-positive results. If ultrasound examination shows injury to the vertebral vessels, arteriography with possible embolization is warranted because surgical exposure of the vertebral artery is difficult. Exposure of the vertebral arteries is discussed later in the section, Surgical Approach and Treatment of Specific Injuries.

Evaluation for Digestive Tract Injuries

If the wound is in proximity to the pharynx or esophagus, the work-up previously described in the section, Evaluation for Digestive Tract Injury, for Zone I Injuries is implemented. Again, this begins with an esophagram. If the results are clearly negative, observation alone is warranted. If the results are positive, the patient is taken to the operating theater. If the results are equivocal, one proceeds with esophagoscopy.

Evaluation for Airway Injuries

If the wound is in proximity to the trachea or larynx, the upper respiratory tract must be studied. Bronchoscopy and laryngoscopy are the mainstays of selective management. Because of the anterior location of the trachea, penetrating tracheal wounds are usually obvious (subcutaneous emphysema and/or bubbling at the site of skin penetration). No large series exist in the literature on the results of using laryngoscopy or bronchoscopy for penetrating injuries, so the sensitivity and specificity of these tests are unknown.

Computed Tomography

Computed tomography has been suggested as the test of choice in patients with penetrating neck wounds, used in lieu of angiography, Doppler ultrasound, esophagography, esophagoscopy, and bronchoscopy and laryngoscopy. It is appealing to replace several tests with just one, but there are insufficient data to justify the recommendation of this approach at this time.

ZONE III INJURY

Initial Steps

Surgical exposure in Zone III is difficult, and most surgeons do not operate regularly in this complex region. Patients who are hemodynamically unstable or have massive hemorrhage require rapid determination of the source. Following the ABCs of ATLS, the airway is rapidly assessed. Loss of the airway may be secondary to a compressive hematoma, aspiration, or altered mental status secondary to exsanguinating hemorrhage. The airway can be secured via the oral route with in-line traction or with nasotracheal intubation. If oropharyngeal trauma is present, an emergent cricothyroidotomy may be necessary.

Breathing is assessed after the airway has been secured. Zone III injuries are

Zone II Algorithm

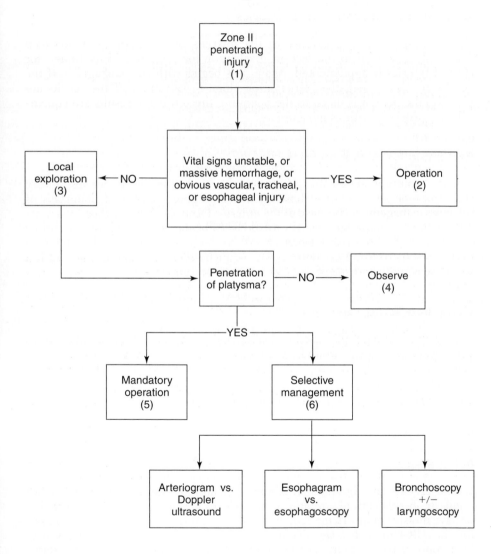

1. Zone II is the area extending from the cricoid cartilage to the angle of the mandible. Structures injured may include the carotid, subclavian, or vertebral vessels, and the trachea, esophagus, or neural structures.
2. Emergent operation is guided mainly by the findings on physical examination. Exploration is directed at the main cause of the hemodynamic instability, which is usually a vascular or airway injury. After the injury has been controlled, exploration should continue to include visualization of the esophagus, pharynx, carotid, jugular, neural structures, and airway.
3. Local exploration should not be done by blind probing. This may dislodge a clot and turn an elective operation into an emergent nightmare. Local exploration should be undertaken using a local anesthetic and good lighting. There should be no reservation about extending the wound to gain adequate exposure. Penetration of the platysma must be determined.
4. Length of time needed for observation varies depending on the extent of injury. For minor force injuries, only a few hours in the emergency department may be necessary. For more formidable injuries proper observation may entail admission.
5. Operative management must encompass a thorough exploration of the neck, that should include visualization of the esophagus, pharynx, carotid, jugular, neural structures, airway, and injury tract.
6. Selective management is an alternative to mandatory exploration. It must include a thorough work-up of all systems in Zone II, including vascular and aerodigestive investigations. If any of these investigations yields an injury, exploration must be undertaken. If any investigations show positive results, a complete neck operative exploration must be undertaken, repairing the injury found and continuing with a thorough search for any other injuries.

Zone III Algorithm

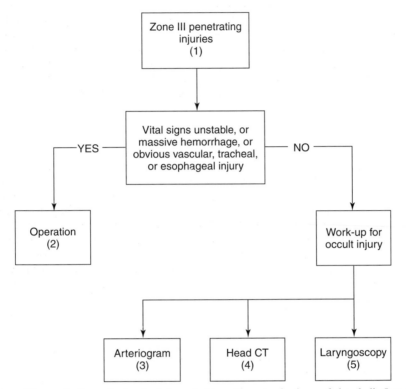

1. Zone III extends from the level of the cricoid cartilage to the base of the skull. Suspected injuries may involve the internal, external, or common carotid vessels, the vertebral artery within the intraosseous canal, the jugular system, esophagus, pharynx, and oral cavity, or they may extend intracranially.
2. Emergent operation for Zone III injuries is at best unnerving for even the most experienced trauma surgeon. Exposure of the vertebral artery or the distal carotid can be quite difficult and may involve unroofing the intraosseous canal or dislocating the mandible to gain exposure.
3. If arteriography demonstrates a lesion of the carotid, operative repair is governed by the location of the lesion and the neurologic status of the patient. Lesions of the vertebral artery are usually best handled by embolization techniques.
4. Neck injuries that extend intracranially or that have intracranial sequelae are usually best managed with neurosurgical consultation.
5. Laryngoscopy is useful in Zone III injuries to evaluate the oropharynx and hypopharynx. There should be no hesitation about combining laryngoscopy with esophagoscopy.

usually some distance from the thorax and should not in themselves lead to intrathoracic injuries, but combined and associated injuries are common. If breath sounds are decreased on one side, the possibility of aspiration, mainstem bronchus intubation, or associated injuries should be considered. In a crisis situation it is better to place an unneeded needle thoracostomy or chest tube than to miss a life-threatening pneumothorax or hemothorax.

Circulatory status should be assessed, and two large-bore (18-gauge or larger) intravenous lines inserted, even if the patient is hemodynamically stable. Obvious external hemorrhage is controlled with external pressure, and emergent operative intervention is warranted. The myriad possible sources of bleeding and their difficult exposure makes operating unnerving even for the most experienced trauma surgeon. For specific operative techniques, see the later section, Surgical Approach and Treatment of Specific Injuries.

Evaluation for Occult Injuries

If the patient presents with stable vital signs and no obvious uncontrolled hemorrhage, a search is made for occult injuries using arteriography, esophagraphy, and, possibly, computed tomography of the head. The great majority of patients with Zone III injuries do not have uncontrolled bleeding. Angiography can be both diagnostic and therapeutic. Embolization can be considered an alternative form of treatment whenever arterial ligation is considered. Embolization is indicated for injuries to expendable arteries or for arteries that are difficult to access surgically.[2] Laryngoscopy and esophagography are indicated to evaluate the mouth and pharynx. Laryngoscopy is added in this group of patients because the injuries are in the region of the pharynx, and laryngoscopy is easily performed.

SURGICAL APPROACH AND TREATMENT OF SPECIFIC INJURIES

Carotid Artery Injuries

Carotid artery injuries can present in the most dramatic fashion, but surprisingly, 90% of these patients are stable enough to undergo arteriography.[14] In 16 series compiled by Asensio and colleagues, the common carotid was the artery most commonly injured in the neck, followed, in order, by the internal and then the external carotid.[15] Carotid artery injuries can present in a myriad of ways. An expanding hematoma can occlude the airway. Massive external hemorrhage can lead to exsanguination. The neurologic status can range from normal to contralateral complete hemiplegia. The diagnosis can be suspected from the physical examination, but this is neither overly sensitive (80%) nor highly specific (58%).[16] Arteriography, on the other hand, is accurate in diagnosing carotid injuries in stable patients. In addition, arteriography can be especially helpful for diagnosing injuries in Zones I and III of the neck, since surgical exploration is difficult and carries significant risk[5, 17, 18] Hiatt and associates have argued that arteriography increases the yield for explorations, but this concept must be tempered by the realization that delays in diagnosis and treatment may increase morbidity and mortality.[17]

In the operating theater, several options are available for managing a carotid injury, and the best procedure is not always clear. Thal and colleagues divided patients into three categories.[19] Based on neurologic deficit, patients were divided into those presenting without neurologic deficits, those with a mild deficit consisting of weakness of the extremity, and those with severe deficits. It was concluded that patients with no deficit or a mild deficit should have the carotid injury repaired. Patients with a severe neurologic deficit present a more difficult treatment dilemma. If the carotid is patent in patients with a severe neurologic deficit, Thal and colleagues recommend repair, but if the vessel is completely occluded, they recommend ligation.[19] Repair of the carotid artery in a patient with a fixed neurologic defect produces poor results and may actually convert an anemic infarct into a hemorrhagic infarct. For this reason, Bradley also recommended against revascularization in patients with severe nerologic deficits.[20] Liekweg and Greenfield in 1978 reviewed over 200 cases and concluded that repair had a better outcome in patients who were not in coma but that results were poor for patients in coma regardless of treatment plan.[21] To counter this conclusion, in 1980 Unger and associates reviewed 722 cases in the literature over a 27-year period and found that 34% of patients with a severe deficit improved with repair, whereas only 14% improved if the carotid was ligated or left alone.[22] In his thorough review of penetrating neck injuries, Asensio and colleagues[15] reviewed seven series from 1970 through 1988[20, 23–26] consisting of 433 patients and recommended primary repair for all injuries except those in patients in profound coma with bilateral fixed and dilated pupils. Clearly, patients with mild to no deficit should have the injury repaired. Conversely, repair should not be performed in patients in profound coma with bilateral fixed and dilated pupils. In the case of a more severe deficit, the mitigating factor should probably be time from injury. If more than 6 hours have passed, revascularization should probably not be attempted.

Surgical exposure of the common carotid artery and its bifurcation is obtained by making an oblique incision along the anterior border of the sternocleidomastoid muscle. The sternocleidomastoid is retracted laterally exposing the carotid sheath. The anatomy is often markedly distorted from a hematoma resulting from the injury. Care is taken not to injure the vagus nerve, which runs along the carotid artery and the internal jugular vein within the carotid sheath. The incision is extended to allow for proximal and distal control. If the proximal carotid artery is injured, the incision may have to be extended transversely along the clavicle to gain proximal control. The carotid artery at its origin can be controlled if the clavicle is resected.

The choice of repair method is determined by the mechanism and location of the injury and any tissue deficit. An intimal flap may only need arteriotomy and tacking of the flap. Tangential injury and complete transection are more difficult to address. Methods of repair include primary repair, ligation, interposition grafting, and arterial transposition. When the common or internal carotid is completely transected and a defect of less than 1 cm is found to be present, enough vessel can usually be mobilized to yield a tension-free primary anastomosis. The same is true for a tangential injury involving less than 1 cm of the vessel. The injured portion is resected, and primary anastomosis performed. Likewise, resection is the best choice for a tangential injury in which more than 15% to 20% of the vessel circumference is injured. In this case, primary repair would result in an unacceptable stenosis and a subsequent flow defect. The external carotid, with few exceptions, can be ligated above and below the injury with no adverse consequences. When more than 1 cm of vessel is missing, whether secondary to injury or resection, grafting or transposition should be considered. The choice of polytetrafluoroethylene (PTFE), Dacron, or vein remains a point of controversy. All form an adequate conduit. Synthetic materials offer the benefits of easy acquisition and handling but are associated with a higher degree of intimal hyperplasia. PTFE may be more resistant to infection than Dacron; it has been used successfully in superficial femoral artery reconstruction after traumatic injury with acceptably low rates of infection.[27] The use of vein taken from ankle versus that from the thigh remains a point of contention. There is usually a better size match with thigh vein, and there have been reports of ankle vein rupture postoperatively.[28] For these reasons, we usually prefer thigh vein over ankle vein. The choice of PTFE versus vein must depend on a given situation. Another option for proximal common carotid injuries is transposition of the carotid to the subclavian. This can be done by extending the incision supraclavicularly to expose the subclavian. Occasionally, in this situation an interposition graft may be needed to obtain adequate length, but this method may avoid sternotomy.

Vertebral Artery Injuries

Vertebral artery injuries are usually missed unless they are considered in the differential diagnosis of penetrating neck injuries. The majority of patients have no clinical findings that suggest an arterial injury other than a neck wound.[29] In Reid and Weigelt's series only 13% of patients presented with overt hemorrhage.[29] In addition, the Glasgow Coma Scale is normal in most patients with this injury. Associated injuries are common in these patients, especially cervical bony injuries, which, occur in approximately three-quarters of the patients.[29] Treatment of these injuries depends on the patient and the institution. If the patient is actively hemorrhaging from the vertebral artery and is unstable, operative intervention is the only acceptable treatment. Proximal and distal ligation can be done safely in the majority of patients based on the Parkland Hospital experience.[19] Exposure is considerably more difficult if the injury is at the level of the first and second cervical vertebrae, and in these instances, it may be possible to obtain only proximal control. If bleeding from the distal vessel remains a problem and control cannot be obtained rapidly, percutaneous transluminal embolization should be considered.[30, 31]

The vertebral artery can be divided into four anatomic sections. Section V1 extends from the origin to the transverse process of C6. V2 is the intraosseous segment of the artery extending from C6 to C2. V3 runs from the transverse process of C2 to the base of the skull. V4 is intracranial.[32] V1 can be exposed through either a supraclavicular or a vertical anterior cervical approach. The supraclavicular approach can be used only for proximal injuries and requires transection of the sternocleidomastoid muscle. If the injury is on the left, the thoracic duct must also be ligated. The vertical anterior cervical approach does not require muscle transection and allows easier exposure of the distal vessel. This is essentially the same approach used for exposure of the carotid artery. The omohyoid muscle may have to be divided for more proximal exposure. The carotid sheath and contents are retracted medially, and the sternocleido-mastoid is retracted laterally. The scalene fat pad is reflected laterally by mobilizing the medial border. The anterior scalene muscle is deep to this fat pad. When the muscle is retracted laterally, the vertebral artery is found just deep it. Care should be taken to avoid injuring the phrenic nerve, which courses on the ventral surface of the anterior scalene. The inferior thyroid artery may have to be ligated to gain adequate exposure.

V2, the intraosseous segment, is exposed using the vertical anterior cervical approach, unroofing the costocervical canal one level above the injury.[33] This allows ligation of the vessel above the injury and also in the V1 region. The sternocleidomastoid is retracted laterally, and the carotid sheath, pharynx, and larynx are retracted medially, exposing the sympathetic ganglia on the prevertebral muscles. The anterior longitudinal ligament is exposed and incised to expose the muscles. A periosteal elevator can be used to separate the prevertebral fascia and muscles from the transverse processes. It is better to expose the vessel within the bony canal than in the intervertebral space because there are myriad venous communications in this space.

Exposure of injuries in segments V3 and V4 is very difficult and is likely to require neurosurgical assistance to ensure intracranial exposure and distal control. It is for this reason that percutaneous embolization has gained such favor.[30, 31]

If the patient is stable, diagnosis and treatment can be performed radiograph-ically. The vertebral artery can be embolized proximally. When the distal vessel is not embolized or ligated, the risk of arteriovenous fistula remains. Although there are no long-term series on patients treated only with proximal ligation or embolization, there are many reports of fistulas occurring in these patients, thus warranting follow-up studies in this select group.[29, 32] Distal control can be obtained with occipital craniectomy if required.

Venous Injuries

Venous injuries are common and usually involve the jugular veins in neck wounds. There is disagreement about the need for surgical treatment of jugular venous injuries. Those advocating selective management allow for missed venous injuries, since this system is not evaluated. There is reason to believe that the low-pressure venous system will tamponade, but external hemorrhage and airway compromise can result from internal jugular injuries. If there is significant active bleeding or an expanding hematoma, surgical intervention is warranted.

Two options exist for treatment of jugular venous injuries. The majority of these injuries are treated with simple ligation. If the internal jugular vein is involved with only partial transection, lateral venorrhaphy can be used.

Esophageal Injuries

Esophageal injuries are difficult to diagnose, as described earlier in this chapter. Once diagnosed, these injuries can usually be treated with primary repair and drainage. Primary repair can be accomplished using a two-layer technique—the inner layer consists of absorbable suture and the outer layer is composed of silk. Some advocate a single-layer closure, which also yields adequate results. Regardless of which method is used, postoperative drainage should be used. Ten to twenty percent of injuries can be expected to leak after repair; thus external drainage is justified. With time, almost all cervical leaks will close. In a review by Asensio, cervical esophageal fistulas closed with conservative management in 15 of 15 patients.[15] After repair, routine esophagography on postoperative day 7 should be considered because 50% of patients with postoperative leaks are asymptomatic.[34]

Tracheal Injuries

Tracheal injuries can be the epitome of true surgical emergencies. Injuries at or above the thyroid cartilage with airway compromise are treated with emergent cricothyroidotomy. This should be performed in the emergency department if there is any suggestion of airway compromise. If the injury is below the cricoid membrane and there is loss or impending loss of the airway, emergent *tracheostomy* can be life-saving. Ideally, the tracheostomy is performed one ring below the injury, but any airway will suffice in the cyanotic patient.

Tracheal injuries can present in a less emergent manner with only hoarseness or tenderness over the trachea or thyroid cartilage. Some patients may have no obvious signs or symptoms, which is the reason why bronchoscopy and laryngoscopy must be used in patients with injuries in proximity to the trachea. Injuries are usually repaired primarily. The need for tracheostomy, which is usually performed one ring below the injury, remains controversial. The need to convert an emergent cricothyroidotomy to a tracheostomy during neck exploration is also controversial, although most surgeons believe it should be done.

Exposure of the trachea can be achieved by means of the vertical anterior cervical incision. This can be brought inferiorly to allow for tracheostomy. Occasionally two incisions are necessary. Tracheal repair can be accomplished with simple interrupted sutures of fine absorbable suture material. Chromic suture is metabolized too quickly to produce a good repair.

Tracheoesophageal Injuries

Combined tracheal and esophageal injuries present a difficult situation. Primary repair with or without tracheostomy is associated with a high complication rate. More than 50% of repairs will leak, resulting in an esophageal or recurrent tracheoesophageal fistula.[35] Placing the sternocleidomastoid or strap muscle between the repairs may decrease fistula formation, but this has not been proved. Drains should also be placed in an attempt to control the probable formation of fistulas. If there is extensive destruction of the esophagus, a cervical esophagostomy can be created to divert oropharyngeal fluids.

References

1. Bailey H: Surgery of Modern Warfare, 3rd ed, Vol 2. Baltimore, Williams & Wilkins, 1944, p. 674.
2. Fogelman MJ, Stewart RD: Penetrating wounds of the neck. Am J Surg 1956;91:581.
3. Ayuyao AM, Kaldezi YL, Parsa MH, et al: Penetrating neck wounds: Mandatory versus selective exploration. Ann Surg 1985;202:563.
4. Bishara RA, Pasch AR, Douglas DD, et al: The necessity of mandatory exploration of penetrating zone II neck injuries. Surgery 1986;100:655.
5. Golueke P, Scalfani SJA, Philips T, et al: Routine versus selective exploration of penetrating neck injuries: A randomized prospective study. J Trauma 1984;24:1010.
6. Narrod JA, Moore EE: Initial management of penetrating neck wounds: A selective approach. J Emerg Med 1984;2:17.
7. Ordog GJ, Albin D, Wasserberger J, et al: 110 bullet wounds to the neck. J Trauma 1985;25:238.
8. Pate JW, Casini M: Penetrating wound of the neck: Explore or not? Am Surg 1980;46:38.
9. Saletta JD, Lowe RJ, Leonardo TL, et al: Penetrating trauma of the neck. J Trauma 1976;16:579.
10. Wood J, Fabian TC, Magianate EC: Penetrating neck injuries: Recommendations for selective management. J Trauma 1989;29:602.
11. Reid JDS, Weigelt JA: Forty-three cases of vertebral artery trauma. J Trauma 1988;28:1007.
12. Weigelt JA, Thal ER, Snyder WH, et al: Diagnosis of penetrating cervical esophageal injuries. Am J Surg 1987;154:619.
13. Montalvo BN, LaBlang SD, Nunez DB, et al: Color Doppler sonography in penetrating injury of the neck. AJNR 1996;17(5):943.
14. Sankaran S, Walt AJ: Penetrating wounds of the neck—Principles and controversy. Surg Clin North Am 1977;57:139.
15. Asensio JA, Valenziano CP, Falcone RD, Grosh JD: Management of penetrating neck injuries: The controversy surrounding zone II injuries. Surg Clin North Am 1991;71:267.
16. McCormick TM, Burch BH: Routine angiographic evaluation of neck and extremity injuries. J Trauma 1979;19:384.
17. Hiatt JR, Busuttil RW, Wilson SE: Impact of routine arteriography on management of penetrating neck injuries. J Vasc Surg 1984;1:860.
18. Reid JD, Weigelt JA, Thal ER, et al: Assessment of proximity of a wound to major vascular structures as an indication for arteriography. Arch Surg 1988;123:942.
19. Thal ER, Snyder WH, Hays RA, et al: Management of carotid artery injuries. Surgery 1974;76:955.
20. Bradley EL III: Management of penetrating carotid injuries: An alternative approach. J Trauma 1973;13:248.
21. Liekweg WG Jr, Greenfield LJ: Management of penetrating carotid arterial injury. Ann Surg 1978;188:587.
22. Unger SW, Tucker WS Jr, Mrdeza MA, et al: Carotid artery trauma. Surgery 1980;87(5):477.
23. Brown MF, Graham JM, Feliciano DV, et al: Carotid injuries. Am J Surg 1982;144:748.
24. Fry RE, Fry WJ: Extracranial carotid artery injuries. Surgery 1990;88:581.
25. Ledgerwood AM, Mullins RJ, Lucas CE: Primary repair vs ligation for carotid artery injuries. Arch Surg 1980;115:488.
26. Richardson JD, Simpson C, Miller FB: Management of carotid artery trauma. Surgery 1988;104:673.
27. Martin LC, McKenney MG, Sosa JL, et al: Management of lower extremity arterial trauma. J Trauma 1994;37(4):591.
28. Riles TS, Lamparello PJ, Ginagola G, et al: Rupture of vein patch: A rare complication of carotid endarterectomy. J Vasc Surg 1990;107:10.
29. Reid JDS, Weigelt JA: Forty-three cases of vertebral artery trauma. J Trauma 1988;28:1007.
30. Bergsjordet B, Strother CM, Crummy AB, et al: Vertebral artery embolization for control of massive hemorrhage. AJNR 1984;5:201.
31. Kobernick M, Carmody R: Vertebral artery transection from blunt trauma treated by embolization. J Trauma 1984;24:854.
32. Berguer R: Vertebral artery reconstruction for vertebrobasilar insufficiency. *In* Ernst CB, Stanley JC (eds): Current Therapy in Vascular Surgery. Toronto, BC Decker, 1987, p. 62.

33. Shumacker HB: Arteriovenous fistulas of the cervical portion of the vertebral vessels. Surg Gynecol Obstet 1946;27:856.
34. Scalfani SJA, Panetta T, Goldstein AS, et al: The management of arterial injuries caused by penetration of zone III of the neck. J Trauma 1985;25:871.
35. Winter RP, Weigelt JA: Cervical esophageal trauma: Incidence and cause of esophageal fistulas. Arch Surg 1990;125:849.
36. Feliciano DV, Bitondo CG, Mattox KL, et al: Combined tracheoesophageal injuries. Am J Surg 1985;150:710.

Chapter 5

Penetrating Chest Trauma

Thoracic trauma accounts for one in four trauma-related deaths in North America and contributes significantly to another 25% of deaths due to trauma.[1-5] Up to 85% of penetrating chest injuries can be adequately treated with tube thoracostomy, with only 15% requiring thoracotomy or other operative intervention.[4] Simple and timely interventions are often life-saving and are the mainstay of the initial treatment of chest wounds. Responsibility for this treatment rests on the shoulders of the physician who initially examines the patient. Trauma to the thorax may cause injuries to the heart, lung, great vessels, tracheobronchial tree, or esophagus. Penetrating thoracic wounds may cause intra-abdominal injuries as well. During exhalation the diaphragm may rise as high as the fourth intercostal space anteriorly and the seventh intercostal space posteriorly. Wounds below this level must be considered potentially to have crossed the diaphragm and are therefore "thoracoabdominal" in nature. Wounds outside the chest, such as penetrating wounds to Zone I of the neck or penetrating abdominal wounds crossing the diaphragm, may involve intrathoracic structures and require a selective work-up to rule out injury to an intrathoracic structure. Penetrating iatrogenic injuries may be caused by a variety of diagnostic and therapeutic procedures. In this chapter we will concentrate on extracardiac chest wounds. Cardiac wounds are discussed in Chapter 6.

INITIAL ASSESSMENT AND MANAGEMENT

Initial assessment of the patient with penetrating thoracic trauma consists of a primary survey followed by resuscitation and then a detailed secondary survey. The primary survey is easily remembered by the acronym ABC, stressed by the Advanced Trauma Life Support (ATLS) course of the American College of Surgeons. *A* is a reminder to evaluate the airway initially and above all else. If the patient does not have an adequate airway, one should be obtained. Oral intubation with in-line traction is acceptable in the great majority of patients; nasotracheal intubation is acceptable also but requires a spontaneously breathing patient.[6, 7] If associated facial or oropharyngeal trauma is present, making oropharyngeal intubation impossible, a cricothyroidotomy may be necessary. This situation usually presents a contraindication to nasotracheal intubation. A final method that can be considered in the stable patient with suspected tracheal or laryngeal disruption (e.g., massive subcutaneous emphysema, hoarseness, voice change, and so on) is transnasal or transoral fiberoptic intubation under direct vision. This minimizes the potential for complete disruption or separation of a severely injured trachea or larynx with loss of the airway. The bronchoscope can be used to "stent" the disrupted airway while the endotracheal tube is passed over it through the area of injury.

After the airway has been secured, attention is turned to the patient's breathing. Lack of breath sounds on one side may be the result of a pneumothorax or hemothorax. On percussion these are identified by tympany (pneumothorax) or dullness (hemothorax) on the affected side. When an associated mediastinal shift is present there is tracheal deviation to the opposite side. Both of these processes can cause respiratory as well as circulatory embarrassment. The latter occurs with tension pneumothorax or hemothorax secondary to kinking of the vena cava with mediastinal shift, resulting in impaired venous return and decreased cardiac output. The patient with a tension hemothorax may not manifest jugular venous distention as seen with a tension pneumothorax due to associated hypovolemic shock.

A third possible cause of absent breath sounds is a mainstem bronchus intubation. This usually occurs on the right side because the right mainstem bronchus branches off the trachea at a less acute angle than the left mainstem bronchus, resulting in right mainstem intubation in the majority of cases. This possibility should be considered in the hemodynamically stable patient when breath sounds are absent on the left following intubation; it results from passing the endotracheal tube too far at the time of intubation. This complication can be minimized by determining the depth of endotracheal tube placement at the time of insertion. As a general guideline, the endotracheal tube should be inserted 21 to 23 cm from the incisors with orotracheal intubation and 25 to 27 cm from the nares with nasotracheal intubation.' This places the tip of the endotracheal tube 2 to 3 cm above the carina in the majority of patients.

If breath sounds are absent in a patient with good endotracheal tube placement, the treatment plan is based on the patient's vital signs. In the patient who is unstable or in extremis, action must be taken without a chest radiograph to aid in diagnosis. An appropriately placed needle thoracostomy in the second intercostal space in the midclavicular line can treat a life-threatening tension pneumothorax. This must be followed by definitive placement of a thoracostomy tube. If the physician has adequate experience and the necessary equipment is readily available, he or she can then proceed directly to chest tube placement in the fifth or sixth intercostal space, anterior to the midaxillary line. The thoracostomy tube is directed posteriorly for pneumothoracies and hemothoracies secondary to penetrating trauma. Almost all pneumothoraces visible on chest radiograph show some degree of associated hemothorax. A large chest tube, preferably 36 Fr or larger, should be used to evacuate blood. Smaller tubes are acceptable for isolated pneumothoraces.

With confirmaion of adequate ventilation one must then ensure circulatory stability. Two large-bore intravenous cannulas should be placed, preferably in a peripheral location. Blood should be sent for type and cross-match, and O-negative blood should be transfused if the patient remains in hypovolemic shock after 2 liters of crystalloid solution have been infused. If the patient remains in extremis, an emergency department anterolateral thoracotomy is indicated. This is performed with minimal prepping and draping because of time constraints. Although it is often futile, this procedure can be diagnostic, therapeutic, and life-saving. The cause of the hypotension is usually a major vascular injury or pericardial tamponade secondary to a cardiac wound. Release of a pericardial tamponade may result in hemodynamic stabilization. A finger placed over a cardiac wound may control bleeding, allowing further resuscitation and transport to the operating room for definitive cardiac repair (see Chapter 6 for further details). If the injury involves a major pulmonary vessel, treatment in the emergency department is usually limited to cross-clamping the pulmonary hilum to control blood loss and prevent air embolism. The descending thoracic aorta may be clamped to increase afterload, thus increasing perfusion to the heart and brain.

The majority of patients with penetrating chest trauma present with stable vital signs, thus allowing time for the physician to obtain a chest radiograph. Even when pneumothorax, hemothorax, or hemopneumothorax is absent on an initial chest radiograph, a repeat chest radiograph should be obtained after 3 to 6 hours. A normal chest radiograph at this time interval allows safe discharge of the patient with close outpatient follow-up provided there is no other reason to admit the patient.[8, 9] A pneumothorax or hemothorax is treated with a chest tube as described earlier. A massive hemothorax is an indication for a thoracotomy (see later section, Surgical Approaches for Penetrating Chest Trauma for details). These patients are in varying stages of hemorrhagic shock; however, individual changes in vital signs vary, if they are present at all. Recommendations of the American College of Surgeons as outlined in the ATLS guidelines indicate that blood loss of 1500 ml is an indication for thoracotomy. A major pulmonary vessel is the usual source of bleeding with this quantity of initial output. This blood may be salvaged and autotransfused in the patient who is hemodynamically unstable.[10–13] If there is initially a major air leak that persists after expansion of the lung, or if the lung cannot be reexpanded, operation is also strongly considered, since this situation is usually the result of a major bronchial injury.[11, 14] Loss of tidal volume through the chest tube, making ventilation difficult, is another indication for emergent operation. If the initial output from the chest tube is less than 1500 ml, if there is no major air leak, and if the patient is stable, a period of observation is warranted. If the output remains greater than 200 to 300 ml/hour for 2 to 3 hours, operative intervention is warranted. The injury in this setting is usually an intercostal vessel, internal mammary vessel, or small parenchymal vessel.

Although the ATLS criteria are excellent guidelines, a clinical approach to patients with hemothorax should also be used. Most patients who have over 1500 m of drainage from a chest tube immediately on insertion have ongoing active bleeding and are hemodynamically unstable, prompting a trip to the operating room. It is dangerous and unwise merely to observe these patients. Patients who drain less than a liter of blood are usually hemodynamically stable or can be stabilized with infusion of crystalloid solution. These patients rarely require blood transfusion if the chest wound is the only injury. These individuals can almost always be observed and require operation only if the chest tube drainage continues at a significant rate (>200 ml/hour) for the next 2 to 3 hours, or if a large air leak is present with failure to expand the lung. Consideration should be given to transfusion requirements in these patients as well. If observation means that a transfusion will be required for a dropping hemoglobin level with its associated physiologic changes, the risk of thoracotomy may be less than that of a blood transfusion.

There is a group of patients in which decisions should be based on the patient's hemodynamic status, taking into account other associated injuries and the patient's premorbid physiologic status. In this group drainage is generally between 1000 and 1500 ml on initial chest tube insertion. Those who are hemodynamically stable may be observed if the drainage slows down quickly, provided no other indication for thoracotomy exists and the patient does not require excessive transfusion. On the other hand, the patient who is hemodynamically unstable may be best served by an early thoracotomy. This is especially true if the patient has other associated injuries, is failing to respond to resuscitation, or has poor physiologic reserve. If the decision is made to observe the patient, a chest radiograph is always performed to confirm reexpansion of the lung and evacuation of the hemothorax. It is also important to ensure good chest tube placement, making sure that there are no kinks in the tube and that the last hole in the chest tube is within the pleural cavity. The drainage system should reflect respiratory variation in the water chamber, confirming a functional chest tube. The chest tube is left in place until drainage decreases to less than 100 ml/day, no air leak is present, and the chest radiograph confirms reexpansion of the lung with evacuation of the hemothorax. The chest tube can be removed immediately after suction is discontinued and a follow-up chest radiograph confirms continued expansion of the lung. No evidence or data suggest that a water-seal trial prior to chest tube removal decreases the incidence of recurrent pneumothorax.

Patients who have a retained hemothorax after 48 to 72 hours of chest tube drainage should be considered for early surgical evacuation of the retained hemothorax.[11, 15, 16] This can be accomplished through a limited muscle-sparing thoracotomy or through thoracoscopy.[17-19] This prevents the potential complication of infected hematoma with progression to empyema and entrapped lung, fibrothorax, and restrictive lung disease.[11, 15, 16, 20]

SURGICAL APPROACHES FOR PENETRATING CHEST TRAUMA

Unlike the situation with abdominal trauma, no single operative approach is ideal for thoracic trauma. The surgeon treating a patient with thoracic trauma has to choose the appropriate incision for the patient. Options include emergency department (anterior) thoracotomy, anterolateral thoracotomy, anterolateral thoracotomy with cross-sternal extension into the contralateral thorax, median sternotomy, sternotomy with right sternocleidomastoid extension, sternotomy with left supraclavicular and left anterolateral thoracic extensions (trap door incision), and the standard right or left posterolateral thoracotomy.[11]

Emergency Department Thoracotomy (Anterior Thoracotomy)

This incision allows access to the hemithorax, pulmonary hilum, descending thoracic aorta, and heart on the left, and to the hemithorax, pulmonary hilum, superior vena cava, and right atrial appendage on the right. This incision is most often used on the left side when thoracotomy must be performed and there is no time to position the patient. These patients are usually moribund on arrival and may show no signs of life; however, vital signs have been present in most in the field, and often signs of life have been witnessed. The presence of electrical activity in the myocardium should be confirmed before one embarks on an emergency department (ED) thoracotomy. The results of ED thoracotomy are uniformly dismal in patients with asystole or agonal rhythms on the electrocardiographic (ECG) tracing following penetrating trauma, especially gunshot wounds.[21, 22] Down times of greater than 20 minutes are also predictive of poor results. Nonintubated trauma patients with more than 5 minutes of prehospital cardiopulmonary resuscitation (CPR) and intubated trauma patients with more than 10 minutes of prehospital CPR rarely if ever survive.[23-25] If narrow complex pulseless electrical activity (PEA) is present, these patients may benefit from ED thoracotomy. Patients with isolated stab wounds to the chest have the best chance of resuscitation, and the most aggressive efforts should be made to salvage these patients.[26-28]

The resuscitative thoracotomy is performed with the patient in the supine position. The chest is rapidly prepped after the airway has been secured and large-bore intravenous access has been placed. Uncross-matched O-negative blood is given immediately to these patients simultaneously with crystalloid infusion. An incision is made from the sternum in the fourth or fifth intercostal space to the posterior axillary line using a scalpel with a No. 10 blade. The exposure and extent of the incision can be significantly improved by placing the patient's left arm above the head, which affords a longer incision with a more posterior extension. One cut with the knife divides the skin, subcutaneous tissues, and chest wall musculature, exposing the intercostal space. Mayo scissors are used to divide the intercostal muscles and pleura, with care taken not to injure the neurovascular bundle on the inferior surface of the rib.

A Finochetti retractor is placed in the incision and opened wide to expose the hemithorax. This exposes the pericardial sac and allows access to the descending thoracic aorta and the pulmonary hilum. Initial maneuvers in the left chest are determined by the presence or absence of a tense pericardium. In the setting of pericardial tamponade the pericardial sac is grasped with forceps and opened sharply. The pericardial incision is then extended parallel and anterior to the phrenic nerve with care taken not to injure this structure. Blood and clot are evacuated from the pericardium, and the heart is delivered from the pericardial sac. Inspection is performed, and digital control of cardiac bleeding is obtained. This is relatively easy when the heart is reparable. Release of the pericardial tamponade often stabilizes the patient; however, if the patient remains moribund, the descending thoracic aorta should be clamped, increasing perfusion of the coronary and cerebral circulation. It should be noted that this increased afterload may worsen bleeding from a cardiac wound, and the surgeon should be prepared for this.

If the patient shows no evidence of a pericardial tamponade, immediate attention should be turned toward the descending thoracic aorta. This should be clamped just above the diaphragm for the reasons previously mentioned. This is accomplished by sweeping one's hand along the posterior left chest until one encounters the vertebral column. The collapsed aorta will be felt anterior and slightly lateral to the spine. The presence of a nasogastric tube is of great help to the surgeon performing this procedure. The tube aids identification of the esophagus and allows the surgeon to bluntly dissect the plane between the aorta and the esophagus, which is located anterior to the aorta in this location. This allows secure complete clamping of the descending thoracic aorta without inadvertent injury to the esophagus, a potentially devastating iatrogenic injury. Great care must be taken during clamping of the aorta not to avulse the intercostal branches from the aorta. Either a straight vascular clamp or a Satinsky clamp may be used depending on the surgeon's preference.

Aortic hemorrhage from a torn intercostal vessel may explain continued bleeding in the thoracic cavity after the primary injury has been repaired. This is best treated by prevention by ensuring careful and accurate placement of the aortic cross clamp. Following clamping of the descending thoracic aorta, the pericardium should be opened as previously described and the heart delivered, allowing open cardiac massage with internal defibrillation should either of these procedures be necessary. The emergency department thoracotomy also allows rapid placement of a Satinsky clamp across the pulmonary hilum should exsanguinating hemorrhage from a major pulmonary vessel be found. This maneuver also affords protection from a fatal air embolism until the injury can be definitively controlled.

If the resuscitative thoracotomy is successful, attention should turn rapidly to control of chest wall bleeding. These patients have systemic acidosis, are frequently hypothermic, and often receive massive transfusion, resulting in significant coagulopathy. Divided muscle and tissues on the chest wall may bleed significantly when systemic perfusion is restored. Early attention to the hemostasis of these tissues will prevent continued blood loss while other injuries are treated.

Anterolateral Thoracotomy

This procedure is very similar to the anterior (ED) thoracotomy just described; however, it is preferable in the patient who is stable enough to be transported to the operating room where simple, rapid positioning is carried out. It is a more focused attack in the patient in whom thoracotomy is indicated. The incision is performed on the right or left side depending on the location of the suspected injury. The incision can be extended posterolaterally by placing a roll parallel to the patient's spine and log rolling the patient 15 to 30 degrees to the side opposite the planned incision. The ipsilateral arm may be positioned on an arm board or suspended from an ether screen at 90 degrees to the chest wall, removing it from the surgeon's field. This procedure is best for suspected injuries to the pulmonary parenchyma and its vasculature, or injuries to the anterior or middle mediastinal structures. It is poorly suited for access to the superior mediastinum. Although the posterior mediastinal structures can be reached through this incision, definitive repair of these structures can be difficult with this approach. Control of the subclavian vessels is also difficult with this approach; however, they can usually be manually compressed through the incision, controlling life-threatening hemorrhage while a more suitable exposure is sought for definitive repair of these vessels.

This remains the approach of choice in patients who are hemodynamically labile or unstable who have indications for thoracotomy. Minimal time is required for positioning, prepping, and draping the patient. This approach allows rapid access to the structures in the thoracic cavity that can result in rapid exsanguination if injured.

Anterior or Anterolateral Thoracotomy with Cross-Sternal Extension

Occasionally one encounters a situation in which the left chest has been opened in a resuscitative effort only to find that the injury producing the moribund state is located in the right chest. The patient may also have life-threatening injuries in both thoracic cavities resulting from a transmediastinal injury. In these cases, the anterior or anterolateral thoracotomy incision can be extended to the contralateral thorax by dividing the sternum transversely. The procedure can be accomplished with rib cutters, a Gigli saw, or a Lebsche knife. Sacrifice of one or both internal mammary arteries is mandatory. These must be ligated proximally and distally on either side of the sternum to prevent significant uncontrolled bleeding.[17] The thoracotomy incision is then extended through an intercostal space on the contralateral side of the chest, providing as much exposure as necessary to control the injury. This approach provides adequate exposure for structures in either hemithorax, the anterior and superior mediastinal structures, the aortic arch, and the arch vessels.

Median Sternotomy

A median sternotomy provides excellent exposure to the heart, superior mediastinal structures, aortic arch, and proximal great vessels. It also allows access to the pulmonary hilum, although not as well as a thoracotomy. The posterior mediastinum cannot be reached through a median sternotomy, and this is a poor choice of incision in patients with a known or suspected injury to a posterior mediastinal structure. The posterior mediastinum is better approached through a posterolateral thoracotomy (in a stable patient) or an anterolaleral thoracotomy (in an unstable patient). The sternotomy is the preferred approach for stable patients with penetrating injuries to the "precordial box" and an echocardiogram that is positive for an effusion and for those with a subxiphoid pericardial window that is positive for blood.[29] Stability should be emphasized because this approach usually requires more time than an anterolateral thoracotomy, especially in the hands of the noncardiac surgeon. The "precordial box" is defined as the square area bordered by the clavicles superiorly, the costal margins inferiorly, and the midclavicular lines laterally. Injuries to this region are dealt with in Chapter 6 and will not be discussed further here. The median sternotomy is also the procedure of choice if it is anicipated that cardiopulmonary bypass will be required for repair of the patient's injuries.

The sternotomy is begun by making an incision from the sternal notch to just below the xiphoid process. This incision is carried down to the manubrium and sternum, dividing the presternal fascia. A plane must then be developed posterior to the sternal notch, and this requires division of the suprasternal ligament, allowing access to the posterior aspect of the sternum with the sternal saw and preventing injury to the left innominate vein, which passes just posterior to the superior aspect of the manubrium. A plane must also be developed posterior to he xiphoid process, freeing the lower end of the sternum. This can be done rapidly with blunt finger dissection. Blunt dissection can now be performed from above and below the sternum, clearing the plane immediately posterior to it. If time permits, it is advisable to mark a line from the sternal notch to the xiphoid process in the center of the sternum, providing a guide for the sternal saw. This can be readily accomplished with electrocautery. Such a line prevents uneven division of the sternum, which can pose significant problems at the time of closure and can compromise wound healing.

Next, the sternum is divided with the sternal saw beginning at the sternal notch and proceeding caudally. It is important to divide the sternum smoothly in the midline, maintaining a constant upward tension on the saw. This step requires communication with the anesthesiologist, who should not ventilate the patient during the sternal splitting. Under suboptimal conditions when a sternal saw is not readily available, a Lebsche knife and mallet may be used to accomplish sternal division. On completion of the sternotomy a sternal retractor is placed in the wound with the sternal edges protected by laparotomy sponges. If time permits, hemostasis of the sternal edges should be obtained because these can be a source of constant blood loss.

The pericardium is now exposed anteriorly. The left innominate vein should be identified at this point and carefully dissected to avoid iatrogenic injury to this structure. If blood is present in the pericardial sac the sac should be opened anteriorly, exposing the anterior surface of the right ventricle. Blood and clot should be evacuated from the pericardium, and digital pressure can be used to control bleeding from the heart as previously described if a cardiac injury is encountered. This approach also allows excellent access to the aortic arch, the great vessels of the upper extremities, and the cerebral circulation if these structures are known to be injured.

Closure of the sternotomy wound is just as important as opening the chest. If the pericardium was opened it is left open and drained. One to two mediastinal chest tubes should be placed prior to closure, and appropriate pleural tubes should be placed if the mediastinal pleura was violated on either side of the chest. The manubrium should be closed with at least two 22-gauge interrupted stainless steel sutures, and the sternum should be closed with four to six interrupted stainless steel sutures of the same size. Care should be taken in placing the sternal wires not to injure the underlying mammary vessels by placing them medial to the mammary vessels. The presternal fascia should be reapproximated using a running continuous absorbable suture. The abdominal fascia should be closed anterior to the xiphoid to prevent a subxiphoid incisional hernia.[30] The subcutaneous layer should be approximated with a running absorbable suture, and the skin should be carefully approximated. Failure to perform meticulous closure of the sternotomy incision creates the potential for disastrous complications including wound dehiscence, sternal osteomyelitis, and mediastinitis that can be life-threatening.[31-34] It is tragic to have a patient survive a lethal injury only to succumb from a wound complication. All efforts should be made to avoid these often preventable disasters.

Median Sternotomy with Right Sternocleidomastoid Extension

There are specific injuries in the chest that are not easily approached from any one incision, and for these injuries superior exposure is provided by using a combination of incisions in continuity. One such example is the median sternotomy used in combination with a right sternocleidomastoid incision. This incision provides access to the innominate artery from its origin at the aortic arch. It allows control of this vessel as well as its major branch vessels, the right subclavian artery and the right common carotid artery (Fig. 5–1). The origin of the right vertebral artery from the first portion of the subclavian artery is also visualized. This exposure is ideally suited for repair or bypass of any of the above named vessels except the vertebral artery.

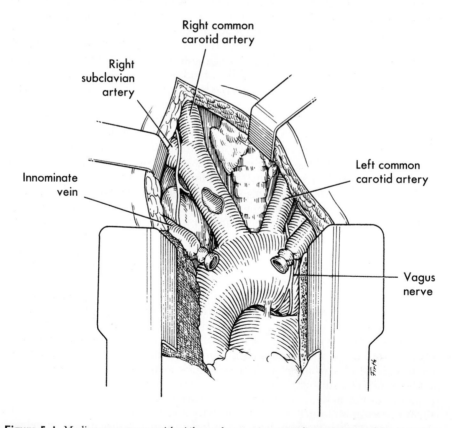

Figure 5–1. Median sternotomy with right neck extension providing exposure of the innominate, right subclavian, and right common carotid arteries. (From Donovan AJ: Trauma Surgery: Techniques in Thoracic, Abdominal, and Vascular Surgery. St. Louis, Mosby, 1994.)

A median sternotomy is performed as described earlier. The sternotomy incision is then joined by an incision that divides the platysma muscle along the anterior border of the sternocleidomastoid muscle and extends to the sternal notch. The sternal and clavicular heads of the sternocleidomastoid muscle are then divided. Division of the innominate vein enhances exposure of the innominate artery if this is necessary and provides adequate exposure of the first part of the right subclavian artery. Care must be taken to protect the right vagus nerve and its recurrent laryngeal branch, which passes around the right subclavian artery at this location.

The subclavian artery is anatomically divided into three portions by the anterior scalene muscle. The first portion extends from its origin to the medial border of this muscle. The second portion passes posterior to the anterior scalene muscle, and the third portion extends from its lateral border to the lateral edge of the first rib. Exposure of the second portion of the subclavian artery is accomplished by making a supraclavicular incision approximately 2 cm above the medial and middle thirds of the clavicle. The anterior scalene muscle is divided, exposing the second portion of the subclavian artery. Great care must be taken to avoid the phrenic nerve, which passes over the anterior scalene muscle. Exposure of the third portion of the subclavian artery is achieved by carrying the supraclavicular incision laterally and performing an infraclavicular incision beneath the middle the lateral thirds of the clavicle, dividing the pectoralis major muscle. At times, exposure of the subclavian artery can be facilitated by resecting the head and medial third of the clavicle. This can be accomplished using a Gigli saw, taking care not to injure the subclavian vein immediately posterior to the clavicle

The axillary artery can be exposed through the same infraclavicular incision, dividing the pectoralis major muscle and the pectoralis minor muscle near its insertion on the coracoid process. The axillary artery is divided into three anatomic portions by the pectoralis minor muscle. The first portion extends from the lateral border of the first rib to the medial head of the pectoralis minor muscle. The second portion lies immediately posterior to the head of this muscle. The third portion extends from the lateral aspect of the pectoralis minor muscle to the medial border of the teres major muscle near its insertion on the humerus. The axillary artery can be repaired without entering the thoracic cavity. The first portion can be exposed through an infraclavicular incision. Exposure of the second portion requires division of the pectoralis minor muscle as well. Exposure of the distal third may require extension of the infraclavicular chest wall incision into the axilla and onto the medial aspect of the upper arm. Great care must be taken when exposing this vessel not to injure the brachial plexus. The medial and lateral cords are identified as the axillary artery is exposed anteriorly, and the posterior cord is intimately related to the posterior aspect of this vessel. As with the median sternotomy, meticulous attention is required to close these wounds to minimize postoperative morbidity.

Median Sternotomy with Left Supraclavicular and Left Anterolateral Thoracic Extension

Injury to the left subclavian artery causing free exsanguination into the thorax challenges even the most skilled thoracic, vascular, and trauma surgeon.

Control of this injury may require a series of operative maneuvers that may begin with an ED thoracotomy for resuscitation of the moribund or lifeless victim of penetrating wound to the chest. A massive left hemothorax may be encountered; however, the left subclavian artery is not easily visualized or controlled through the anterior left thoracotomy. A skilled surgeon can recognize this injury but can do little to repair it through this approach. It may be possible to place an occluding vascular clamp proximal to the injury. If not, manual compression can be applied through the left chest, tamponading free bleeding into the thorax while anesthesia personnel replace the patient's blood volume and restore perfusion. Preparations are then made to further expose the injured vessel while manual occlusion is maintained through the thoracotomy incision.

A combination of incisions provides the best exposure of this vessel. A supraclavicular incision over the proximal and middle thirds of the clavicle may be all that is necessary to control the vessel and provide adequate exposure for repair. Resection of the head and medial third of the clavicle may improve this exposure as described for exposure of the right subclavian artery. If this does not prove adequate, a "trap door" exposure may be required. This involves the use of a sternotomy incision to connect the supraclavicular incision above and the thoracotomy incision below, creating a window that provides exposure of the entire course of the subclavian artery. A sternal retractor may provide exposure. If this is inadequate, the clavicle and first several ribs can be divided at the lateral margin of the exposure, allowing the surgeon to fold back a trap door in the anterior chest wall (Fig. 5–2). Care must be taken to protect the vagus nerve and its recurrent laryngeal branch, which pass in an anterior to posterior direction around the aortic arch just posterior to the ductus arteriosus on this side of the chest. The origins of the left common carotid and vertebral arteries are also exposed with this approach.

Although this incision may be life-saving, it is fraught with wound healing problems and postoperative pain syndromes and causalgias.[35–37] It should be used only when other attempts to control the subclavian artery have failed. It should not be used for primary exposure of the left common carotid or the left vertebral artery. Adequate exposure of these vessels can usually be obtained extrathoracically. The left axillary artery can be exposed for repair without entering the thorax in the same way as that described for the right axillary artery.

Posterolateral Thoracotomy

The structures of the posterior mediastinum on both the right and left sides of the chest are not easily exposed through any of the incisions previously discussed. While they can be approached and bleeding can be controlled, definitive repair can be difficult. These structures are best approached through a standard right or left posterolateral thoracotomy. These incisions provide access to the pulmonary hilum, the lung parenchyma, and the diaphragm on both sides of the chest. The left posterolateral thoracotomy also provides exposure of the lateral aspect of the heart and left ventricle, the left subclavian artery, the descending thoracic aorta, the lower third of the esophagus, and

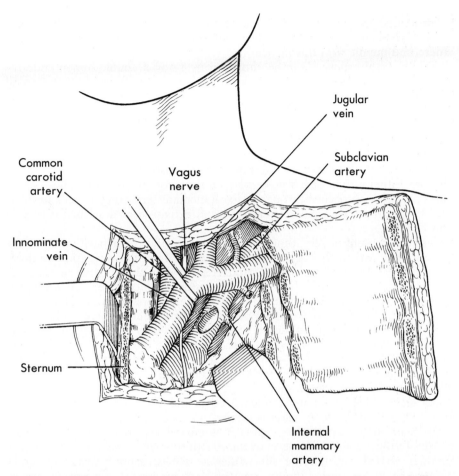

Common
carotid
artery

Vagus
nerve

Jugular
vein

Subclavian
artery

Innominate
vein

Sternum

Internal
mammary
artery

Figure 5–2. "Trap door" exposure of the left subclavian artery. (From Donovan AJ: Trauma Surgery: Techniques in Thoracic, Abdominal, and Vascular Surgery. St. Louis, Mosby, 1994.)

the left mainstem bronchus. The right posterolateral thoracotomy incision exposes the azygous vein, the superior vena cava, the right atrium, the upper thoracic esophagus, the intrathoracic trachea, the carina, and the right mainstem bronchus. The posterolateral thoracotomy incision is used primarily in stable patients because it takes time to position the patient properly, and it is not wise to take this time in an unstable patient. Consideration must also be given to the integrity of the thoracic and cervical spine before positioning these patients in the lateral decubitus position.

Ideal exposure for a known or suspected injury can be achieved by adjusting the intercostal space entered to the appropriate level of the injured structure. If the nature of the injury is unknown, the best overall exposure is achieved through the fourth or fifth intercostal space. Subperiosteal resection of a rib may facilitate exposure. Posterior transection of a rib without resection often provides adequate exposure and avoids rib resection and iatrogenic rib fracture caused by opening the rib spreader. Caution must be used not to injure the intercostal bundle with this maneuver.

Finally, ideal exposure can be enhanced by using a double-lumen endotracheal tube or an endobronchial blocker, which allows collapse of the ipsilateral lung intraoperatively once the chest has been opened. It also protects the dependent lung from blood and secretions during the operation. This tube requires significant preoperative time for insertion and experienced personnel familiar with its use.[38] If it is used, correct placement should be confirmed before positioning the patient for the operation.

Exposure of the anterior and superior mediastinal structures is difficult through either a right or left posterolateral thoracotomy incision. These structures are best approached through either a median sternotomy or an anterolateral thoracotomy with possible cross-sternal extension as described earlier in this chapter.

Successful posterolateral thoracotomy begins with proper positioning of the patient. The patient should be placed in the lateral decubitus position, preferably on a bean bag to aid in stabilization. A soft roll is placed between the axilla and the operating room table to avoid compression neuropathy of the upper extremity. The upper arm is supported on a Mayo stand or an airplane splint. Care should be taken to avoid compression of the median nerve at the elbow. The lower leg is bent at 90 degrees and the top leg is kept straight. Padding or pillows are placed between the legs at the knees and beneath the ankles to relieve pressure points. The pelvis is stabilized by taping the region of the anterior iliac spine to the operating room table on both sides. The patient is then prepped and draped widely.

An incision beginning at the midclavicular line of the interspace desired for exposure is made. This incision is carried posteriorly, and approximately 1 to 2 cm beneath the tip of the scapula it is curved cephalad along the medial border of the scapula to the level of the fourth thoracic vertebrae. The incision is then carried through the subcutaneous tissues, exposing the auscultory triangle on the posterior thorax near the sixth interspace. This triangle is so named because it is an area devoid of muscular tissue and is ideal for auscultation of the chest. Its borders are the trapezius, latissimus dorsi, and rhomboid major muscles. This provides an ideal area in which to develop an avascular plane between the muscles of the chest wall. It allows one to isolate the latissimus dorsi muscle anteriorly and the trapezius posteriorly. These muscles are divided with the electrocautery, achieving careful hemostasis. The serratus muscle anteriorly and the rhomboid major muscle posterioly are now divided in similar fashion. This exposes the rib cage and the intercostal spaces. The scapula is lifted off the chest wall with the use of the scapular retractor, and the ribs are counted to select the interspace for entering the thorax. This can be done in two different ways. The first is to count from the first rib; the second is to count from the second rib that can be identified by palpating the insertion of the middle scalene muscle. The intercostal muscles are divided in the selected interspace, exposing the pleura. If a rib is to be taken, a periosteal elevator is used to elevate the intercostal muscle superiorly. After separating the neurovascular bundle from the inferior aspect of the rib, the rib is then divided with a rib cutter. The remaining rib ends may be trimmed with a

Sauerbruch, enhancing the extent of rib resection. The rib may be cut posteriorly to allow better exposure without formal rib resection as discussed earlier. The pleura is divided, and the thoracic cavity, is entered.

Ideal exposure involves selecting the appropriate interspace for the injury to be repaired. If this is unknown, the fourth to fifth interspace provides optimal exposure for the majority of structures in either hemithorax. It is often a preoperative study such as an angiogram, esophagram, esophagoscopy, or a bronchoscopy that has identified the injury that brings the stable patient to the operating room. In this situation, preoperative knowledge of the level of injury dictates the interspace incised, and optimal exposure can be achieved. On the right side of the chest an injury to the thoracic esophagus or trachea is best approached through the fourth or fifth intercostal space. Repair of the carina or right mainstem bronchus is best accomplished through the fifth interspace. Most other injuries in the right chest are not identifiable preoperatively and are approached through the fourth to fifth interspace. On the left side, injuries to the left subclavian artery or high descending thoracic aorta are best approached through the third intercostal space. Repair of the left mainstem bronchus can be accomplished through an incision in the fourth or fifth intercostal space.[39] Injuries to the lower thoracic aorta or the esophagus in the left chest are best exposed through the seventh intercostal space.

Following repair of the injured thoracic structures, wide drainage should be employed. The thoracic cavity should be inspected for chyle to ensure that the thoracic duct has not been violated. Two 36-Fr chest tubes should be placed, one in the apex and one in the posterior sulcus, to evacuate blood and air, and they should be brought through the anterior and midaxillary lines. The chest wall is then closed in layers. The ribs are first approximated with interrupted pericostal sutures. A rib approximator facilitates tying these sutures. The intercostal muscles are then closed with a running absorbable suture, providing an airtight seal of the pleural cavity. The rhomboid major and serratus anterior muscles are approximated with a running absorbable suture, as are the latissimus dorsi and trapezius muscles. The skin is closed in all cases. The chest tubes are hooked to suction after the intercostal muscles have been closed.

The patient is then placed in a supine position on the operating table. If the patient requires continued intubation and a double-lumen tube was used, it is changed to a standard endotracheal tube at this point. If a standard endotracheal tube was used during the operation it is a good idea to perform a bronchoscopy prior to leaving the operating room. This removes blood and secretions from the lung that was dependent during the operation, minimizing the chance of postoperative lobar collapse due to retained blood and secretions.

These patients all require aggressive pulmonary toilet postoperatively as well as adequate analgesia. This incision is one of the more painful surgical incisions for patients. A properly placed epidural catheter provides excellent postoperative pain relief with a low incidence of narcotic-related side effects.[40–50] This should be considered in all patients if there is no contraindication to placing one.

Thoracoscopy

Thoracoscopy has been used increasingly in elective thoracic surgery, and further applications are being realized.[51] Thoracoscopy has a role in the patient with penetrating thoracic trauma as well. It is an excellent and minimally invasive method of diagnosing diaphragmatic injuries resulting from penetrating trauma. It is also a very effective way of evacuating a retained hemothorax if it is done early in the postinjury period, preventing potential infection, empyema, and associated morbidity.[16, 51-54] These patients should all be intubated with a double-lumen endotracheal tube because collapse of the lung on the operative side is required for adequate visualization in the chest. Minimal pain is associated with this procedure and most patients do well with minimal compromise of pulmonary status. As further experience with this technique is gained, its usefulness in patients with penetrating thoracic trauma may increase.

THE PENETRATING CHEST WOUND

The patient presenting with a penetrating chest wound requires resuscitation in an organized fashion beginning with the ABCs as outlined in the American College of Surgeon's Advanced Trauma Life Support (ATLS) course. This begins with evaluation of the airway, which is secured if it is compromised (see text). Evaluation of breathing and assessment of the patient's ability to ventilate follows. This begins with checking the patient's breath sounds. If breath sounds are adequate, a radiograph is performed to ensure that no pneumothorax or hemothorax is present. In the absence of these findings stabilization of the circulation, assessment of neurologic disability, and complete exposure of the patient are performed next. If a pneumothorax or hemothorax is present, a chest tube is placed on the appropriate side. If breath sounds are absent, rapid assessment for respiratory distress and hemodynamic stability is required.

The patient who is stable without respiratory distress may be evaluated radiographically. Position of the endotracheal tube should be checked if the patient is intubated. If the tube is inserted too far, it should be repositioned and breath sounds reassessed. The chest radiograph should be examined for the presence of a pneumothorax or hemothorax. If either of these is present a chest tube should be inserted on the appropriate side. Following either intervention, breath sounds are reassessed, and the chest radiograph is repeated. Intervention must be performed without a chest radiograph in the patient with respiratory distress or hemodynamic instability. A chest tube should be placed on the side on which breath sound are absent. If the patient stabilizes, breath sounds are reassessed, and a chest radiograph is performed.

If the patient remains unstable, intervention is based on the output from the chest tube. If the chest tube output is massive (see text) and the patient is moribund, an emergency department thoracotomy should be performed on the left side of the chest. In the unstable patient who is not moribund, rapid transport to the operating room for anterolateral thoracotomy is indicated. If the chest tube output is low one must ensure that the tube has been properly positioned. This is accomplished clinically by assessing the thoracic drainage system for respiratory variation. The tube is improperly positioned if no respiratory variation is present; in this case, the tube should be repositioned or replaced. If there is good respiratory variation in the system, the tube is properly placed, and instability is likely to be secondary to another cause.

The physician should obtain a chest radiograph to confirm the clinical impression of a properly placed chest tube while searching for other causes of instability. Possible sources that should be considered include: pericardial tamponade, hemoperitoneum, retroperitoneal or pelvic hemorrhage, spinal shock, and cardiac contusion. Diagnostic tests such as echocardiography, subxiphoid pericardial window, diagnostic peritoneal lavage, rectal examination, spinal radiographs, and computed tomography may be useful adjunctive studies to help clarify the cause of the problem.

PENETRATING CHEST WOUND THAT REQUIRES OPERATION

The operative approach to the patient with penetrating chest trauma depends on the hemodynamic stability of the patient. The moribund patient requires urgent emergency department thoracotomy if he or she is to be salvaged. This allows pericardial decompression in the setting of cardiac tamponade. Cross-clamping of the descending thoracic aorta can be performed to improve cardiac and cerebral blood flow. The pulmonary hilum can be cross-clamped to prevent exsanguination and air embolism. Open cardiac massage and defibrillation may be performed if necessary. The incision may be carried across the sternum if the patient is in extremis from a right-sided thoracic injury. The unstable patient who has an obtainable blood pressure also requires urgent operative intervention. These individuals are rapidly transported to the operating room for anterolateral thoracotomy on the side of injury.

Hemodynamically stable patients require assessment of the area of injury. There are four injury patterns to be considered: precordial (anterior cardiac box), zone I of the neck, posterior thorax, and transmediastinal injuries. Wounds to the anterior cardiac box (see text) place the patient at risk for pericardial tamponade. Pericardial fluid can be identified by either echocardiography or a subxiphoid pericardial window.[29, 55–57] If either of these studies is positive, the patient should undergo median sternotomy for repair of the injury leading to fluid (blood) in the pericardial sac.

The patient who has an injury to zone I of the neck (the area below the cricoid cartilage) is at risk for injury to the great vessels, esophagus, and intrathorcic trachea and mainstem bronchi. These individuals should undergo evaluation including esophagram, esophagoscopy, bronchoscopy, and aortic arch study of the great vessels. If abnormalities are found on the esophagram, esophagoscopy, or bronchoscopy, the patient requires a posterolateral thoracotomy for repair. If the aortic arch study is positive, the patient requires an operation. The aortic arch can be repaired through a median sternotomy. Injury to the innominate, right subclavian artery, or origin of the right common carotid artery also requires median sternotomy with extension along the right sternocleidomastoid muscle for repair. Injuries to the left subclavian artery may be repaired through a supraclavicular incision; clavicular resection may enhance exposure. If exposure remains inadequate, a "trap door" approach may be utilized (see text).

The patient with an injury confined to the posterior thorax requires a workup that includes esophagram, esophagoscopy, and aortogram of the descending thoracic aorta. Positive results on any of these studies require posterolateral thoracotomy for repair (see text).

The person with a transmediastinal wound is at greatest risk for injury and requires extensive evaluation. Work-up should consist of echocardiography or a subxiphoid pericardial window, esophagram and esophagoscopy, bronchoscopy, and an aortogram of the aortic arch, proximal great vessels, and descending thoracic aorta. If the echocardiogram or the subxiphoid pericardial window is positve, the patient requires a median sternotomy. If the esophagram, esophagoscopy, or bronchoscopy reveals injuries, the patient requires a posterolateral thoracotomy to repair these structures. If the arteriogram reveals injury to the descending thoracic aorta, a posterolateral thoracotomy is also required. If the arteriogram reveals injury to the aortic arch or proximal great vessels, a median sternotomy with possible sternocleidomastoid extension is required for repair on the right. A supraclavicular incision with possible "trap door" exposure is required to repair the left subclavian artery.

References

1. LoCicero J, Mattox KL: Epidemiology of chest trauma. Surg Clin North Am 1989;69:15.
2. Mattox KL, Wall M: Thoracic trauma. *In* Baue AE, Geha AS, Hammond GL, et al (eds): Glenn's Thoracic and Cardiovascular Surgery, 6th ed. Stamford, Appleton and Lange, 1996, p. 91.
3. Wilson RF, Murray C, Antonenko DR: Nonpenetrating thoracic injuries. Surg Clin North Am 1997;57:17.
4. Mattox KL, Wall MJ, Pickard LR: Thoracic trauma: General considerations and indications for thoracotomy. *In* Feliciano DV, Moore EE, Mattox KL (eds): Trauma, 3rd ed. Stamford, Appleton and Lange, 1996, p. 345.
5. Nagy KK, Barrett J: Diaphragm. *In* Ivatury RR, Cayten GC (eds): Textbook of Penetrating Trauma. Baltimore, Williams & Wilkins, 1996, p. 564.
6. Iverson KV: Blind nasotracheal intubation. Ann Emerg Med 1981;10:468.
7. Benumof J: Conventional (laryngoscopic) orotracheal and nasotracheal intubation (single lumen type). *In* Benumof J (ed): Clinical Procedures in Anesthesia and Intensive Care. Philadelphia, JB Lippincott, 1992, p. 115.
8. Kerstein KJ: Role of three hour roentgenogram of the chest in penetrating and non-penetrating injuries of the chest. Surg Gynecol Obstet 1992;175(3):249.
9. Kerr TM, Sood R, Buckman RF: Prospective trial of the six hour rule in stab wounds of the chest. Surg Gynecol Obstet 1989;169:233.
10. Mattox KL: Autotransfusion in the emergency department. J Am Coll Emerg Physicians 1975;4:218.
11. Mattox KL: Indications for thoracotomy: Deciding to operate. Surg Clin North Am 1989;69:47.
12. Van Way CW: Advanced techniques in thoracic surgery. Surg Clin North Am 1989;69:143.
13. Symbas PN, Levin JM, Ferrier FL et al: A study of autotransfusion from hemothorax. South Med J 1969;62:671.
14. Grover FL, Ellestad C, Arom KV et al: Diagnosis and management of major tracheobronchial injuries. Ann Thorac Surg 1979;28:384.
15. Coselli JS, Mattox KL, Beall AC: Reevaluation of early evacuation of clotted hemothorax. Am J Surg 1984;148:786.
16. Milfeld DJ, Mattox KL, Beall AC: Early evacuation of clotted hemothorax. Am J Surg 1978;136:686.
17. Siegel T, Steiger Z: Axillary thoracotomy. Surg Gynecol Obst 1982;155:725.
18. Hazelrigg SR, Landreneau JL, Boley TM, et al: the effect of muscle sparing versus standard posterolateral thoracotomy on pulmonary function, muscle strength, and postoperative pain. J Thorac Cardiovasc Surg 1991;101:394.
19. Ginsberg RJ: Alternative (muscle-sparing) incisions in thoracic surgery. The First International Symposium of Thoroscopic Surgery. Ann Thorac Surg 1993;56:752.
20. Symbas PN, Gott JP: Delayed sequela of thoracic trauma. Surg Clin North Am 1989;69:135.

21. Moore EE, Moore JB, Galloway AC, et al: Postinjury thoracotomy in the emergency department: A critical evaluation. Surgery 1979;86:590.
22. Harnar TJ, Oreskovich MR, Copass MK, et al: Role of emergency thoracotomy in the resuscitation of moribund trauma victims. Am J Surg 1981;142:96.
23. Mattox KL: Prehospital care of the patient with an injured chest. Surg Clin North Am 1989;69:21.
24. Copass MK, Oreskovich MR, Bladergroen MR: Prehospital cardiopulmonary resuscitation of the critically injured patient. Am J Surg 1984;148:20.
25. Mattox KL, Feliciano DV: Role of external cardiac compression in truncal trauma. J Trauma 1982;22:934.
26. Baxter BT, Moore EE, Cleveland HC, et al: Emergency department thoracotomy following injury: Critical determinants for survival. World J Surg 1988;12:671.
27. Washington B, Wilson RF, Steiger Z, et al: Emergency thoracotomy: A four-year review. Ann Thorac Surg 1985;40(2):188.
28. Ivatury RR, Rohman M: The injured heart. Surg Clin North Am 1989;69:93.
29. Nagy KK, Lohmann C, Kim D, et al: Role of echocardiography in the diagnosis of occult penetrating cardiac injury. J Trauma 1995;38:859.
30. Davidson BR, Bailey JS: Repair of incisional hernia after median sternotomy. Thorax 1987;42:549.
31. Demmy TL, Park SB, Liebler GA, et al: Recent experience with major sternal wound complications. Ann Thorac Surg 1990;49:458.
32. Grossi EA, Culliford AT, Krieger RH, et al: A survey of 77 major infectious complications of median sternotomy: A review of 7,949 consecutive operative procedures. Ann Thorac Surg 1985;40:214.
33. Miller J, Nahai F: Repair of dehised median sternotomy incision. Surg Clin North Am 1989;69:1091.
34. Molina E: Primary closure for infected dehiscence of the sternum. Ann Thorac Surg 1993;55:459.
35. Graham JM, Feliciano DV, Mattox KL, et al: Management of subclavian vascular injuries. J Trauma 1980;20:537.
36. Graham JM, Feliciano DV, Mattox KL: Innominate vascular injury. J Trauma 1982;22:647.
37. Mattox KL: Approaches to trauma involving major vessels of the thorax. Surg Clin North Am 1989;69:77.
38. Slinger PD: Fiberoptic bronchoscopic positioning of double-lumen tubes. J Cardiothorac Anesth 1989;3:486.
39. Pate JW: Tracheobronchial and esophageal injuries. Surg Clin North Am 1989;69:111.
40. Johnston JR, McCaughey W: Epidural morphine. A method of management of multiple fractured ribs. Anaesthesia 1980;35:155.
41. Mackersie RC, Shackford SR, Hoyt DB, et al: Continuous epidural fentanyl analgesia: Ventilatory function improvement with routine use in treatment of blunt chest injury. J Trauma 1987;27:1207.
42. Wisner DH: A stepwise logistic regression analysis of factors affecting morbidity and mortality after thoracic trauma: Effect of epidural analgesia. J Trauma 1990;30:799.
43. Worthley LIG: Thoracic epidural in the management of chest trauma. Intens Care Med 1985;11:312.
44. Moss G, Regal ME, Lichtig L: Reducing postoperative pain, narcotics, and length of hospitalization. Surgery 1986;99:206.
45. Shulman M, Sandler AN, Bradley JW, et al: Postthoracotomy pain and pulmonary function following epidural and systemic morphine. Anesthesiology 1984;61:569.
46. James EC, Kolberg HL, Iwen GW, et al: Epidural analgesia for post-thoracotomy patients. J Thorac Cardiovasc Surg 1981;82:898.
47. El-Baz NM, Faber LP, Jesnik RJ: Continuous epidural infusion of morphine for treatment of pain after thoracic surgery: A new technique. Anesth Analg 1984;63:757.
48. Gray JR, Fromme GA, Nauss LA, et al: Intrathecal morphine for postthoracotomy pain. Anesth Analg 1986;65:873.
49. Logas WG, El-Baz N, El-Ganzouri A, et al: Continous thoracic epidural analgesia for postoperative pain relief following thoracotomy: A randomized prospective study. Anesthesiology 1987;67:787.
50. Salomaki TE, Laitinen JO, Nuutinen LS: A randomized double-blind comparison of epidural

versus intravenous fentanyl infusion for analgesia after thoracotomy. Anesthesiology 1991;75:790.

51. Simmon RJ, Ivatury RR: Current concepts in the use of cavitary endoscopy in the evaluation and treatment of blunt and penetrating truncal injuries. Surg Clin North Am 1995;75:157.
52. Eddy AC, Luna GK, Copass M: Empyema thoracis in patients undergoing emergent closed tube thoracostomy for thoracic trauma. Am J Surg 1989;157:494.
53. Mancini M, Smith LM, Nein A, et al: Early evacuation of clotted blood in hemothorax using thoracoscopy: Case reports. J Trauma 1993;34:144.
54. Branco JMJ: Thoracoscopy as a method of exploration in penetrating injuries of the thorax. Dis Chest 1946;12:330.
55. Miller FB, Bond SJ, Shumate CR, et al: Diagnostic pericardial window: A safe alternative to exploratory thoracotomy for suspected heart injuries. Arch Surg 1987;122:605.
56. Brewster SA, Thirlby RC, Synder WH: Subxiphoid pericardial window and penetrating cardiac trauma. Arch Surg 1988;123:937.
57. Mayor-Davies JA, Britz RS: Subxiphoid pericardial windows: Helpful in selected cases. J Trauma 1990;30:1399.

Chapter 6

Penetrating Injuries to the Precordium

Penetrating injury to the precordium demands rapid, focused diagnostic maneuvers to answer the essential question, "Is the injury a cardiac injury or a great vessel injury?" The algorithm presented here depicts the course recommended for the patient who arrives in the emergency center alive or with recently lost vital signs.

Rates of prehospital mortality for patients with penetrating precordial trauma vary in reports from different centers, but they are invariably high.[1-6] Baker and colleagues reported that 51% of patients with a cardiac injury were dead on arrival at the hospital[1] whereas Demetriades and associates reported a 76.5% mortality before reaching medical attention.[3] Saadia and colleagues categorized the arrival condition of patients with penetrating precordial wounds into five groups. These are (1) lifeless, (2) critically unstable, (3) cardiac tamponade, (4) thoracoabdominal injury, and (5) benign.[7] We have used these categories in the algorithm in this chapter. In all cases, one must remember to follow the ABCs (airway, breathing, circulation) while minimizing time-wasting maneuvers and institutional procedures. Most patients require only a blood specimen for type and cross-match, which is drawn while intravenous access is established. Other patients may be stable enough to obtain further laboratory and radiologic studies as needed for the clinical situation.

HISTORY

The first successful cardiorrhaphy in a human was performed by Rehn in 1896.[8] Although enthusiasm for thoracotomy for the treatment of penetrating cardiac injuries increased during the following decades, the high complication rate of thoracotomy led to a report by Blalock and Ravitch in 1943[32] supporting definitive treatment of tamponade by repeated aspiration and observation. In 1959 Isaacs[9] reported on 60 cases of penetrating injury to the heart and advocated a selective approach to the choice of operative versus nonoperative management. Further advances occurred with the introduction of emergency room thoracotomy,[34] the subxiphoid window,[26] and echocardiography for penetrating cardiac trauma.[29]

PATHOPHYSIOLOGY

Two pathophysiologic phenomena dominate the presentation of penetrating precordial injury. The first is cardiac tamponade. If the pericardial laceration seals with fat or clotted blood, the pericardial sac rapidly fills with blood. The

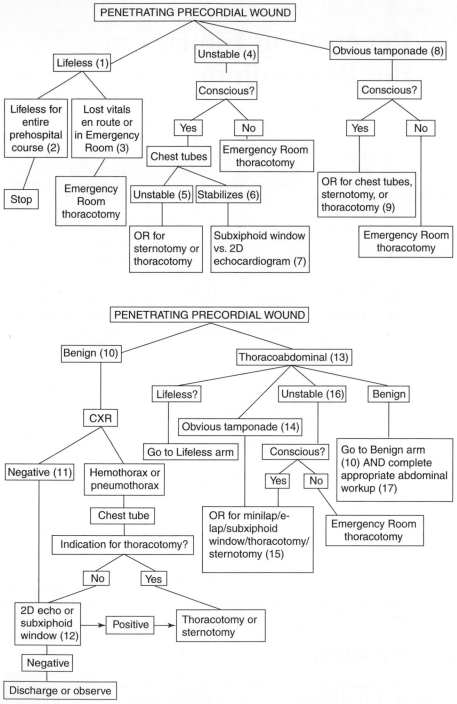

1. The lifeless patient shows no pupillary response or vital signs. Lifeless patients who regain signs of life after initial resuscitative efforts in the field move to the "unstable" arm.
2. Patients who exhibit no signs of life during the entire prehospital course and arrive at the hospital with no signs of life are usually not salvageable, and thoracotomy or other resuscitative efforts are futile.
3. Patients who have vital signs but lose them en route to the hospital or in the emergency room are the best candidates for emergency room thoracotomy. See text for details of technique.
4. This arm of the algorithm is for patients who exhibit hypotension (systolic blood pressure [SBP]<90) or, in the absence of severe hypotension, signs of shock (diaphoresis, altered sensorium). Patients with obvious tamponade move to the "obvious tamponade" arm of the algorithm. Note that no time is spent getting chest x-rays (CXR) in these unstable patients, although portable CXR can be done in patients who become stable after insertion of a chest tube as long as this does not become the rate-limiting step in getting the patient to the OR or delay echocardiography.
5. If the patient remains unstable after placement of appropriate chest tubes, a cause for the instability must be sought. If the chest tube output does not meet the criteria for performing a thoracotomy, the heart must be explored through a sternotomy or thoracotomy. If chest tube output does meet criteria for performing a thoracotomy, one must remember to explore the heart at the time of thoracotomy (do not be distracted by other injuries found at thoracotomy).
6. Stabilization at this point does not mark the end of the algorithm. Although a hemothorax or pneumothorax may have been treated, the heart still must be evaluated.
7. Either a subxiphoid window or two-dimensional echocardiography is acceptable. The choice depends on institutional availability of resources. If resources for cardiac repair are not available, the patient should be transferred.
8. Obvious tamponade indicates that the patient has an injury over the cardiac silhouette, hypotension or narrow pulse pressure, and one or more of the remaining components of Beck's triad (jugular venous distention, muffled heart notes). Uncertainty about the diagnosis should prompt a move to the "unstable" arm of the algorithm.
9. It is necessary to place appropriate chest tubes to determine the need for thoracotomy (e.g., combined bleeding pulmonary injury and cardiac injury). Although the heart can be addressed through a thoracotomy, the pleural cavity cannot be approached well through a sternotomy.
10. Patients in this arm of the algorithm are hemodynamically stable, have no respiratory distress, and are without signs of shock.
11. Negative results on CXR does not preclude the need for cardiac work-up.
12. Cardiac work-up remains necessary. The choice between two-dimensional echocardiography and subxiphoid window depends on the institutional capabilities available and the surgeon's preference.
13. Patients in the "thoracoabdominal" arm have either multiple penetrating injuries to the precordium and abdomen, or a single injury due to an object whose trajectory may have involved the chest and the abdomen.
14. See Number 8.
15. The myriad of possibilities of combined injuries make it impossible to categorize every possibility. Our practice in cases of combined injuries and hemodynamic instability is to make an upper midline incision just large enough to determine if there is ongoing intraperitoneal exsanguinating hemorrhage. If this is the case, full laparotomy must be performed at this time. If not, the thorax should be addressed. See text for further discussion.
16. This arm of the algorithm is for patients who exhibit hypotension (SBP<90) or, in the absence of severe hypotension, signs of shock (diaphoresis, altered sensorium). Patients with obvious tamponade move to the "obvious tamponade" arm of the algorithm.
17. These patients need a work-up for each component of the injury. If the abdominal component is to be worked up with exploratory laparotomy, the pericardium can be addressed by pericardial window or echocardiography in the operating room.

normally noncompliant pericardium does not expand to accommodate the increased volume, and the heart can no longer fill during diastole because the pressure in the pericardial sac is greater than the central venous pressure. Increasing the central venous pressure with volume infusion can temporarily compensate for the increased pericardial pressure, but unrelieved, tamponade soon causes severe hypotension and death. Blood filling the pericardium occupies space needed to fill the heart during diastole. Initially, signs of elevated central venous pressure (CVP) are noted, particularly jugular venous distension (JVD), because the right atrium cannot fill. Cardiac output is reduced as stroke volume is reduced because the heart cannot refill during diastole. Pulse pressure becomes narrowed as tamponade worsens, reflecting the decreased stroke volume; ultimately, there is little difference between systolic and diastolic size and pressure when the heart is compressed by blood within the pericardium. Catecholamines are released in an attempt to maintain blood pressure. The vasoconstriction induced by the catecholamines, in combination with the decrease in cardiac output, lead to a profound metabolic acidosis.

The second major pathophysiologic phenomenon is hemorrhage. Uncontrolled hemorrhage from the heart obviously leads to hypotension and death. Tamponade more frequently results from stab wounds. Hemorrhage more frequently results from gunshot wounds.[4]

INCIDENCE

Rising rates of civilian violence are leading to rising rates of penetrating cardiac injury.[10, 11] Cardiac injuries are the cause of approximately 10% of deaths due to gunshot wounds. Although most patients with penetrating cardiac injuries die before they reach the hospital, improvements in prehospital life support are causing more patients to reach the hospital alive.[12] The frequency of injury of the chambers of the heart is right ventricle 43%, left ventricle 33%, right atrium 15%, left atrium 6%, and intrapericardial great vessels 3%.[13]

DIAGNOSIS

Techniques

Diagnosis of the injured heart can be difficult[14] in the asymptomatic patient. Suspicion should be high if the precordium has been penetrated. Nagy and others have described the "cardiac box," delimited by the clavicles superiorly, the midclavicular lines laterally, and the costal margins where they intersect the midclavicular lines inferiorly, as an area that should raise great diagnostic suspicion when penetrated.[15, 16] In one series, 85% of patients with penetrating injuries in the area of the heart required operative treatment; 73% of these had cardiac injuries.[17] The diagnosis of pericardial tamponade can be difficult. Electrocardiography has been found to be normal in 87% of patients with penetrating cardiac injuries and is therefore not useful in making the diagnosis.[18–20] Chest radiography is normal in more than 80% of patients with cardiac tamponade.[21] The classic findings in Beck's triad (distended neck veins, muffled heart tones, and hypotension) are not found commonly[3, 21, 22] and were present in less than 10% of patients in Demetriades' series.[3] This finding may reflect concurrent hemorrhage and difficulty in recognizing muffled heart sounds during a noisy resuscitation. Central venous pressure monitoring is not useful in the combative agitated patient and is associated with a high percentage of errors.[19, 20, 23, 53] Although pericardiocentesis is commonly thought to be a useful tool in the diagnosis of traumatic pericardial tamponade, this belief has *not* been supported by data. There is a high incidence of false-positive and false-negative results in the use of this procedure in trauma patients.[3, 5, 21–25]

In 1970 Fontenelle and colleagues[26] revisited the subxiphoid pericardial window first described by Larrey in the nineteenth century.[27] They described patients who had tamponade secondary to trauma and other medical conditions. Their simple technique remains essentially unchanged to this day. Through a vertical incision over the xiphisternum, the musculofascial attachments to the xiphoid are taken down (this is most easily accomplished using electrocautery). The xiphoid is then elevated with a heavy clamp and excised with scissors. Finger dissection through the prepericardial adipose tissue reveals the diaphragm and pericardium. A bloodless field should be created to avoid causing a false-positive result, and the pericardium is then grasped with Kocher clamps. Scissors are then used to incise the pericardium. If the effluent is clear, no cardiac injury is presumed to have occurred (Miller and associates[28] had one false-positive and one false-negative result in a series of 104 subxiphoid pericardial windows). If the fluid has any tinge of blood, sternotomy and cardiac exploration are performed. This procedure should be performed only by a surgeon who is capable of proceeding to sternotomy and cardiac repair.

The significant rate of true negative subxiphoid pericardial windows procedures performed[20] led to a search for noninvasive methods of diagnosing pericardial tamponade. Jimenez and associates 1990[29] prospectively compared subxiphoid window to two-dimensional echocardiography in the diagnosis of occult penetrating cardiac injury and found no difference in the reliability of echocardiography versus subxiphoid window in the diagnosis of pericardial tamponade. The utility of echocardiography was shown again in 1991 by Freshman and colleagues,[30] who went on to suggest that stable patients with small (i.e., physiologically normal amounts of pericardial fluid) pericardial effusions could safely be admitted for observation and repeat echocardiography.

TREATMENT

The treatment of penetrating cardiac injury is surgical repair. Repeated aspiration or simple observation,[31] which was recommended by Blalock and Ravitch over 50 years ago,[32] are not options for definitive therapy today. Patients whose condition is classifed as "benign" can be taken to the operating room expeditiously for median sternotomy. With the sternum divided, the pericardium is opened, clot is evacuated, and the defect in the heart is controlled by a well-placed finger. Lateral application of a Satinsky clamp may be useful in obtaining hemostasis, particularly in patients with atrial wounds. The wound is directly sutured using pledgeted nonabsorbable suture. After successful repair of the anterior wound, the heart must be rotated (after warning the anesthesiologist that this maneuver can lead to hypotension and arrhythmias), and inspection is performed for posterior wounds. When a posterior nonbleeding injury is found, and rotation of the heart leads to arrhythmias, it may be necessary to place the patient on cardiac bypass to repair the posterior injury safely.

When aortic, tracheal, esophageal, or posterior cardiac wounds are suspected, an anterolateral thoracotomy is preferred, with extension of the incision across the sternum as needed to expose the anterior surface of the heart. The posterior mediastinal structures are not well exposed through sternotomy or anterolateral thoracotomy. However, this discussion assumes the presence of precordial penetration, which means the most likely injury is to the anterior surface of the heart. It is not necessary to seek intracardiac injuries during the initial operation; they should be evaluated postoperatively with echocardiography or angiography.

Lifeless or Critically Unstable Patients

Those patients in the "lifeless" or "critically unstable" category raise the issue of emergency center thoracotomy.[1, 14, 15, 31, 33–51] Patients who have no signs of life before they arrive at the hospital can usually not be saved, and efforts at resuscitation via thoracotomy are futile.[31] Patients who are agonal or who have lost vital signs en route to the emergency center are the best candidates for emergency center thoracotomy. Reported rates of survival range from 9%[52] to 72%.[48] Patients who are critically unstable should be given crystalloid or blood to stabilize them during transport to the operating room. When transport time is long, emergency center thoracotomy should be considered instead. The Ryder Trauma Center technique involves a left fifth intercostal space incision to the level of the intercostal muscles using a scalpel. This incision is carried across the sternum in case it should become necessary to perform a transverse sternotomy. A pair of blunt-tipped scissors are used to enter the left pleural space, and these scissors are then used to divide the intercostal muscles and latissimus dorsi all the way back to the table. The rib spreader is then placed with the open side of the U created by the spreader facing the sternum, so that the closed end will not interfere with transverse sternotomy should it become necessary. The aorta is cross-clamped with a DeBakey aortic aneurysm clamp. The empty aorta can be difficult to identify; a nasogastric tube placed by an assistant will help to differentiate it from the esophagus. The pericardium is incised with scissors in a longitudinal fashion anterior to the phrenic nerve, and the pericardiotomy is extended with scissors. Cardiorrhaphy is performed, but the patient is not transported to the operating room until a measurable blood pressure is obtained. Further details of the procedure and its indications can be found in the review by Feliciano and Mattox.[42]

Cardiac Tamponade

Patients who are obviously in cardiac tamponade but are not critically unstable should be transported to the operating room expeditiously for median sternotomy. No time should be wasted on additional diagnositc procedures or further resuscitative attempts.

Benign Injuries

Although these patients appear to be clinically stable, it is still necessary to rule out cardiac injury. Andrade-Alegre and Mon[53] performed subxiphoid pericardial window in 76 patients with penetrating wounds in proximity to the heart (unstable patients and patients with obvious signs of tamponade were excluded). Sixteen patients (21%) were found to have hemopericardium.[53] A high index of suspicion cannot be overemphasized. These patients should be evaluated with subxiphoid pericardial window or echocardiography.

Thoracoabdominal Injuries

Multiple penetrating injuries to the thorax and abdomen raise diagnostic and therapeutic dilemmas. However, most dilemmas can be resolved by using a structured approach. The first question is, "Which injury is most immediately life-threatening?" Emergency center thoracotomy is the only hope for the patient who has lost vital signs en route to the hospital. The patient who is obviously in tamponade but is not critically unstable must have the tamponade relieved first, and the abdomen addressed secondarily. The critically unstable patient is the most difficult to manage. Our approach is to begin with a small upper midline abdominal incision to answer the question, "Does this patient have massive intra-abdominal hemorrhage?" If the answer is "yes," the incision is extended, the abdomen is packed for hemostasis, and a subxiphoid pericardial window is performed. Definitive therapy of the abdominal wounds is delayed until tamponade or cardiac hemorrhage can be corrected. If the answer is "no," a subxiphoid window is performed. If the window is positive, sternotomy is performed. If the window is negative, another cause for the patient's condition must be found (i.e., reassess for missed injuries to the extremities, head, or thorax), and proceed to laparotomy to search for retroperitoneal hemorrhage.

Sequelae

Intracardiac lesions must be reevaluated in the postoperative period. High incidences of pathologic lesions have been found postoperatively in many series, including intracardiac shunts, valvular lesions, ventricular aneurysms, retained foreign bodies, and aortocaval and aortopulmonary fistulas.[54-56] These reports led Mattox and colleagues to suggest that echocardiography be performed in all symptomatic patients and in asymptomatic patients with any physical, radiographic, or electrocardiographic abnormalities in the postoperative period.[57]

SUMMARY

Although penetrating precordial trauma is potentially devastating, a rational approach to these patients can result in survivors. The ABCs must be followed, the index of suspicion should remain high, and the threshold for operation should remain low. The key to success is mental preparation on the part of the surgeon for the complex decisions that need to be made in a timely fashion.

References

1. Baker CC, Thomas AN, Trunkey DD: The role of emergency center thoracotomy in trauma. J Trauma 1980;20:848.
2. Cooley DA, Dunn RJ, Brockman ML, et al: Treatment of pericardial wounds of the heart: Experimental and clinical observations. Surgery 1955;37:882.
3. Demetriades D, VanderVeen PW: Penetrating injuries of the heart: experience over two years in South America. J Trauma 1983;23:1034.
4. Ivatury RR, Rohman M, Steichen FM, et al: Penetrating cardiac injuries: Twenty year experience. Am Surg 1987;53:310.
5. Sugg W, Rea W, Ecker R, et al: Penetrating wounds of the heart: An analysis of 459 cases. J Thorac Cardiovasc Surg 1968;56:531–545.
6. Naughton M, Brissie R, Bessey P, et al: Demography of penetrating cardiac trauma. Ann Surg 1989;209:676–681.
7. Saadia R, Levy D, Degiannis E, Velmahos GC: Penetrating cardiac injuries: Clinical classification and management strategy. Br J Surg 1994;81:1572–1575.
8. Rehn L: Ueber penetrirende Herzwunden and Hervalt. Arch Klin Chir 1897;55:315.
9. Isaacs JP: Sixty penetrating wounds of the heart: Clinical and experimental observations. Rec Adv Surg 1959;45:696–708.
10. Symbas PN: Cardiac trauma. Am Heart J 1976;92:387.
11. Symbas PN: Traumatic heart disease. Curr Probl Cardiol 1982;7:3.
12. Ivatury RR: Injury to the heart. In Feliciano DV, Moore EE, Mattox KL (eds): Trauma, 3rd ed. Stamford, Appleton & Lange, 1996, p. 409.
13. Karrel R, Shaffer MA, Franaszek JB: Emergency diagnosis, resuscitation, and treatment of acute penetrating cardiac trauma. Ann Emerg Med 1982;1:504.
14. Rohman M, Ivatury RR, Steichen FM, et al: Emergency room thoracotomy for penetrating cardiac injuries. J Trauma 1983;23:570–576.
15. Sumida MP, Ciraulo DL, Lewis PL, Barker DE: Penetrating injury to the "cardiac box:" diagnostic options for evaluation of this potentially fatal injury. Tenn Med 1998;91(2):65–68.
16. Nagy KK, Lohman C, Kim DO, Barrett J: Role of echocardiography in the diagnosis of occult penetrating cardiac injury. J Trauma 1995;38:859–862.
17. DeGennaro VA, Bonfils-Roberts EA, Ching N, et al: Aggressive management of potential penetrating cardiac injuries. J Thorac Cardiovasc Surg 1980;79:833.
18. Marshall WG, Bell JL, Kouchoukos NT: Penetrating cardiac trauma. J Trauma 1984;24:147.
19. Brewster SA, Thirby RC, Snyder WH: Subxiphoid pericardial window and penetrating cardiac trauma. Arch Surg 1988;123:937–941.
20. Duncan AO, Scalea TM, Scalfani SJ, et al: Evaluation of occult cardiac injuries using subxiphoid pericardial window. J Trauma 1989;29:955–960.
21. Arom KV, Richardson JD, Webb G, et al: Subxiphoid pericardial window in patients with suspected traumatic pericardial tamponade. Ann Thorac Surg 1977;23:545–549.
22. Shoemaker WC, Carey JS, Yao ST, et al: Hemodynamic alterations in acute cardiac tamponade after penetrating injuries of the heart. Surgery 1970;67:754–764.
23. Miller FB, Bond SJ, Shumate SR, et al: Diagnostic pericardial window. Arch Surg 1987;122:605–609.
24. Demetriades D: Cardiac wounds. Experience with 70 patients. Ann Surg 1986;203:315–317.
25. Trinkle JK, Toon RS, Franz JL, et al: Affairs of the wounded heart: Penetrating cardiac wounds. J Trauma 1979;19:467–472.
26. Fontenelle LJ, Cuello L, Dooley BN: Subxiphoid pericardial window. Am J Surg 1970;120:679–680.
27. Larrey DJ: Clinique chirurgicale, exercee particulierement dans les camps et les hospitaux militaires, depuis 1792 jusqu'en 1836. 5v.,8⁰;atlas,4⁰. Paris, Gabon, 1829–1836.
28. Miller FB, Bond SJ, Shumate CR, et al: Diagnostic pericardial window. Arch Surg 1987;122:605–609.
29. Jimenez E, Martin M, Krukenkamp I, Barrett J: Subxiphoid pericardiotomy versus echocardiography: A prospective evaluation of the diagnosis of occult penetrating cardiac injury. Surgery 1990;108:676–680.

30. Freshman SP, Wisner DH, Weber CJ: 2-D echocardiography: Emergent use in the evaluation of penetrating precordial trauma. J Trauma 1991;31:902–906.
31. Ivatury RR, Rohman M: The injured heart. Surg Clin North Am 1989;69:93–110.
32. Blalock A, Ravitch M: A consideration of the nonoperative treatment of cardiac tamponade resulting from wounds of the heart. Surgery 1943;14:157–162.
33. Steichen FM, Dargan EL, Efron G, et al: A graded approach to the management of penetrating wounds of the heart. Arch Surg 1971;103:574.
34. Mattox KL, Beall AC Jr, Jordan GL Jr, et al: Cardiorrhaphy in the emergency center. J Thorac Cardiovasc Surg 1974;68:886.
35. Mattox KL, Espada R, Beall AC Jr: Performing thoracotomy in the emergency center. J Am Coll Emerg Physicians 1974;3:313.
36. Mattox KL, VonKoch L, Beall AC Jr, et al: Logistic and technical considerations in the treatment of the wounded heart. Circulation 1975;52:210.
37. MacDonald JR, McDowell RM: Emergency department thoracotomies in a community hospital. J Am Coll Emerg Physicians 1978;7:423.
38. Bodai BI, Smith JP, Blaisdell FW: The role of emergency thoracotomy in blunt trauma. J Trauma 1982;22:487.
39. Bodai BI, Smith JP, Ward RE, et al: Emergency thoracotomy in the management of trauma: A review. JAMA 1983;249:1891.
40. Cogbill TH, Moore EE, Millikan JS, et al: Rationale for selective application of emergency department thoracotomy in trauma. J Trauma 1983;23:453.
41. Danne PD, Finelli F, Champion HR: Emergency bay thoracotomy. J Trauma 1984;24:796.
42. Feliciano DV, Mattox KL: Indications, techniques, and pitfalls of emergency center thoracotomy. Surg Rounds 1981;4:32.
43. Feliciano DV, Bitondo CG, Cruise PA, et al: Liberal use of emergency center thoracotomy. Am J Surg 1986;152:654.
44. Flynn TC, Ward RE, Miller PW: Emergency room thoracotomy. Ann Emerg Med 1982;11:413.
45. Ivatury RR, Rohman M: Emergency department thoracotomy for trauma: A collective review Resuscitation 1987;15:23.
46. Moore EE, Moore JB, Galloway AC, et al: Post-injury thoracotomy in the emergency department: A critical evaluation. Surgery 1979;86:590.
47. Roberge RJ, Ivatury RR, Stahl WM, et al: Emergency department thoracotomies for penetrating injuries: predictive value of patient classification. Am J Emerg Med 1986;4:129.
48. Schwab CW, Adcock OT, Max MH: Emergency department thoracotomy (EDT): A 26-month experience using an "agonal" protocol. Am Surg 1986;52:20.
49. Tavares S, Hankins JR, Moulton AL, et al: Management of penetrating cardiac injuries: The role of emergency room thoracotomy. Ann Surg 1984;38:183.
50. Vij D, Simoni E, Smith E, et al: Resuscitative thoracotomy for patients with traumatic injury. Surgery 1983;94:554.
51. Washington BW, Wilson RF, Steiger Z, et al: Emergency thoracotomy: A four-year review. Ann Thorac Surg 1985;40:188–191.
52. Demetriades D: Cardiac penetrating injuries: Personal experience of 45 cases. Br J Surg 1984;71:95–97.
53. Andrade-Alegre R, Mon L: Subxiphoid pericardial window in the diagnosis of penetrating cardiac trauma. Ann Thorac Surg 1994;58:1139–1141.
54. Symbas PN, DiOrio DA, Tyras DH, et al: Penetrating cardiac wounds: Significant residual and delayed sequelae. J Thorac Cardiovasc Surg 1973;66:526.
55. Fallah-Nejad M, Kutty ACK, Wallace HW: Secondary lesions of penetrating cardiac injuries: A frequent complication. Ann Surg 1980;191:228.
56. Fallah-Nejad M, Wallace HW, Su CC, et al: Unusual manifestations of penetrating cardiac injuries. Arch Surg 1975;110:1357.
57. Mattox KL, Limacher MC, Feliciano DV, et al: Cardiac evaluation following heart injury. J Trauma 1985;25:758.

Chapter 7

Blunt Thoracic Trauma

Two thirds of victims of major blunt trauma suffer thoracic injury. Thoracic injuries directly account for 20% to 25% of deaths due to trauma, and most of these are secondary to motor vehicle accidents.[1, 2] Furthermore, major thoracic trauma is associated with multisystem injuries in 70% of cases.[3] Immediate and early deaths (minutes to hours) postinjury are typically due to cardiac tamponade, major laceration to the aorta and its great vessels, airway obstruction, tension pneumothorax, or exsanguinating hemorrhage.[4-8] Late occurring deaths (beyond 5 days) following blunt thoracic trauma are often related to respiratory complications, pulmonary infections, or missed injuries.

All patients sustaining significant blunt thoracic trauma must be managed to safeguard against a cervical spine injury. A cervical collar must be placed; orotracheal intubation employing in-line traction or nasotracheal intubation is employed to avoid possible injury secondary to neck motion if tracheal intubation is required. Eighty-five percent of patients with blunt thoracic trauma can be managed by simple tube thoracostomy, and the great majority of early or late deaths can be minimized by paying attention to the ABCs of trauma care. At least two large-bore intravenous catheters are inserted to initiate hemodynamic resuscitation, and a central venous line (i.e., internal jugular vein, subclavian vein, or femoral vein) permits monitoring of central venous pressure.

The chest x-ray is fundamental to the initial examination. The anteroposterior chest x-ray should be among the initial radiographs obtained in the emergency room. Chest tubes (36 to 40 Fr) are inserted for radiographic or clinical evidence of hemothorax or pneumothorax. The chest tube is placed through the fourth or fifth intercostal space between the mid and anterior axillary lines, following finger inspection to confirm that the pleural space is free of adhesions. Most chest tubes can be removed in 2 to 3 days when there is no further air or fluid leak. It is safe to remove the thoracostomy tube if the pleural output is less than 150 ml every 24 hours and there is no air leak.

Life-threatening conditions such as a tension pneumothorax may require urgent needle thoracentesis before an x-ray film is taken. In the great majority of cases of blunt cardiorespiratory arrest, open cardiac massage is not appropriate. In these situations, bilateral chest tubes, pericardiocentesis, and correction of hypovolemia are high-priority measures.[2] The only indications for emergency room thoracotomy after blunt thoracic trauma are (1) suspected cardiac tamponade, (2) witnessed emergency room cardiac arrest, and (3) suspected vascular injury to the pulmonary hilum or thoracic inlet, massive air leaks, or an exsanguinating hemothorax. Indications for a thoracotomy in a patient in the nonacute postresuscitation setting include (1) an unevacuated clotted or infected hemothorax, (2) traumatic diaphragmatic hernia, (3) traumatic thoracic aortic aneurysm, (4) nonclosing thoracic duct fistula, (5) missed tracheal or bronchial injury, (6) tracheal esophageal fistula, (7) innominate artery to trachea fistula, (8) empyema refractory to chest tube or percutaneous drainage, and (9) traumatic arteriovenous fistula.[3]

Computed tomography of the chest is highly sensitive in detecting thoracic injuries after blunt trauma and is superior to routine chest x-ray in visualizing lung contusions, pneumothorax, and hemothorax. The use of thoracic computed tomography is recommended in the initial diagnostic work-up of patients with multiple injuries and suspected chest trauma because early and exact diagnoses of these injuries often result in significant therapeutic consequences and reduce the incidence of complications.

STERNAL FRACTURE

The importance of a sternal fracture is not the fracture itself but its association with other more serious injuries such as aortic and great vessel injury, pulmonary contusion, and myocardial trauma.[1] Chest pain is an almost universal finding in patients with sternal fracture. Physical examination may reveal chest bruising and deformity, and palpation often elicits tenderness and crepitus. If a sternal fracture is suspected, a lateral chest x-ray is diagnostic. Management of the patient depends on the associated injuries and the presence of an associated myocardial or pulmonary contusion. Operative reduction is usually not necessary.[3] Hospitalization is not mandatory if the electrocardiogram (ECG) is normal and the patient's vital sign are stable. The victim can be discharged home with adequate oral analgesics.

FLAIL CHEST

A flail chest represents the loss of stability of the chest wall because of multiple rib fractures; it is defined by fracture of two or more consecutive ribs in two places each. Ventilatory insufficiency and hypoxemia are related to associated pulmonary contusion, paradoxical movement of the chest wall (which results in inefficient expansion of the thorax and a significant increase in energy expenditure for the work of breathing), and pain from the fractures leading to splinting.[2] Optimal pain relief can usually be achieved with thoracic epidural anesthesia or an intercostal nerve block. Aggressive pulmonary toilet is essential to the management of the patient because it facilitates the clearance of secretions and optimizes alveolar recruitment to maintain functional residual capacity.[1] Optimal pulmonary toilet includes frequent tracheobronchial suctioning, incentive spirometry, postural drainage, chest physiotherapy, and bronchoscopy. Endotracheal intubation and positive pressure ventilation are indicated for decompensating levels of the work of breathing and for hypoxemic or hypercarbic ventilatory failure. The likelihood of adult respiratory distress syndrome (ARDS) is increased 20% to 30% in the presence of a flail chest.[1] In selected patients noninvasive ventilatory techniques (i.e., continuous positive airway pressure [CPAP] or bilateral positive airway pressure [BIPAP]) can be applied as a method of improving functional residual capacity (FRC) and decrease the work of breathing, with the intent of avoiding intubation. Fluid administration should be monitored closely.

Blunt Thoracic Trauma

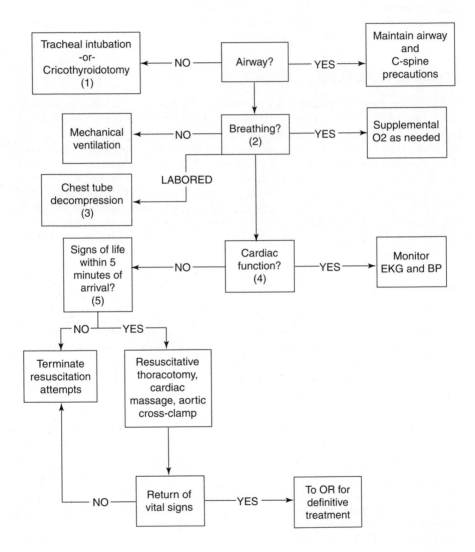

1. Unless cervical spine injury can be excluded with certainty, nasaotracheal intubation, orotracheal intubation with in-line traction, or surgical cricothyroidectomy is performed to control the airway and avoid cord injury by neck motion.
2. Pulmonary contusion is managed by aggressive pulmonary toilet and incentive spirometry. End-expiratory volume support, using a noninvasive modality (continuous positive airway pressure [CPAP], bilateral positive airway pressure [BIPAP]) or, if the patient requires intubation, positive pressure ventilation with positive end-expiratory pressure (PEEP), may be required to reverse atelectasis. The use of intravenous crystalloid resuscitation should be restricted in the hemodynamically stable patient. Supplemental oxygen and pain relief by thoracic epidural or intercostal nerve block are essential in the management of patients with multiple rib fractures or flail chest and underlying pulmonary contusion. Pulse oximetry or serial blood gas determinations are obtained to determine the need for mechanical ventilation and expiratory pressure support.
3. An admission chest x-ray is mandatory. Thoracostomy tube placement must be considered for all patients with a traumatic pneumothorax or hemothorax. Moreover, the clinician should strongly consider tube thoracostomy in the presence of multiple rib fractures and subcutaneous emphysema, particularly if urgent general anesthesia is required (≤24 hours from injury). In patients with isolated subcutaneous emphysema, a follow-up chest x-ray is necessary.
4. Aggressive resuscitation with large-bore intravenous lines is essential in the hemodynamically unstable patient. Cardiac tamponade is characterized by shock, distended neck veins, and elevated central venous pressures. Pericardiocentesis is performed by aiming a large-bore needle from the right of the subxiphoid process toward the left shoulder. If fluid is aspirated from the pericardium and the patient improves, the patient is transported to the operating room for median sternotomy with the needle left in place. However, if no improvement occurs, immediate left thoracotomy is performed. Cardiac contusion is suggested by electrocardiographic (ECG) changes of right bundle branch block, right axis deviation, or supraventricular tachyarrhythmias. Echocardiogram is the study of choice for confirming this diagnosis. Patients with significant contusions may require right heart catheter monitoring to optimize left ventricular filling. Treatment is largely supportive and expectant (i.e., bed rest, monitoring, and fluid restriction).
5. Emergency room thoracotomy should be considered in blunt traumatic arrest victims only if some signs of life are present in the emergency room. Emergency room thoracotomy is universally unsuccessful in patients who lose all signs of life for longer than 5 minutes before arrival in the emergency room because closed chest CPR is not effective in traumatic arrest patients and permanent brain damage occurs after 3 to 5 minutes if adequate circulation is not restored.

PULMONARY CONTUSION

Lung contusion is considered one of the most important factors contributing to increased morbidity and mortality from thoracic injuries.[2] Pulmonary contusion can lead to respiratory failure and ARDS and is associated with an increased incidence of pulmonary septic complications and multiple organ system failure. Histologically, pulmonary contusion is seen as the leakage of blood and protein into the alveolar and interstitial space of the lung. Computed tomographic scanning of the chest is the most accurate imaging modality for determining the extent of pulmonary contusion, but it should be considered a luxury and not a necessity because injuries not evident on chest radiographs are typically not clinically important. Although the classic radiologic findings of pulmonary contusion become manifest within several hours of injury, these findings often lag behind arterial blood gas abnormalities. Chest x-ray findings may range from minimal interstitial infiltrates to extensive lobar consolidation.

Treatment of pulmonary contusion is similar to the management of flail chest. Attention is concentrated on analgesia and pulmonary toilet; patients are selectively intubated strictly for excessive work of breathing, hypoxemia, and hypercarbic ventilatory failure. As in the management of flail chest, noninvasive positive pressure ventilation (CPAP, BIPAP) may be beneficial in avoiding intubation. Overhydration should be avoided; prophylactic antibiotics and steroids have not proved beneficial.[2]

INJURY TO THE LARYNX, TRACHEA, AND BRONCHI

The incidence of injuries to the larynx, trachea, and major bronchial airways has dramatically increased in this century, paralleling the increase in modern high-speed motor vehicle transportation.[6] The reported incidence is 1% to 6% of all cases of thoracic trauma. The primary mechanism is typically a nonpenetrating crushing or compressive trauma to the thorax. The prognosis of patients with tracheobronchial injuries depends on the location and extent of the lesion. About a third of patients with tracheal injuries die, 50% of these succumbing in the first hour.[9] The high mortality rate is often secondary to associated injuries to the azygous vein or heart or to the presence of tension pneumothoraces. In contradistinction to death in the prehospital setting, approximately 90% of those who are transported alive to the hospital survive.

Causative mechanisms include shearing forces caused by rapid deceleration, direct compression between the sternum and vertebral bodies, and barotrauma due to build-up of pressure within the major airways against the closed glottis.[5] Early diagnosis and primary repair of these injuries yield few complications and the best long-term results. Missed injuries can be devastating and can lead to bronchial stricture with postobstructive pneumonitis, bronchiectasis, pneumonia, or lung collapse.[5] Crepitus and subcutaneous emphysema of the neck suggest cervical laryngeal or tracheal injuries. Pneumothorax with an air leak and mediastinal emphysema suggest intrathoracic tracheal or bronchial rupture. Injury to the distal trachea or bronchus may cause hemoptysis or airway obstruction. A tension pneumothorax should always be treated emergently with needle thoracentesis followed by thoracostomy tube placement. Upper airway obstruction or suspicion of tracheal disruption should be treated with fiberoptic intubation, and if unsuccessful, emergent cricothyroidotomy. A significant persistent air leak may require selective intubation of the uninvolved bronchus and operative repair of the injury. Fiberoptic bronchoscopy is the diagnostic study of choice; bronchography is not beneficial in a patient with an acute injury but may be helpful when a strong suspicion of an injury exists but bronchoscopy is negative.

Patients with isolated laryngeal trauma not requiring immediate airway control can be managed conservatively provided they are closely observed with sequential, flexible fiberoptic laryngoscopy.[10] Computed tomography is helpful for identifying and staging laryngeal injuries but is not accurate for injuries to the more distal airways. Intravenous steroids to decrease edema are most effective in the acute phase of the injury. Once edema and ecchymosis are established, the benefits of steroids are questionable. Laryngeal trauma that is managed conservatively should be reevaluated in 10 to 14 days to avoid cricoarytenoid joint dysfunction that may become permanent when edema subsides. Vocal cord edema from hematomas is slow to resolve and is the cause of persistent dysphonia. Most laryngeal or proximal tracheal injuries are easily addressed through a transverse (collar) incision.

Treatment of tracheal injuries depends on the location of the lesion and the patient's clinical condition. Cervical tracheal injuries are treated by neck exploration and repair using absorbable sutures in either one or two layers. A right posterior lateral thoracotomy is the preferred incision for repair of intrathoracic tracheal lacerations as well as right mainstem bronchial injuries. The fact that more than 80% of major bronchial injuries occur within 2 cm of the carina also allows the repair of proximal injuries to the left mainstem bronchus through this approach.[5, 6] A standard left posterolateral thoracotomy through the fifth intercostal space is the approach used to manage a complete transection of the left mainstem bronchus, particularly if it is further than 1 cm from the carina. The principles used for all tracheobronchial injuries include adequate debridement of healthy tissue and a mucosal to mucosal closure using interrupted nonabsorbable sutures. Reinforcement with cervical neck strap muscles, pleura, pericardium, or a pedicle intercostal muscle flap may be necessary, particularly for injuries to the posterior membranous aspect of the trachea.

ESOPHAGEAL RUPTURE

Initial symptoms of blunt esophageal rupture are nonspecific. Early signs of esophageal rupture may include findings of pneumothorax or pneumomediastinum. If mediastinal air dissects into the pericardium, it can be heard as a rhythmic "Hamman's crunch" (the sound generated with compression of air within the pericardial sac with each heart beat).[3, 4] Chest x-ray may demonstrate a pneumothorax or pleural effusion. Cervical air may be visible on a cervical spine film. Diagnosis is typically confirmed by dilute Gastrografin or ciné esophagography. Endoscopy is less specific and has the potential to extend the injury. Initial treatment of esophageal disruption includes isotonic fluid resuscitation, nasogastric decompression, and use of broad-spectrum antibiotics. Patients should be taken to the operating room as soon as possible because delay in repair results in increased mortality.

Esophageal perforation remains a difficult operative problem.[11, 12] Although the traditional adage has been that 24 hours represents a finite cut-off time between performing a buttressed primary repair or an esophageal exclusion procedure, recent reviews now support the concept that time from diagnosis is less important than the appearance of the esophagus and mediastinal tissues at the time of operation. Accurate intraoperative evaluation and precise repair based on fundamental surgical principles remain the most important determinants of the need for esophageal repair versus exclusion and proximal diversion.[11-13] In patients with noncontained thoracic esophageal perforations, debridement of necrotic tissue, generous mediastinal and pleural irrigation, and complete mediastinal drainage are essential. Identification of the mucosal and muscularis wall layers (because the mucosal tear is usually longer) is important, and a two-layer closure (inner absorbable, outer interrupted nonabsorbable suture) with enforcement (buttressing) of the primary repair (i.e., with intercostal, pleural, gastric fundus, or pericardial flap) is performed.[13] Some advocate esophageal exclusion, proximal diversion, decompressive gastrostomy, and placement of a feeding jejunostomy for the management of delayed esophageal perforations.

Proximal diversion is established by creating a lateral cervical esophagostomy or placing a proximal nasogastric tube. Creation of a controlled fistula using a T-tube to divert all secretions has been advocated. The T-tube is brought out through a separate stab incision and secured in a lateral position away from the aorta. The T-tube remains in place for 2 to 3 weeks to allow development of an artificial tract. The need for a second operation to reestablish esophageal continuity and the potential for esophageal stricture remain undesirable consequences of exclusion and diversion of the esophagus. An intensive care unit environment is usually required postoperatively.

Delayed tracheoesophageal fistula is an uncommon complication. Tracheoesophageal fistulas are often suggested by uncontrolled coughing with swallowing and the presence of subcutaneous and mediastinal air; diagnosis is made by bronchoscopy.[14] Treatment is accomplished with right thoracotomy and fistula take-down. The trachea is closed with nonabsorbable sutures, and the esophagus is repaired in two layers with an interposition pleural flap or intercostal pedicle flap placed between the repaired trachea and the esophagus, which is secured with interrupted nonabsorbable sutures.

CARDIAC TRAUMA

In patients with closed thoracic trauma, the incidence of cardiac damage is reported to be between 10% and 16%. Cardiac injuries accompanying blunt thoracic trauma as a result of motor vehicle accidents, falls, assaults, or sporting injuries result from rapid deceleration or damage due to direct impact on intrathoracic structures. Blunt cardiac injuries include myocardial contusion, lacerations of the atrium and ventricle, pericardial laceration, coronary vessel injury, valvular damage, arrhythmias, and conduction abnormalities.[7] An adequate level of clinical awareness and timely use of diagnostic techniques are essential for rapid identification of cardiac trauma of blunt origin. Routine tests include baseline chest x-ray, ECG, and echocardiography.[8] A cardiac cause of shock should be suspected in any patient with severe chest trauma and hypotension that is disproportionate to the estimated blood loss or with an inadequate hemodynamic response to conventional fluid resuscitation.

MYOCARDIAL CONTUSION

Myocardial contusion is the most common injury to the heart following blunt trauma.[3, 7, 8] Autopsy findings demonstrate a range of lesions from subepicardial and subendocardial bruising to full-thickness myocardial necrosis. Diagnosis is extremely difficult. Supraventricular arrhythmias are characteristic and range from sinus tachycardia to supraventricular tachyarrhythmias (i.e., atrial flutter, atrial fibrillation, paroxysmal supraventricular tachycardia). Conduction abnormalities or nonspecific ST–T-wave changes may also be seen. However, the presence of ventricular ectopy should lead the investigator to suspect ischemic (occlusive) myocardial damage.

An elevated CPK-MB isoenzyme level is sensitive for myocardial cell injuries but not specific enough to suggest a diagnosis of myocardial contusion. The dilemma is whether the enzyme elevation is due to myocardial cell damage or occlusive myocardial injury. A new serum assay, cardiac troponin, appears to be a more reliable marker for blunt myocardial cell damage.

Echocardiography has emerged as the imaging test of first choice because it shows abnormal myocardial contractility, regional wall motion abnormalities, intracardiac shunt, and valvular irregularities. Unfortunately, transthoracic two-dimensional echocardiography does not provide a satisfactory image in up to 25% of patients sustaining blunt cardiac trauma. Transesophageal echocardiography is far more sensitive but is operator dependent.

Treatment of myocardial contusion is expectant and supportive.[15] The need for hospitalization and monitoring is based on the presence of arrhythmias and hemodynamic instability. If the details of the accident, physical examination, or continuous bedside ECG monitoring suggest myocardial contusion, a 12-lead electrocardiogram should be obtained. If the patient remains stable and has no persistent ECG abnormalities and no other reasons for admission, he or she can be safely discharged home after a brief period of observation. However, if there are persistent ECG abnormalities (nonspecific changes in the ST segment or P waves), minor arrhythmias (sinus tachycardia, premature atrial contractions, or premature ventricular beats), or anginalike chest discomfort, the patient should be admitted to a telemetry unit and evaluated with echocardiography, particularly if these signs and symptoms persist for longer than 12 hours. Patients with progressive dyspnea, signs of congestive heart failure, ischemia on ECG, complex arrhythmias (e.g., a conduction defect, atrial fibrillation, multifocal premature ventricular beats, or periods of ventricular tachycardia) or hemodynamic instability must be admitted to an intensive care environment. Treatment of cardiogenic shock requires adequate intraventricular volume, inotropic support, and reduction of afterload to optimize cardiac performance. If these measures fail, intra-aortic balloon counterpulsation should be considered to enhance cardiac output.[7] Myocardial rupture and cardiac tamponade may occur either at the time of injury or several weeks later when the myocardium softens. Ventricular wall aneurysm formation is a late event.

BLUNT CARDIAC RUPTURE

Blunt cardiac trauma can result in rupture of the free atrial or ventricular wall (typically the right ventricular wall), intraventricular septum, heart valves, papillary muscles, or chordae tendineae.[7] The event can be dramatic or delayed (for up to 2 weeks) owing to myocardial necrosis. In most cases of free-wall rupture, death ensues rapidly. Those who survive often manifest symptoms of cardiac tamponade characterized by Beck's triad (hypotension, elevated central venous pressures [e.g., jugular venous distention], and distant [muffled] heart sounds). If the diagnosis of myocardial rupture is suspected, further diagnostic studies are superfluous. Pericardial aspiration may be attempted en route to emergent median sternotomy, but a negative study does not exclude tamponade. Echocardiography can be used to detect pericardial fluid. Treatment must be operative repair because mortality in patients with signs of myocardial rupture or tamponade on arrival in the emergency department exceeds 50%. The patient should be prepped prior to induction of anesthesia to facilitate rapid median sternotomy if acute hypotension occurs. The right ventricle is repaired using pledgeted nonabsorbable sutures. In patients who develop severe congestive heart failure or a new holosystolic murmur, rupture of the anterior ventricular septum or its valvular apparatus (papillary muscle, or chordae tendineae) must be ruled out. Diagnosis of intraventricular septal rupture or papillary muscle disruption can be made accurately with transesophageal echocardiography.[7, 15, 16] Confirmation, if necessary, requires cardiac catheterization. The need and timing of surgical repair depend on the severity of the congestive heart failure and the patient's overall physiologic stability. If cardiogenic insufficiency results in medically refractory hypotension, cardiopulmonary bypass is essential.

PERICARDIAL INJURY

Blunt trauma to the pericardium ranges from small lacerations that heal spontaneously to large rents that may allow herniation of the heart and subsequent entrapment with impaired filling.[7, 15] The diagnosis can be suspected on routine chest x-ray, which demonstrates displacement of the heart. The presence of pneumomediastinum, ECG evidence of a shift in axis, or a new bundle branch block is suggestive. Treatment consists of median sternotomy with repositioning of the heart and pericardial repair.

CORONARY ARTERY INJURY

Coronary artery laceration, dissection, fistulization and rupture, thrombosis, and myocardial infarction can follow blunt cardiac trauma.[7] The proposed mechanism of coronary artery thrombosis is increased sympathetic activity during and immediately after the trauma, resulting in coronary spasm, platelet aggregation, and thrombosis. Intracoronary thrombolysis, systemic thrombolysis, and percutaneous angioplasty with stent placement have been successfully used to manage these injuries.

BLUNT AORTIC AND GREAT VESSEL INJURIES

Acceleration and traction forces are the causative mechanisms underlying injuries to the thoracic aorta and its great vessels. Horizontal deceleration creates shear forces at the aortic isthmus. Vertical deceleration displaces the heart caudally, displacing it into the left pleural cavity, and acutely strains the ascending aorta–innominate artery junction. Thirty-five to ninety percent of patients with thoracic aortic rupture die at the scene. The few survivors owe their lives to a fragile contained perivascular hematoma. Although the natural history of the contained hematoma is rupture, the time elapsed before free-rupture is not predictable. Recent information based on the nonoperative management of contained aortic ruptures in high-risk patients with severe intracranial injuries demonstrates that the immediate prognosis for patients who initially survive to reach the hospital is less dismal than that previously suggested from extrapolation of autopsy reports (30% die within 24 hours, and 50% die within 1 week). Death from hemorrhage during the first hours of admission occurs in only 18% to 30%. However, no prospective evidence validates routine delay of operative repair beyond the time required to complete evaluation and treatment of associated emergency life-threatening conditions (e.g., hemorrhagic shock due to bleeding from injuries to the abdomen or major vascular structures of the extremities). Therefore, nonthoracic sources of hemorrhage should be sought and treated rapidly (e.g., laparotomy, embolization of pelvic arterial lacerations, ligation or repair of major extremity artery injuries, and so on) before the thoracic aorta is evaluated. More than 80% of injuries rupture through the intima, media, and adventitial tissue, resulting in exsanguinating hemorrhage and death at the accident site.[15] In survivors the integrity of the adventitial tissue is maintained, but transmural rupture remains a risk.[15] More than 80% of ruptures occur in the descending aorta distal to the left subclavian artery (ligamentum arteriosum). The ascending aorta is the second most common site involved.

The clinical presentation varies from traumatic arrest to normal vital signs. Coarctation syndrome with hypotension of the extremities and diminished pulses has been described but is absent in most cases. The chest radiograph is first inspected for mediastinal widening, a finding that has about 90% sensitivity and 10% specificity for traumatic aortic rupture. In approximately 20% of patients with blunt aortic disruption the chest radiograph is normal initially. Remember, mediastinal widening is in the eye of the beholder and not in the yardstick. Relative values have been suggested (8 to 12 cm at the aorta-pulmonary window), but no direct measurement is better than the clinician's subjective assessment of the mediastinum.

The second most predictive radiographic finding is loss of the aortic knob.

Other findings include displacement of the trachea and esophagus to the right, an apical cap, pleural effusion, downward displacement of the left mainstem bronchus, and associated upward displacement of the right mainstem bronchus. Dynamic contrast-injected computed tomography can often confirm the diagnosis, but aortography remains the gold standard of diagnosis. A normal computed tomogram almost certainly rules out an injury to the aorta or its great vessels. Eighty-five percent of cases of mediastinal widening are secondary to mediastinal venous bleeding. Transesophageal echocardiography has become the method of choice for the diagnosis of traumatic aortic disruptions and dissection in some medical centers.[16] However, because of its dependence on operator skill and experience, most centers continue to use contrast-injection (dynamic) CT and aortography, which should be considered the gold standard work-up.

Transesophageal echocardiography is far more sensitive than transthoracic echocardiography in detecting these injuries. Medical therapy with beta-blockers and vasodilators aims at controlling or reducing shear stress in the aortic wall and should be initiated immediately in any patient with a suspected or confirmed aortic tear. Surgical management of aortic isthmus tears can be performed with or without partial circulatory support, although repair with circulatory support appears to be safer.

Sudden extension of the neck or traction on the shoulder can overstretch the arch vessels and produce tears of the intima or a complete rupture of the arterial wall. The injuries may range from dissection, thrombosis, and pseudoaneurysm to free hemorrhage. Minor lesions of the arterial wall (e.g., mural hematoma or a limited intimal flap) have a benign course and frequently regress spontaneously. These lesions can be followed with serial transesophageal echocardiography, Doppler duplex ultrasonography, or angiography. All pseudoaneurysms should be resected because very few remain stable (even those less than 0.5 cm); they tend to expand and rupture. Moreover, they may lead to thrombosis embolization, fistulas to adjacent organs, or compression of nearby structures. Lacerations of the great vessels require mandatory repair or ligation. Primary repair is sometimes possible, but frequently a prosthetic graft is necessary. Repair of the aorta and aortic arch often necessitates circulatory support with extracorporeal circulation. Hypothermic circulatory arrest may be required for repair of injuries to the arch.

DIAPHRAGM

Diaphragmatic rupture occurs in 1% to 3% of patients with blunt chest trauma, usually as the result of a motor vehicle accident.[3] The injury occurs most commonly on the left side because of the protective effect of the liver on the right diaphragm. Almost all patients have associated injuries, and mortality commonly ranges from 15% to 12%. The negative intrathoracic pressure caused by the bellow effect of ventilation pulls the abdominal contents into the chest. Chest radiographs are most useful as the initial study, but less than half of patients with documented rupture have chest radiographic findings that are diagnostic, and 25% have normal radiographs. Chest thoracoscopy has been used but is not particularly helpful. Other diagnostic studies include contrast studies, failure to recover peritoneal lavage fluid, and CT scan. Operative repair of the diaphragm is mandatory but should not precede more pressing diagnostic and therapeutic measures. Use of pneumatic antishock garments is to be avoided because they increase intra-abdominal pressure and may aggravate the condition. Delayed recognition increases mortality (i.e., 30%) in patients who present in the late obstructive phase.

References

1. Ciravlo D, Elliott D, Mitchell K, et al: Flail chest as a marker for significant injuries. J Am Coll Surg 1994;178:466–470.
2. Trupka A, Waydhas C, Hallfeldt K, et al: Value of thoracic computed tomography in the first assessment of severely injured patients with blunt chest trauma: Results of a prospective study. J Trauma 1997;43:405–412.
3. Jackimczyk K: Blunt chest trauma. Emerg Med Clin North Am 1993;11:8l–95.
4. Martín de Nicholás J, Gámez A, Cruz F, et al. Long tracheobronchial and esophageal rupture after blunt chest trauma: Injury by airway bursting. Ann Thorac Surg 1996;62:269–272.
5. Tull D, Hailston D, Fulda G, et al: Tracheobronchial disruption following low-energy trauma. J Emerg Med 1996;14:579–583.
6. Lin M-Y, Wu M-H, Chan C, et al: Bronchial rupture caused by blunt chest injury. Ann Emerg Med 1995;25:412–415.
7. Olsovsky MR, Wechsler AS, Tapaz O: Cardiac trauma: Diagnosis, management, and current therapy. Angiology 1997;48:423–432.
8. Brown J, Grover F: Trauma to the heart. Chest Surg Clin N Am 1997;7:325–345.
9. Lee R: Traumatic injury of the cervicothoracic trachea and major bronchi. Chest Surg Clin N Am 1997;7:285–304.
10. Chagnon F, Mulder D: Laryngotracheal trauma. Chest Surg Clin N Am 1996;6:733–748.
11. Bufkin B, Miller J, Mansour K: Esophageal perforation emphasis on management. Ann Thorac Surg 1996;61:1447–1452.
12. Bastos R, Graeber G: Esophageal injuries. Chest Surg Clin N Am 1997;7:357–371.
13. Reeder L, De Filippi V, Ferguson M: Current results of therapy for esophageal perforation. Am J Surg 1995;169:615–617.
14. Weber S, Schurr M, Pellett J: Delayed presentation of a tracheoesophageal fistula after blunt chest trauma. Ann Thorac Surg 1996;62:1850–1852.
15. Pretre R, Chilcott M: Blunt trauma to the heart and great vessels. N Engl J Med 1997;336:626–632.
16. Cohn S: Transesophageal echocardiography for exclusion of traumatic aortic tear. Trauma Q 1997;13:199–203.

Chapter 8

Rib Fractures and Hypoxemia

The delicate and life-sustaining organs of the thoracic cavity are protected by the encompassing bony structures of the chest wall—namely, the spine, ribs, and sternum. This skeletal "cage" also protects the upper abdominal structures, especially the liver and spleen. Penetrating projectiles may or may not be deflected by the bones, and in fact, fractured bones or fragments may cause additional injury beyond that induced by the projectile itself. Lacerations of the lung, spinal cord, heart, or even major vascular structures such as the intercostal or subclavian artery or vein, may result from these bone fragments.

Blunt forces applied to the chest can result in injury to a variety of organs with different degrees of severity.[1] Contusion of the right ventricle can be so insignificant that it is detectable only by cardiac isoenzyme determinations. More significant tissue damage can produce dysrhythmias, usually in the form of ventricular extrasystolic contractions, or injury patterns seen on electrocardiography (ECG). Abnormal ventricular wall contractions may be viewed on echocardiography, and with severe blunt injury, disruption of the cardiac valves or papillary muscles can occur.

The structures absorbing the largest share of the forces applied to the thorax are the ribs, and therefore they are the structures most commonly injured. Because of the deep and protected position of the first and second ribs, fracture of these ribs suggests a severe force, and if present, this should raise the question of an associated deceleration-type aortic injury. Fractures of the lower ribs should raise a suspicion of underlying splenic or hepatic injuries; further work-up should include computed tomographic (CT) examination of the abdomen to evaluate these organs.

Like any other fracture, broken ribs are painful and require approximately 6 weeks to heal. However, unlike other bones, fractured ribs cannot be treated with immobilization to reduce pain and hasten healing. On the contrary, attempts to strap the chest in the past resulted in a significant incidence of pneumonia on the affected side. Obviously the human organism must breathe, and while the diaphragm participates to a large extent in reducing intrathoracic pressure during inspiration, expansion of the chest cavity requires elevation of the ribs. Attempts to prevent full movement of the chest wall result in limited expansion of the lung and alveoli and result in atelectasis. Persistent segmental collapse of the lung causes secretions to pool in the area, which eventually become infected, converting a patient with rib fractures to one with rib fractures and pneumonia.

Pneumothorax is frequently seen in patients with fractures of the ribs and may be due either to laceration of the lung from the fractured bone ends or to the compressive force of the injury applied during maximal pressure within the lungs. These are usually closed pneumothoraces and have the potential to develop into tension pneumothorax because air escapes into the intrapleural space, and has no means of escape. Hemothorax is also frequently associated with rib fractures and may vary in degree. The most common source of bleeding is lacerations of the pulmonary parenchyma, intercostal muscles, and pleura. This bleeding is usually small and self-limited. Lacerations of the intercostal artery, however, may require thoracotomy and operative ligation to stop the ongoing significant bleeding.

Flail chest is defined as multiple adjacent ribs fractured in at least two places, creating a free-floating segment of ribs. This unsupported segment collapses in response to the negative intrathoracic pressure change of inspiration, yielding the clinical finding of "paradoxical respiration." Hypoxemia resulting from flail chest injury is usually not secondary to altered inspiratory mechanics from the discontinuous ribs but to (1) inability to inspire fully secondary to pain, resulting in atelectasis or subsegmental collapse, (2) hemothorax or pneumothorax, and (3) underlying pulmonary contusion.[2]

As with blunt injuries to the heart, liver, and spleen, forces applied to the chest wall can be transmitted to the lung, resulting in pulmonary contusion. As with any contusion, blood from broken vessels is released into the soft tissue. However, blood in the pulmonary parenchyma means space lost for alveolar gas exchange. Hypoxemia can be so profound that it prevents oxygenation, and death follows. Even less severe pulmonary contusions cause some degree of alveolar hypoventilation, which is usually seen as a decrease in peripheral arterial oxygen saturation (SaO_2). Measures to correct hypoventilation must be instituted quickly to prevent a progressive decline that may be difficult to reverse subsequently.

TREATMENT

Rib Fractures

As mentioned previously, fractured ribs are painful, but the ribs cannot be immobilized during the healing process. In fact, full excursion is to be encouraged, and this, of course, only exacerbates the pain. Therefore, the primary objective of therapy for patients with fractured ribs is to alleviate the associated pain and encourage activities that will prevent atelectasis. Young healthy patients with only one or two fractured ribs often do well with oral narcotic analgesics for pain control. On the opposite end of the spectrum are elderly patients who, with even one or two ribs broken, frequently have limited pulmonary and/or cardiac reserve and are often unable to tolerate the added insult. More aggressive analgesia must be supplied without further reducing the patient's respiratory drive with large doses of narcotics. A catheter placed percutaneously in the intrapleural space,[3] through which is infused bupivacaine, can produce continuous pain control during the early days following the injury to allow initial healing, after which safe narcotic doses can be given that will effectively reduce the pain. This catheter can also be inserted into the pleural space through an existing chest tube; however, continuous suctioning of a hemothorax or pneumothorax can evacuate some, if not all, of the anesthetic

Text continued on page 100

Hypoxia Algorithm

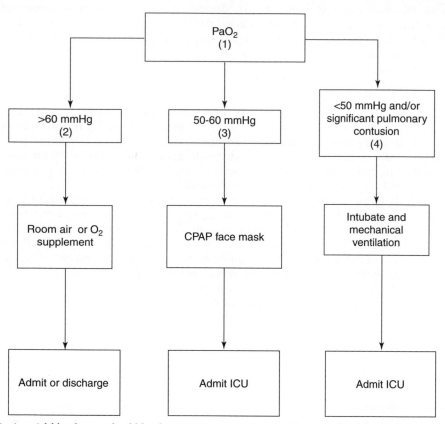

1. Arterial blood gases should be drawn on room air. An arterial oxygen level drawn on patients receiving supplemental oxygen is virtually indecipherable.
2. Most patients with a PaO_2 of >60 mmHg on room air will do well with adequate pain relief. If any doubt exists, the patient should be admitted for 24 to 48 hours of observation and pulmonary toilet.
3. These patients are bordering on significant hypoxemia, usually secondary to a mild to moderate pulmonary contusion and/or atelectasis as a result of hypoexpansion of the ipsilateral hemithorax secondary to pain. Positive pressure ventilation, usually in the form of continuous positive airway pressure (CPAP) via a nasal or face mask, along with aggressive pain relief, is required to prevent worsening of the hypoxemia. This form of ventilation should be administered in a monitored setting with a pulse oximeter and usually requires 2 to 5 days of therapy. For CPAP pressures of greater than 10 mmHg, one should be aware of the possibility of the introduction of gastric air and should consider a nasogastric tube during the time period in which CPAP is applied. Supplemental oxygen alone is contraindicated and is potentially dangerous (see text).
4. These patients are in serious trouble and require expeditious intubation and positive pressure ventilation. Inspired oxygen (FiO_2) should be maintained at less than 0.50, and positive end-expiratory pressure (PEEP) should be sequentially increased to attain adequate oxygenation (PaO_2 of >65 mmHg). Pain control is important, but mechanical ventilation is required until the pulmonary contusion resolves sufficiently to allow alveolar ventilation of the affected lung to resolve the hypoxemia.

Analgesia Algorithm

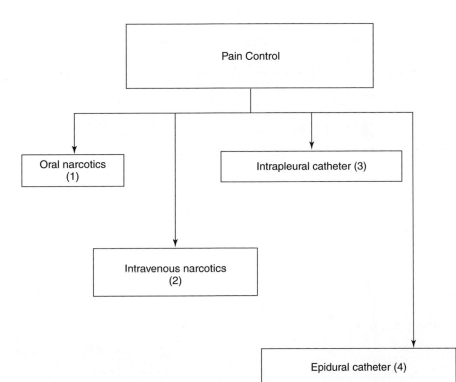

1. Oral analgesics are adequate for minor rib fractures or contusions. Examples include acetaminophen with or without codeine, ketorolac tromethamine, and oxycodone.
2. Intravenous analgesic agents such as morphine sulfate and meperidine are sometimes adequate but may have undesirable systemic side effects (e.g., respiratory depression or somnolence) at doses that are adequate to control pain.[8]
3. Intrapleural catheters[3, 9] can be placed percutaneously or through existing chest tubes. Complications include pneumothorax and inadvertent intra-abdominal placement. Bupivacaine is usually the agent of choice and should be titrated to effect. This route is significantly less effective in the presence of a hemothorax.
4. Thoracic epidural anesthesia is the most effective method of delivering analgesia for chest wall pain.[4] The catheter should be placed at the thoracic level whenever possible, though lumbar catheters can be effective in special circumstances (see text).

Rib Fracture Algorithm

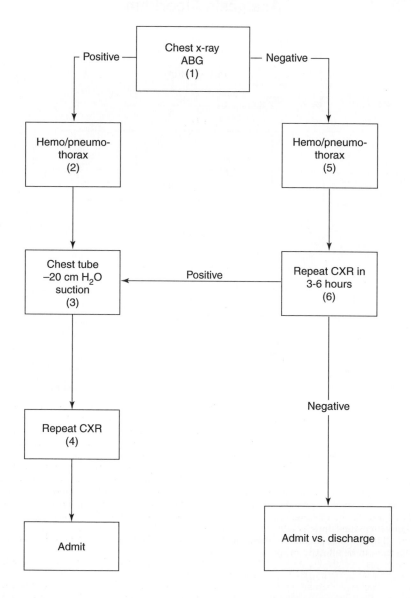

1. Chest roentgenograms confirm the presence or absence of rib fractures, pneumothoraces, hemothoraces, or pulmonary contusions, and should be an integral part of the initial radiographic evaluation of the trauma patient. Arterial blood gases (ABG) not only reveal the oxygenation and ventilation status of the patient but may also reveal a degree of hypoperfusion, usually as a result of hypovolemia, as reflected in the base deficit.
2. Hemothorax and pneumothorax resulting from a fractured rib are usually due to lacerated lung parenchyma or occasionally to a lacerated intercostal vessel. Tube thoracostomy is almost always required. Occasionally a pneumothorax is demonstrated on computed tomography studies but is not evident on chest roentgenogram. These lesions may be treated by observation unless they enlarge or the patient is to undergo an operative procedure or general anesthesia, or will receive positive pressure mechanical ventilation.[6]
3. A large-bore chest tube (36 to 40 Fr) should be placed in the mid or anterior axillary line, level with the inframammary fold.
4. If the lung is fully expanded and the pleural cavity is drained of fluid, suction should be continued until the air leak is resolved and fluid output is less than 100 ml/day.
5. Blood or air in the pleural space may develop in the early hours after injury and may be missed on the initial supine anteroposterior chest x-ray (CXR). If the index of suspicion is high, a repeat chest x-ray should be obtained in 3 to 6 hours.[7, 10]
6. If repeat chest x-rays remain normal, patients may be discharged. One may consider admission for other injuries or for patients in whom thoracic injury is strongly suspected.

agent. A word of caution is needed about continuous intrapleural bupivacaine infusion: Since the amount of systemic absorption of bupivacaine from the pleural space is unknown, the risk of toxicity may be a concern after a few days.

Regional blockade of the intercostal nerves is an alternative method of pain control but is of only marginal value. In general, each fractured rib requires blockade at the levels above and below it. Each injection provides analgesia for as long as the analgesic duration of the agent used, which is usually only about 8 hours. Additionally, each injection carries the risk of laceration of an intercostal blood vessel as well as pneumothorax. For these reasons, rib blocks are infrequently used to manage the pain of an acute rib fracture.

Probably the most technically demanding method of pain control is thoracic epidural analgesia. However, this is probably also the most effective means of providing optimal pain relief while allowing good pulmonary toilet.[4] It also has the advantage over other methods of providing pain relief to both sides of the chest if they are injured. A fine catheter is placed, usually by an anesthesiologist, percutaneously into the epidural space at the thoracic level. Although lumbar epidural anesthesia will control rib pain, a diffusible agent such as morphine sulfate or meperidine,[5] or larger doses of more lipophilic agents such as fentanyl, must be used. The larger doses of fentanyl required may become systemic, thus negating the advantages of epidural anesthesia. At the thoracic level, a continuous infusion of an analgesic agent such as fentanyl, along with bupivacaine, is titrated to effect. It must be remembered that because agents given into the thoracic epidural space can occasionally also attain therapeutic levels in the bloodstream, additional oral or parenteral narcotics should not be given because this compounded effect may result in toxicity. The more diffusible agents must be used with caution because they can cause respiratory depression. If these agents are used, patients should be observed in an intensive care setting.

Hypoxia

Ultimately, whichever analgesic method is chosen, the goal is to obtain good pain control to allow vigorous pulmonary toilet. Although general anesthesia may be the ultimate in pain control, it obviously does nothing to allow spontaneous, patient-directed deep breathing, coughing, and other methods of eliminating or preventing atelectasis. With good pain control, incentive spirometry, and patient education about the importance of pulmonary toilet, most cases of hypoxia can be prevented or reversed. More extensive rib fractures, flail chest, co-morbid conditions, including advanced age, or underlying lung injury require more aggressive approaches.

Frequently, in the initial evaluation of these patients the hypoxia is treated with supplemental oxygen. This is a mistake, for several reasons. Oxygen saturation will improve, leaving medical personnel with a false sense of security and a lessened awareness, a potentially lethal mistake. Because the pathophysiology behind the hypoxia is inadequate ventilation due to inadequate respiratory excursion due to chest wall pain, the resulting atelectasis will rapidly progress to subsegmental collapse. Early appropriate intervention consists of pain control and pulmonary toilet, not oxygen, which only hides the problem.

Alveolar collapse can also be worsened by a process known as "absorption atelectasis." Ambient air, or room air, is composed of 21% oxygen and approximately 79% nitrogen. Although oxygen is readily absorbed through the alveolar membrane, nitrogen is not, and therefore it acts to stent open the alveoli, preventing total collapse. An inspired FiO_2 of 100% oxygen potentially leads to total absorption of inspired gas and collapse of the alveoli. Therefore, minimal inspired supplemental oxygen should be supplied to produce an adequate PaO_2 (65 to 100 mmHg).

More severe hypoxia requires more aggressive ventilatory support. As the oxygen saturation reaches 91% on the oxygen saturation curve, further desaturation results in a significant decrease in PaO_2. If pain control is insufficient to allow pulmonary toilet or improvement in oxygenation, positive pressure ventilation will be needed. The simplest means of providing this support is through a continuous positive airway pressure (CPAP) face mask. CPAP can be provided to an awake patient with no need for airway intubation. A pressure of 10 to 15 mmHg can be delivered, and this is often enough to provide alveolar expansion. It must be mentioned that although a pressure of 10 mmHg is usually well tolerated, pressures higher than this can cause gastric distention, and in such cases a nasogastric tube should be placed. The mask should be left in place for 24 hours, and interruptions of the pressure support should be infrequent. Removing the mask only allows the damaged alveoli to collapse, and some time is required to re-recruit them.

Patients with severe hypoxia require intubation and mechanical ventilation. One should not hesitate to control the airway in a patient who is in significant respiratory distress. Oral endotracheal intubation is safe in experienced hands and can certainly be life-saving. Oxygenation can be obtained simply by the addition of positive end-expiratory pressure (PEEP) and can be boosted with supplemental oxygen.

Flail chest injury sometimes presents a dilemma in terms of management, but if one keeps in mind the pathophysiology of the hypoxia in patients with flail chests, the proper management is apparent. Although the paradoxical motion of the flail segment can be impressive, one must not be led astray. The hypoxia results from underlying pulmonary parenchymal damage, which should be treated to attain the normal endpoint, i.e., an arterial oxygen saturation of over 91%. Attempts to stop the motion of the flail segment may result in overventilation and serve only a cosmetic purpose. As with any rib fracture, pain control is the key, even for patients receiving mechanical ventilation. The goal is to support respiratory activity and encourage patient activity. This goal can be attained only when the patient can inspire deeply without feeling significant pain.

References

1. Ziegler DW, Agarwal NN: The morbidity and mortality of rib fractures. J Trauma 1994;37(6):975.
2. Shackford SR, Virgilio RW, Peters RM: Selective use of ventilator therapy in flail chest injury. J Thorac Cardiovasc Surg 1981;81(2):194.
3. Rocco A, Reiestad F, Gudman J, et al: Intrapleural administration of local anesthetics for pain relief in patients with multiple rib fractures: Preliminary report. Reg Anesth 1987;12:10.

4. Luchette FA, Radafshar SM, Kaiser R, et al: Prospective evaluation of epidural versus intrapleural catheters for analgesia in chest wall trauma. J Trauma 1994;36(6):865.
5. Glynn CJ, Mather LE, Cousins MJ, et al: Peridural morphine in humans: Analgesic response, pharmacokinetics, and transmission into CSF. Anesthesiology 1981;55:520.
6. Enderson BL, Abdalla R, Frame SB, et al: Tube thoracostomy for occult pneumothorax: A prospective randomized study of its use. J Trauma 1993;35(5):726.
7. Coselli JS, Mattox KL, Beall AC: Reevaluation of early evacuation of clotted hemothorax. Am J Surg 1984;148(6):786.
8. Bachmann-Mennenga B, Biscoping J, Kuhn DF: Intercostal nerve block, intrapleural analgesia, thoracic epidural block or systemic opioid application for pain relief after thoracotomy. Eur J Cardiothorac Surg 1993;7:12.
9. Schneider RF, Villamena PC, Harvey J, et al: Lack of efficacy of intrapleural bupivacaine for postoperative analgesia following thoracotomy. Chest 1993;103:414.
10. De la Pedraja J, Erbella J, Vail SJ, Shatz DV: Efficacy of follow-up radiologic evaluation in penetrating thoracic injuries: 3- vs. 6-hour roentgenograms of the chest. J Trauma 1999;46:200.

Chapter 9

Acute Injury to the Spinal Cord

Traumatic spinal cord injury can result from a variety of mechanisms. These injuries can be primary or secondary. Primary injuries may result from direct blunt external trauma due to automobile accidents, falls, diving, or other recreational or sporting activities. Penetrating injuries result from gunshot or knife wounds. Secondary injuries include neuronal damage resulting from hypoxia, hypotension, electrolyte abnormalities, accumulation of neurotransmitters, free radicals, edema, and inflammation. Iatrogenic secondary injuries to the spinal cord may also result from poor immobilization of the unstable vertebral column. The goal of management of these injuries is to diagnose or identify which victims are at greatest risk of having a spinal cord injury and then to immobilize and transport those patients to a hospital facility as quickly as possible, minimizing further neurologic loss. These goals can be attained with a multidisciplinary spinal cord injury system and a specialized facility that includes health care professionals trained in the management of these injuries.

EPIDEMIOLOGY

Approximately 8000 to 12,000 traumatic spinal cord injuries occur each year in the United States.[1] The prevalence of individuals with chronic paralysis due to spinal cord injury varies from 250,000 to 500,000. Others have reported the prevalence of partial paralysis caused by accidents to be 80 in 100,000 population and of quadriparesis to be 20 in 100,000.[2] Of the 12,000 victims who sustain a spinal cord injury each year, about 4200 die before they reach the hospital, and 1500 die during the initial hospitalization.[2] As reported by the National Spinal Cord Statistical Center, 48% of all spinal cord injuries result from motor vehicle accidents, 21% from falls, 15% from penetrating wounds, and 14% from sporting activities. The National Crash Service study reported that in vehicles damaged severely enough to be towed from the scene, approximately 1 in 300 occupants are likely to have sustained a severe neck injury. In addition, the incidence of neck injury increases to 1 in 14 for occupants ejected from an automobile.[3] Nationally, 85% of patients with acute spinal cord injuries are male, and 15% are female. Also, 61% of these injuries occur in patients between the ages of 16 and 30 years, whereas fewer than 15% occur in patients older than 46 years. The level most commonly injured is the middle to lower cervical spine followed by the thoracolumbar junction; these spinal segments are biomechanically more mobile. In addition, it is important to note that head injury of varying degree and severity occurs in approximately 25% to 50% of persons with acute spinal cord injuries.[4, 5] Multisystem trauma in

Acute Spinal Cord Injury

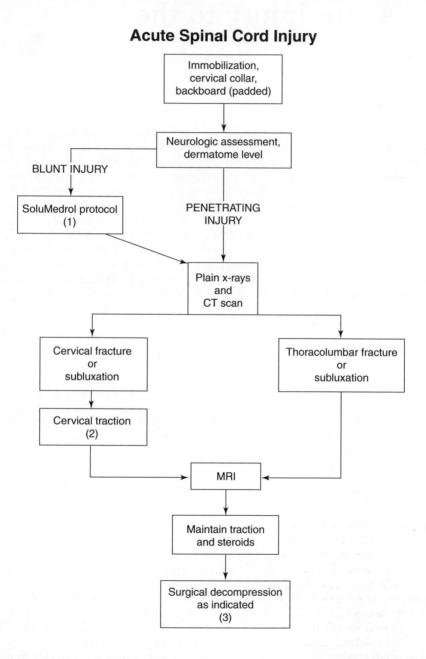

1. At present, there is no support for using the SoluMedrol protocol for patients with penetrating spinal cord injury. For blunt injury, the initial loading dose of SoluMedrol is 30.1 mg/kg, given over 30 minutes. The maintenance dose is then 5.4 mg/kg/hour. For injuries treated within the first 3 hours of the traumatic event, the maintenance dose should continue for 23 hours. For injuries treated 3 to 8 hours after the trauma, the SoluMedrol maintenance infusion should continue for 47 hours.
2. Cervical alignment should be maintained with cervical traction, particularly when there is subluxation or compression of the spinal cord. Traction, however, is contraindicated in patients with cervicocranial dislocation. Cervical reduction may at times require manual reduction under fluoroscopy, particularly when there is evidence of a unilateral or bilateral jumped facet; however, this should be done with extreme caution by highly trained personnel. A follow-up magnetic resonance imaging (MRI) scan is required after reduction to rule out a recurrent herniated nucleus pulposus.
3. MRI is an essential tool to determine the degree of cervical compression resulting from a fracture segment versus disc herniation or epidural hematoma. Acute decompression is considered when significant disc herniation or cervical compromise exists in an incompletely paralyzed patient.

victims of spinal cord injury includes musculoskeletal (18%), head (16%), lung (10.5%), abdominal (2.5%), and cardiovascular (1.5%) injuries.[6]

CLASSIFICATION

Spinal cord injury can be classified as either complete or incomplete. According to the American Spinal Injury Association (AISA), the level of injury is the most caudal segment of the spinal cord in which motor and sensory function is preserved (Table 9–1). For an injury to be classified as complete, there must be an absence of motor and sensory function including function in segments S4–S5.

There are several categories of incomplete injuries according to the ASIA impairment scale. Patients may have sensory function but no motor function below the neurologic level, or they may have motor function below the neurologic level with antigravity strength or greater, whereas some patients may have antigravity strength or less.

Table 9–1. Spinal Nerve Root Motor Innervation

Spinal Cord Level	Muscle Innervation	Function	Reflex
C1–5	Neck muscles		
C3,4,5	Diaphragm	Inspiration	
C5,6	Deltoid	Abduct arm >90 degrees	
C5,6	Biceps	Flexion @ elbow	Biceps
C6,7	Extensor carpi radialis	Extension @ wrist	Supinator
C7,8	Triceps, extensor digitorum	Elbow and finger flexion	Triceps
C8,T1	Flexor digitorum profundus	Flexion @ distal phalanx	
C8,T1	Hand intrinsics	Abduct fifth digit, adduct thumb	
T2-9	Intercostals	Intercostal expansion	
T9,10	Upper abdominals	Beevor's sign	Abdominal cutaneous
T11,12	Lower abdominals	Beevor's sign	Abdominal cutaneous
L2,3	Iliopsoas, adductors	Flexion @ hip	Cremasteric
L3,4	Quadriceps	Extension @ knee	Knee jerk
L4,5	Medial hamstrings, tibialis anterior	Ankle dorsiflexion	Medial hamstrings
L5,S1	Lateral hamstrings, posterior tibialis, peroneals	Flexion @ knee	
L5,S1	Extensor digitorum, EHL	Great toe extension	
S1,2	Gastrocnemius, soleus	Ankle planterflexion	Ankle jerk
S2,3	Flexor digitorum, flexor hallucis		
S2,3,4	Bladder, lower bowel, anal sphincter	Constriction of anal sphincter, maintenance of pelvic floor	Anal cutaneous Bulbocavernosus

ACUTE MANAGEMENT

The first step in management of patients with possible cervical injuries is appropriate management at the accident scene and resuscitation of the patient. Proper spinal immobilization and the ABCs of life support are crucial for survival in these patients. Prehospital personnel at the scene should maintain cervical alignment using a cervical collar and should use a board to maintain spinal immobilization. During transport, sandbags should be placed along the head and neck of the patient, and tape is placed across the forehead and secured to the backboard. The mouth should be well exposed and unobstructed. Administration of oxygen by nasal cannula for adequate oxygenation and placement of at least two intravenous lines to provide hemodynamic support is crucial. Intubation may be required, particularly in patients with cervical injuries that may have compromised the patient's respiratory function. Whether traction of the cervical column is necessary and whether nasal, oral, or fiberoptic intubation is necessary is controversial. Regardless of controversy, intubation depends on the skill as well as the availability of highly trained personnel. The important point is to maintain adequate immobilization of the cervical spine and secure the appropriate airway. Ideally, fiberoptic intubation is recommended; however, both the nasotracheal and orotracheal routes are acceptable. In patients with multiple facial trauma or severe basilar skull fractures, cricothyroidotomy may be necessary.[7-11] Placement of a Foley catheter is essential to monitor urine output, and in patients with cervical injuries, a nasogastric tube is important to prevent air swallowing and gastric rupture.

Hypotension may occur. It is important to differentiate between neurogenic and hemorrhagic shock. Neurogenic shock is characterized by sympathetic denervation, somatic paralysis, urinary retention, areflexia, and hypothermia. The degree of shock is correlated with the severity of injury; however, rarely is the systolic pressure lower than 70 mmHg. In addition, the sensorium does not seem to be altered unless there is an associated head injury or intoxication. Hemorrhagic shock, on the other hand, is characterized by hypotension, tachycardia, altered sensorium, and low urine output. It is important to recognize these differences early because they require different therapeutic strategies.

To prevent secondary spinal cord injury during spinal shock, patients require placement of an arterial line and a pulmonary artery catheter to optimize cardiac output. Use of vasopressors is recommended when necessary to maintain the mean blood pressure at higher than 90 mmHg; this has been shown by Levi and colleagues to help prevent secondary ischemic damage.[12]

Once the patient has been stabilized, the level of neurologic injury must be determined by means of a rapid but careful neurologic examination. This consists of a sensory examination using light touch, pinprick, and proprioception. It is important to test sacral sensation including sensation in the perianal area. In addition, muscular strength should be graded according to the ASIA methodology. A score of 5 represents normal strength, 4 represents strength against resistance, 3 represents strength against gravity, 2 indicates strength within a horizontal plane with no gravity control, 1 indicates palpable or visible contraction, and 0 represents paralysis. Reflexes tested include the biceps, triceps, brachioradialis, Hoffman's, abdominal, knee, ankle, cremasteric, bulbo-cavernosus, and anal wink (Fig. 9–1).

Once a baseline examination level has been established and evidence of a spinal cord injury has been found, steroid treatment should be started as dictated by the National Acute Spinal Cord Injury Study (NASCIS) II study. This study showed that a statistically significant improvement in neurologic function occurred with high-dose intravenous steroid treatment within an 8-hour window in patients with acute spinal cord injury when treatment was given over a period of 24 hours. An initial bolus of 30 mg/kg of methylprednis-olone is given over a period of 15 minutes, followed 45 minutes later by a

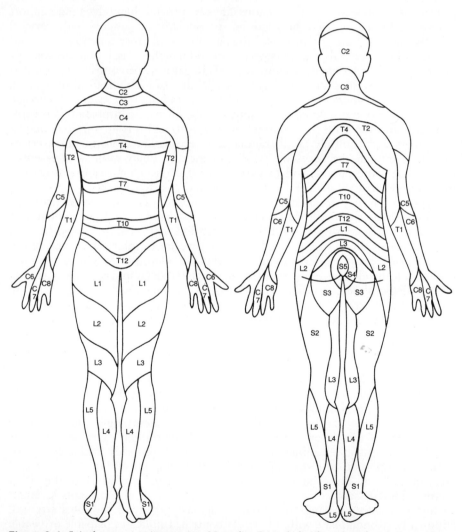

Figure 9–1. Spinal nerve root innervation. Note that C4 includes the upper chest just superior to T2. (From Browner B, et al. [eds]: Skeletal Trauma, 2nd ed. Philadelphia, WB Saunders, 1997.)

continuous infusion of 5.4 mg/kg/hour for 23 hours.[13, 14] Moreover, the most recent (1997) recommendations, according to the NASCIS III study, are as follows: patients with acute spinal cord injury who receive methylprednisolone within 3 hours of injury should be maintained on the high-dose regimen for 24 hours. When patients receive methylprednisolone 3 to 8 hours after injury, they should be treated for 48 hours. Patients treated with methylprednisolone for 48 hours showed improved motor scores compared to the 24-hour group at 6 weeks and 6 months post-injury. Although the 48-hour group had a slightly higher risk of sepsis and pneumonia, mortality among all the groups was similar. Patients treated with tirilazad for 48 hours showed motor recovery similar to that of patients treated for 24 hours with methylprednisolone.

RADIOGRAPHIC STUDIES

The initial radiographic evaluation consists of plain lateral x-rays of the cervical, thoracolumbar, and sacral spine. Visualization of the C7–T1 junction is essential to avoid missing lower cervical fractures or subluxation. This is followed by an anteroposterior view to assess the rotational components, alignment, and pedicle integrity. Oblique views are used to assess the foramen, and open mouth views are useful for assessing the integrity of the dens and articular masses of C1–C2. Computed tomography (CT) provides excellent resolution of the bony anatomy and is indicated in all patients with fractures or subluxations, particularly those with negative results on plain x-rays. It is also helpful in viewing the C7–T1 junction, which may be difficult to visualize on plain x-rays.

CT may miss fractures in the axial plane. This shortcoming can be overcome by performing helical CT scanning and axial reconstruction. Magnetic resonance imaging (MRI) is an essential tool and is indicated in patients with a fixed deficit or significant neurologic dysfunction. Modern MRI gives excellent soft tissue resolution and can help in identifying compression resulting from an acute herniated disc or epidural hematoma. One can also visualize the integrity of the spinal cord. CT myelography has become a less favored procedure and has been replaced by CT and MRI owing to the increased resolution and availability of these techniques. Mechanism of injury and subsequent stability of the spine can be predicted from the radiographic findings (Table 9–2).

CLINICAL SYNDROMES

Brown-Sequard Syndrome

Brown-Sequard syndrome was described in 1850. It may occur after penetrating injuries to the spinal cord and is characterized by a physiologic hemisection of the spinal cord.[16] Patients present with ipsilateral paralysis, ipsilateral loss of proprioception, and contralateral pain and temperature loss. This syndrome is uncommon as an isolated finding and may occur with other spinal cord injuries as well as nerve root or brachial plexus injury. It is most often seen in patients with cervical spine injuries and less frequently in those with

Table 9–2. Fractures and Dislocations of the Spine: Mechanism and Stability

Type	Mechanism	Stability* Immediate	Late
Atlanto-occipital dislocation	Twisting force to head	Poor	Poor
Atlanto-axial dislocation	Flexion	Poor	Poor
Fractures of the base of the odontoid	Flexion (rarely extension)	Poor	Fair
Jefferson's fracture	Axial load to head	Good	Good
Hangman's fracture	Hyperextension and distration	Poor	Good
C3–T1 ant. dislocation with jumped facets	Flexion	Poor	Fair
Unilateral jumped facets	Flexion and rotation	Good	Fair
Simple wedge fracture	Flexion and axial rotation	Good	Fair
Burst fracture	Flexion and axial compression	Good	Good
Teardrop fracture with subluxation	Flexion and axial compression	Fair	Good
Hyperextension fractures	Extension	Good in flexion	Good
Thoracic fractures	Direct trauma or flexion	Good	Good
Thoracolumbar fractures	Flexion	Poor	Poor
Open fractures	Penetrating injuries	Good	Good

*Immediate, stability at the time of injury; late, the potential for future stability after an appropriate period of immobilization.

thoracic lesions. It carries a relatively good prognosis for recovery; however, when the deficit results from a penetrating injury, the recovery is less favorable.

Bell's Cruciate Paralysis

Cruciate paralysis was described in the 1970s by Bell based on some of the initial postulates of Wallenberg. After a hyperextension cervical force or traumatic injury at the cervicomedullary junction, patients present with upper extremity weakness out of proportion to the strength of the lower extremities. The present concept explaining this syndrome assumes the presence of a lesion affecting the cephalad decussating upper extremity fibers in the corticospinal tract and sparing the more caudal decussating lower extremity fibers. However, to date, somatotopic organization of the lateral corticospinal tract has never been demonstrated. It is difficult to differentiate this syndrome from central cord syndrome; however, radiographic studies, plain x-rays, and MRI may reveal a cervicomedullary lesion in Bell's cruciate paralysis, whereas an upper, mid to lower cervical spinal cord injury exists in central cord syndrome.[17]

Central Cord Syndrome

The central cord syndrome was first described by Schneider in 1954. The most common mechanism of injury is neck hyperextension in a patient with cervical canal stenosis and spondylosis.[18] It is one of the most common spinal cord syndromes, and patients present with weakness in the upper extremities greater than that in the lower extremities as well as with urinary retention.

The typical patient is elderly and has sustained a frontal laceration or subgaleal hematoma suggesting a hyperextension force applied to the cervical spine. This syndrome is also seen less commonly in young football players with a congenitally narrowed cervical canal who are injured while tackling an opponent head first. The cause was once thought to be related to central hematomyelia and selective injury to upper extremity fibers situated medially in a somatotopically organized corticospinal tract. New radiographic evidence with histopathologic correlates suggests that a diffuse white matter tract injury exists in the lateral columns.[19] This injury carries a relatively good prognosis for improvement if the injury does not involve the entire column. Recovery of hand function may be minimal, and this is one of the most disabling sequelae.

Anterior Spinal Cord Syndrome

The anterior spinal cord syndrome was first described by Schneider in 1955. It is characterized by a physiologic ventral section of the spinal cord that spares the posterior columns. Patients present with motor paralysis, pain, and temperature loss, but proprioception is spared.[19] This syndrome may be seen in hyperflexion and axial loading injuries as well as in central disc herniation, "tear drop" fractures, and compression fractures that compromise the ventral aspect of the spinal canal. It is an uncommon manifestation of spinal cord injury but can present after a vascular insult.

Conus Medullaris Syndrome

The conus medullaris is found between T11 and L1–L2. Almost all of the sacral spinal cord segments are found between L1–L2 and the lumbar segments at T11–T12. This area is prone to injury because it is at the thoracolumbar junction, which is injured frequently owing to its hypermobility. These patients present with symptoms of upper as well as lower motor root findings. In the acute phase, paralysis of the lower extremities as well as flaccid rectal tone and urinary retention are present. In the chronic phase, evidence of atrophy and hyperreflexia are prominent.

Cauda Equina Syndrome

The cauda equina syndrome is a peripheral nerve injury associated with lesions below the conus (Ll–L2). Patients present with asymmetric and incomplete paralysis and areflexia including loss of bowel and bladder control. These patients have a potentially good recovery. A very dangerous acute syndrome may result from a central disc herniation at L4–L5 or L5–S1, which may permanently damage some of the sacral roots that control rectal and urinary continence. These patients may or may not present with motor weakness. A high index of suspicion requires an emergency MRI followed by acute surgical decompression.

Spinal Cord Injury Without Radiographic Abnormality (SCIWORA)

This syndrome is generally seen in children and is characterized by lack of radiographic evidence of a fracture or subluxation on plain x-rays or CT scan. It is a rare syndrome that is presumed to occur in children as a result of increased ligamentous laxity; it needs reevaluation in the MRI era because MRI provides more detailed resolution and may show evidence of edema or shear injuries not evident on CT scans. In addition, Keith and colleagues described a syndrome of secondary spinal cord injury in adults and children who sustain severe abdominal, thoracic or limb trauma leading to injuries that compromise the radicular and spinal arteries.[20]

CERVICAL SPINE TRAUMA

Whiplash

Whiplash is a colloquial term used to describe a hyperflexion-hyperextension cervical soft tissue injury associated with automobile accidents. This term itself carries legal implications and is associated with chronic pain and disability. However, there have been multiple reports in the literature of cervical ligamentous injuries, laryngeal and pharyngeal trauma, and cervical musculature tears and avulsions.[24] Treatment of these injuries requires soft collar immobilization for comfort, physical therapy, and administration of nonsteroidal anti-inflammatory agents.

Cervical Fractures

Atlanto-Occipital Dissociation

This type of injury occurs in about 1% of patients with cervical spine injuries and is found in 19% of autopsies of persons with fatal cervical spine injuries (see Table 9–2).[22] The presentation varies, and patients may present without symptoms or with immediate respiratory or cardiopulmonary arrest. The dislocation may present longitudinally, anteriorly, or posteriorly, and is the result of severe ligamentous disruption between the occipital condyles and the lateral masses of C1. Disruption of the tectorial membrane and alar and apical ligaments also occurs. Traction is contraindicated in these patients.

Jefferson's Fracture

Jefferson's fractures are fractures through the arches of C1 that result from axial loading. In approximately 50% of patients they are associated with C2 fractures. These fractures do not usually result in a neurologic deficit, and most of them heal with use of a cervical orthosis. They rarely require traction or surgical decompression. Transverse ligamentous disruption must be suspected when there is more than a 7-mm overhang of both C1 lateral masses over C2. MRI may confirm this pathology. Surgery is indicated if fusion fails after more than 12 weeks of cervical immobilization or when there is evidence of transverse ligamentous rupture.[23]

Hangman's Fracture (Traumatic Spondylolisthesis)

This fracture results from axial loading and hyperextension, which result in fracture through the isthmus or pars interarticularis of C2. The fracture differs from the mechanism that occurs in judicial hangings because in executions the mechanism is that of distraction and hyperextension. These injuries are highly unstable when the degree of displacement is greater than 2 mm and angulation is present, indicating severe ligamentous disruption. If there is displacement, these injuries require cervical traction to reduce the misalignment. These injuries heal with use of a cervical orthosis for a period of 8 to 12 weeks. Nonsurgical treatment with a cervical orthosis produces adequate healing and bone fusion in more than 95% of cases. Surgical intervention is indicated if there is (1) acute disc herniation or evidence of an epidural hematoma on MRI causing neurologic deficit, (2) inability to reduce or maintain reduction of the fracture, or (3) nonunion or lack of fusion after more than 12 weeks of use of an external orthosis.[24]

Odontoid Fracture

Odontoid fractures most commonly result from a hyperflexion force. These fractures are commonly missed on routine cervical x-rays. Patients can present with occipital pain and may have a tendency to hold their heads with their hands when walking upright. Type I fractures are rare and occur through the tip of the odontoid. Little is known about this fracture because of its rarity. Type II fractures occur through the base of the odontoid and are considered unstable. Type III fractures occur through the body of C2; they are acutely unstable but have a better potential for healing than Type II fractures. Type I fractures require no treatment, whereas Type III fractures are generally treated with a cervical orthosis. Treatment for Type II fractures is controversial. Treatment options include use of a Halo-Vest or surgical fusion. Some practitioners believe that in patients with displacement of more than 6 mm, those older than 65 years, those who are chronic smokers, and those with posterior subluxations or neurologic deficit (which implies ligamentous disruption at some time), the risk of nonunion is high after Halo-Vest immobilization, and therefore they advocate surgery. In 40% of patients these fractures fail to fuse after a course 8 to 12 weeks of use of a cervical orthosis, and they then become candidates for surgical fusion.[25-27]

Cervical Hyperflexion Injuries

Severe hyperflexion injuries result in posterior ligamentous disruption. The degree of disruption is associated with the severity of neurologic deficit, the lower cervical spine at C5–C6 and C6–C7 being the most vulnerable. According to Panjabi and colleagues,[28] horizontal subluxation of more than 3 mm and/or 11 degrees of angulation as well as a neurologic deficit is associated with significant ligamentous instability. These injuries are acutely unstable, have a poor potential for healing, and require surgical stabilization.

Hyperflexion with a rotational or lateral bending component results in a unilateral locked facet. This results when the inferior facet of the vertebrae above jumps and locks in front of the superior facet of the vertebrae below. These vertebrae are typically displaced less than 25% (occasionally there is little or no displacement).[29] Also, on the anteroposterior x-ray view, the spinous process of the superior vertebrae may deviate from the midline to the side of the disruption. Unilateral locked facets may be difficult to diagnose, and approximately 40% of patients may present up to 2 weeks after the initial injury.[30–32] Bilateral locked facets result from severe hyperflexion and represent the worse degree of ligamentous injury and disruption. Radiographically, subluxation of more than 50% occurs from the vertebrae above to that below. However, because of the severe ligamentous disruption, the hypermobile subluxation may reduce, resulting in minimal radiographic malalignment. This hypermobility, if not recognized, may result in worsening of an already compromised neurologic state. One must have a high index of suspicion in cases with a severe neurologic deficit and minimal to no malalignment on lateral cervical x-ray.[29, 31]

Treatment of these injuries requires closed reduction or open reduction. Patients are placed in tongs traction with 3 to 5 pounds per level, up to a total of 70 pounds for locked facets. Care, however, must be taken when performing sequential cervical lateral x-rays and neurologic examination to prevent overdistraction or a worsening neurologic state. The success rate with closed reduction may be as low as 25% for patients with unilateral locked facets to about 50% for those with bilateral locked facets.[30] If cervical traction does not reduce the subluxation some have advocated manual distraction under fluoroscopy and controlled conditions including intubation if necessary. Closed reduction, however, may lead to a worsening of the neurologic status. There have been isolated reports of acute disc herniations that cause worsening cord compression that result in a worse outcome.[33] These patients require emergency MRI to rule out an acute disc herniation, which may be surgically decompressed. Surgical reduction is indicated if attempts at closed reduction fail, if closed reduction seems dangerous owing to worsening of the neurologic state, if there is evidence of cord compression due to a herniated disc fragment, displaced bone fragment, or hematoma and worsening of the neurologic state, and if the neurosurgeon prefers to operate to prevent long-term instability.

Cervical Hyperextension Injuries

Cervical hyperextension injuries result in anterior longitudinal ligament disruption. Lesions range from no fracture to disruption of the posterior elements including laminar fractures and ligamentous disruption. Anterior and inferior vertebral body surface avulsions may also occur. These injuries are commonly seen in elderly patients with a history of significant cervical spondylosis. Clinically the patients may present with a central cord syndrome.

These injuries are stable in flexion and require cervical fusion if a laminectomy is done for decompression.

Compression Fractures

Compression fractures of the cervical spine include wedge fractures, burst fractures, and teardrop fractures. Wedge fractures result from axial loading and a flexion component. The anterior column of the cervical spine is compromised, resulting in collapse of the anterior vertebral body with preservation of the middle and posterior elements (Fig. 9–2). These fractures are relatively stable and have a good prognosis for healing with use of a cervical orthosis device and 6 to 12 weeks of cervical immobilization. The greater the degree of compression and angulation, the greater the degree of middle and posterior

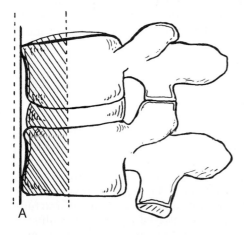

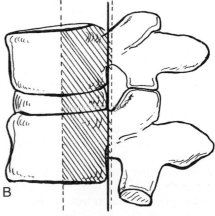

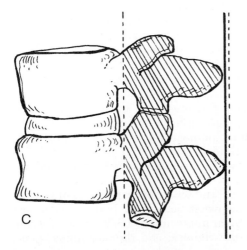

Figure 9–2. Schematic diagram of the components of the three columns of the thoracolumbar spine. *A,* The anterior column corresponds to the anterior third of the vertebral body and the anterior longitudinal ligament (ALL). *B,* The middle column contains the posterior half of the vertebral body and the posterior longitudinal ligament (PLL). *C,* The posterior column contains all bone and ligamentous elements posterior to the PLL. Instability is defined as disruption of two or more columns. (From Bucholz RW, Gill K: Classification of injuries of the thoracolumbar spine. Orthop Clin North Am 1986; 17:70.)

column compromise and the higher the risk of cervical instability. Burst fractures result from axial loading and result in compromise of the anterior and middle column with preservation of the posterior elements. There is also retropulsion of bone into the cervical canal. These fractures may be associated with severe neurologic compromise and may require surgical decompression in patients with acute disc herniation and bony compromise along with a fixed neurologic deficit. These fractures are acutely unstable and have the potential for healing with use of a cervical orthosis and cervical immobilization for several weeks. Surgical stabilization may be required in patients with severe angulation or those in whom conservative treatment has failed.

Clay Shoveler's Fracture

Clay shoveler's fracture is a fracture of the spinous process of C7 or T1 that results from an avulsion of the spinous process during active extension of the arms and hyperflexion of the cervical spine. It was initially described in Australia in patients who shoveled clay. It may also result from a direct injury to the spinous process. This fracture is stable and requires no orthosis, although a cervical collar may be used for comfort.[34]

THORACOLUMBAR TRAUMA

Thoracic and thoracolumbar fractures include compression fractures, burst fractures, seat belt fractures, and fracture dislocations. Fractures through the thoracic spine from T2 to T10 indicate the application of a severe force but may be stable owing to the stability provided by the rib cage. However, the thoracolumbar junction is a transition zone from the rigid thoracic spine to the more mobile lumbar spine, and it sustains a higher percentage of fractures and angulation. Compression fractures result from axial loading and failure of the anterior column with preservation of the middle and posterior columns. Burst fractures also result from axial loading and failure of both the anterior and middle columns with retropulsion of vertebral body fragments into the central canal. Seat belt fractures result from hyperflexion and failure of both posterior and middle columns. Fracture dislocations result from rotation, shear, and compression forces and failure of all three columns. Failure of two or more columns, as reported by Denis, is associated with instability, particularly if the posterior column is involved.[35]

Simple wedge fractures, compression fractures, and burst fractures may present with either no neurologic sequelae or a focal neurologic deficit. If the fracture is stable, it is treated with a thoracolumbar brace. If, however, progressive angulation occurs or if there is evidence of a fixed neurologic deficit from a disc or bone fragment, surgical intervention may be indicated for decompression and stabilization.[35]

Fracture dislocations, seat belt fractures, and severe burst fractures are highly unstable fractures and present with the worst neurologic findings including paraplegia. These fractures require surgical intervention. Different approaches are used to decompress and stabilize the thoracic and thoracolumbar spine;

these include anterior decompression via a transabdominal or transthoracic approach, and anterolateral and posterior approaches, depending on the site of compression. Stabilization techniques are fashioned depending on the mechanism of fracture and the preference of the neurosurgeon; these techniques may include the use of "rods," pedicle screws and hooks, and autologous or cadaveric bone fusion.[35]

Penetrating Injuries

Penetrating injuries may be explored surgically if there is evidence of gross contamination or progressive neurologic decompensation. Low-velocity penetrating injuries such as stab wounds or gunshot wounds are explored electively, if necessary, after the patient has been stabilized from other injuries or surgical lesions. These injuries may include dural tears or fixed neurologic deficits for which prophylactic treatment may prevent future tethering or pain syndromes. Gunshot wounds involving a hollow viscus and spinal cord or roots are in themselves not an indication for surgical exploration. The methylprednisolone protocol is not recommended for patients with a penetrating spinal cord injury, particularly when the patient requires a laparotomy or other major surgical procedure. In addition, methylprednisolone does not appear to provide any significant benefit for patients with spinal cord trauma from gunshot injuries.[36]

CONCLUSION

Acute spinal cord injury can result in significant neurologic morbidity. It requires a team effort of highly trained personnel to ensure expeditious recognition and prevention of secondary spinal cord injury and to administer the proper treatment. This aggressive approach guarantees the best chance of gaining some functional recovery.

References

1. Green BA, Edgar R: Spinal injury pain. *In* Long DM (ed): Current Therapy in Neurological Surgery. Philadelphia, Decker, 1989, p. 294.
2. Krous JF, Fronti CE, Riggins RS: Incidence of traumatic spinal cord lesions. J Chron Dis 1975;28:471.
3. Huelke DF, O'Day J, Mendlesohn RA: Cervical injuries suffered in automobile crashes. J Neurosurg 1981;54:316.
4. Davidoff GN, Roth EJ, Richards JS: Cognitive deficits in spinal cord injury: Epidemiology and outcome. Arch Phys Med Rehabil 1992;73:275.
5. Davidoff GN, Morris J, Roth EJ, Bleightberg J: Closed head injury in spinal cord injured patients: Retrospective study of loss of consciousness and post traumatic amnesia. Arch Phys Med Rehabil 1985;66:41.
6. Eisenburg HM, Cayard CC, Papancolaua FF: The effects of three potentially preventable complications on outcome after severe closed head injury. *In* Ishar S, et al (ed): Intracranial Pressure, 5th ed. New York, Springer-Verlag, 1983, pp. 549–553.
7. Rhee RJ, Green W, Holcraft JW, Mangili JA: Oral intubation in the multiply injured patient: The risk of exacerbating spinal cord damage. Ann Emerg Med 1990;9:511.
8. Talucci RC, Shaiuh KA, Schwab CW: Rapid sequence induction with oral endotracheal intubation in the multiply injured patient. Am Surg 1988;54:1851.

9. Wright SW, Robinson GG, Wright MB: Cervical spine injuries in blunt trauma in patients requiring emergent endotracheal intubation. Am J Emerg Med 1992;10:104.

10. Mulder DS, Wallace DH, Woolhouse FM: The use of the fiberoptic bronchoscope to facilitate endotracheal intubation following head and neck trauma. J Trauma 1975;15:638.

11. Meschimo A, Devitt JH, Koch JP, Szalki JP, Schwartz MC: The safety of acute tracheal intubation in cervical spine injury. Can J Anesth 1992;39:114.

12. Levi L, Wolf A, Belzberg H: Hemodynamic parameters in patients with acute cervical cord trauma: Description, intervention, and prediction of outcome. Neurosurgery 1993;33:1007.

13. Bracken MB, Shephard MJ, Collins WF, et al: Methylprednisolone or naloxone in the treatment of acute cervical cord injury. J Neurosurg 1992;76:23.

14. Bracken MB, Shephard MJ, Collins WF, et al: A randomized controlled trial of methylprednisolone or naloxone in the treatment of acute cervical cord injury. N Engl J Med 1990, 322:1405.

15. Bracken MB, Shephard MJ, Holford TR, et al: Administration of methylprednisolone for 24 or 48 hours or tirilazad mesylate for 48 hours in the treatment of acute cervical cord injury: Results of the Third National Acute Spinal Cord Injury Randomized Controlled Trial. JAMA 1997;277:1597.

16. Brown-Sequard CE: Course of Lectures on the Physiology and Pathology of the Central Nervous System. Philadelphia, Collins, 1860.

17. Dickman CA, Hadley MN, Pappas CT, Sonntag VK, Geisler FH: Cruciate paralysis: A clinical and radiographic analysis of injuries to the cervicomedullary junction. J Neurosurg 1990;73:850.

18. Schneider RC, Cherry GL, Pantek HF: The syndrome of acute central cervical spinal cord injury. J Neurosurg 1954;11:546.

19. Quencer RM, Bunge RP, Egnor M, et al: Acute traumatic central cord syndrome: MRI and pathological correlations. Neuroradiology 1992;34:85.

20. Keith WS: Traumatic infarction of the spinal cord. Can J Neurol Sci 1974;1:124.

21. Evans R: Some observations on whiplash injuries. Neurol Clin 1992;18:10.

22. Alker GJ, Leslie EV: High cervical spine and craniocervical junction injuries in fatal traffic accidents: A radiological study. Orthop Clin North Am 1978;9:1003.

23. Hadley MN, Dickman CA, Browner CM, Sonntag VK: Acute traumatic atlas fractures: Management and long term outcome. Neurosurgery 1988;23:31.

24. Effendi B, Roy D, Cornish B, Dussault RG, Laurin CA: Fractures of the ring of the axis: A classification based on the analysis of 131 cases. J Bone Joint Surg 1981;63B:319.

25. Hadley MN, Dickman CA, Browner CM: Acute axis fractures: A review of 229 cases. J Neurosurg 1989;71:642.

26. Apuzzo ML, Heiden JS, Weiss MH, Ackerson TT, Harvey JP, Karze T: Acute fractures of the odontoid process: An analysis of 45 cases. J Neurosurg 1978;48:85.

27. Ekong CEU, Schwartz ML, Tator CH, Rowed DW, Edmonds VE: Odontoid fracture: Management with early mobilization using Halo device. Neurosurgery 1981;9:631.

28. Panjabi MM, White AA, Johnson RM: Cervical spine mechanics as a function of transection components. J Biomech 1975;8:327.

29. Key A: Cervical spine dislocations with unilateral facet interlocking. Paraplegia 1975;13:208.

30. Rorabeck CH, Rock MG, Hawkins RJ, Bourne RB: Unilateral facet dislocation of the cervical spine: An analysis of the results of treatment of 26 patients. Spine 1987;12:23.

31. Beatson TR: Fractures and dislocations of the cervical spine. J Bone Joint Surg 1963;45B:21.

32. Braakman R, Vinken PJ: Unilateral facet interlocking in the lower cervical spine. J Bone Joint Surg 1967;60B:165.

33. Doran SE, Papadopoulos SM, Ducker TB, Lillehei KO: Magnetic resonance imaging documentation of coexistent traumatic locked facets of the cervical spine and disc herniation. J Neurosurg 1993;79:341.

34. Hall RDM: Clay shoveller's fracture. J Bone Joint Surg 1940;22:63.

35. Denis F: The three column spine and its significance in the classification of the acute thoracolumbar spinal injuries. Spine 1983;8:817.

36. Heary RF, Vaccaro AR, Mesa JJ, Northrup BE, Albert TJ, Balderston RA: Steroids and gunshot wounds to the spine. Neurosurgery 1997;41:576.

Chapter 10

Penetrating Abdominal Trauma

HISTORY

For many years surgeons steadfastly adhered to the basic principle that laparotomy was central to the management of penetrating abdominal injuries. The experience of the two World Wars further reinforced this concept. As more and more laparotomies were performed for penetrating trauma, mortality from these injuries gradually declined to single digit figures over the course of almost a century, a decline that was primarily attributed to the use of laparotomy.

In the early 1900s, surgeons relied mostly on history taking and physical examination to diagnose intra-abdominal injuries; in retrospect, it is estimated that approximately 40% to 45% of these injuries were missed.[1] Policies of mandatory exploratory laparotomy for penetrating abdominal injuries were followed in most centers as recently as 15 years ago. Although the rate of missed injuries declined, these liberal policies led to an increase in the number of nontherapeutic laparotomies. In 1960 Shaftan proposed using a selective nonoperative approach to manage penetrating abdominal injuries.[2] Application of these principles has continued to receive support, and the long-held surgical maxim of mandatory laparotomy for penetrating abdominal injury has been systematically disproved. Questions of negative laparotomy rates, nontherapeutic laparotomy rates, mortality and morbidity, and discussions of the relative merits of different diagnostic modalities and technologies have preoccupied trauma surgeons in their quest for the lowest mortality with the fewest unnecessary and nontherapeutic laparotomies.

In 1965 Root and colleagues described diagnostic peritoneal lavage (DPL) as a diagnostic test for blunt abdominal trauma. This technique helped reduce the rate of missed injuries significantly, and DPL was quickly added to the armamentarium in the evaluation of stab wounds.[3] Diagnostic peritoneal lavage has some drawbacks because it is able only to detect the presence of blood in the peritoneum, not to quantitate or qualify it. Small lacerations to the liver or spleen that spontaneously cease bleeding may result in a positive test. In addition, DPL is not able to address retroperitoneal injuries but instead allows evaluation of only the peritoneal compartment. With time, DPL has become more popular, and more surgeons have relied on it for the work-up of abdominal stab wounds.

The use of computed tomography (CT) as an adjunct in the diagnosis of abdominal trauma came about in 1981, when Federle and colleagues first discussed the value of CT specifically in diagnosing abdominal trauma.[4] Raptopoulus reviewed the usefulness of CT in patients with abdominal trauma.[5]

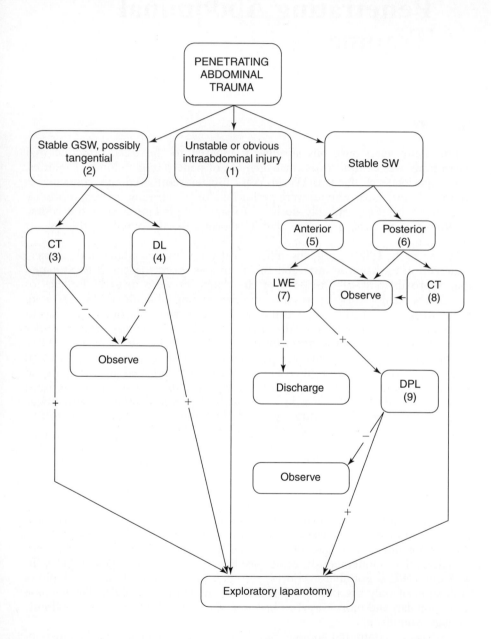

1. Patients with obvious intra-abdominal injury following penetrating trauma must go directly to the operating room. Such injury is suggested by hemodynamic instability, peritonitis, evisceration, and the track of the missile.
2. Potentially tangential gunshot wounds (GSWs) (i.e., missiles that never penetrate the peritoneum) are usually flank wounds, but any wound in which the track of the projectile is suspected to be tangential can fall under this category. If the extraperitoneal track can be confirmed, negative laparotomy can be avoided.
3. In very select cases, patients with suspected tangential GSWs of the abdomen may be evaluated with computed tomography (CT). It should be used only by those with considerable experience in treating abdominal gunshot wounds. If the missile track is clearly identified as extraperitoneal, no further surgical intervention is required.[85, 86]
4. Diagnostic laparoscopy (DL) is another evaluation technique that can be used to determine peritoneal violation, or lack thereof, by a missile. If blood or penetration of the peritoneum is found on laparoscopy, immediate laparotomy is indicated to properly examine the rest of the abdominal contents and repair any injuries. However, if no such violation is found, the patient can be discharged home from the recovery room, avoiding the morbidity associated with a negative laparotomy. Diagnostic peritoneal lavage (DPL) may be considered.[87]
5. The anterior abdomen is defined as the area bounded by the posterior axillary lines laterally, the nipple line superiorly, and the inguinal crease inferiorly. Since the diaphragm (and therefore the abdominal viscera) rises to the level of the nipple line during expiration, thoracoabdominal injuries must be evaluated for both thoracic and abdominal injuries.
6. The posterior abdomen, or flank and back, is bordered by the posterior axillary lines, the tips of the scapulae, and the iliac crest.
7. More than 25% of abdominal stab wounds (SW) fail to penetrate the peritoneal cavity, and because of this, selective management of stable patients is recommended. Anterior abdominal wounds can be locally explored (LWE = local wound exploration), and if no fascial penetration is present, the patient can be discharged. Posterior stab wounds are difficult to explore locally.
8. Computed tomographic scanning with intravenous, oral, and rectal contrast (triple contrast CT) may identify retroperitoneal bowel (duodenum and ascending and descending colon), kidney, and vascular injuries that are not accessible by diagnostic peritoneal lavage (DPL).
9. If fascial penetration is suspected or evident, DPL should be performed to identify those patients requiring laparotomy. See Table 10–1 for criteria indicating positive results of lavage.

With CT, the retroperitoneum, pancreas, kidneys, and duodenum can be evaluated, and the hemoperitoneum can be roughly quantified. Injury to the solid organs can be graded and followed over time, and bony and vascular injuries can be diagnosed. However, computed tomography has proved to be very insensitive in detecting small bowel or diaphragmatic injuries. Another significant drawback is that it takes time to complete the diagnostic work-up and can potentially delay laparotomy. Furthermore, the patient's condition can deteriorate during the course of scanning, and this can create an uncontrolled situation in the radiology suite. Because of these factors, if a patient is unstable and an abdominal injury is suspected, he or she is better served by undergoing immediate laparotomy with no further work-up.

In further attempts to find a more precise and practical modality for the diagnosis of penetrating abdominal trauma, considerable attention has been devoted in recent years to the use of ultrasound and diagnostic laparoscopy. As a result, a number of articles have appeared in the literature about ultrasound as yet another diagnostic tool, although most of these reports deal with its use in blunt trauma (see later section in this chapter on ultrasound).[6-10] Likewise, laparoscopy has been evaluated in many centers as another diagnostic modality that is useful in cases of suspected tangential wounds of the abdomen. It has proved to be a very promising diagnostic and therapeutic tool for patients with penetrating abdominal injuries (see later section on Diagnostic Laparoscopy).[11-14]

ANATOMY

For the purposes of evaluating and treating penetrating abdominal wounds, the torso should be considered as one cavity divided by the diaphragm. This concept is useful because it keeps in perspective the rather common finding of combined thoracic and abdominal injuries. It is easily understood that injuries that penetrate the chest can cross the diaphragm and inflict damage on organs in the abdominal cavity proper. In addition, the diaphragm is a domelike structure, the apex of which can extend to just about the level of the nipples. In fact, the lower rib cage actually overlies most of the liver on the right and the entire spleen on the left. In addition, the pelvic organs lie within the "hollow" of the pelvis and inferior to the symphysis. It is therefore important to rule out abdominal injury in any wound to the chest or perineum. Accordingly, any penetrating wound between the nipples and the gluteal crease should be considered a potential intra-abdominal injury.

ABDOMINAL STAB WOUNDS

Initial Management

Any injured patient should be evaluated initially according to the guidelines of the American College of Surgeons Advanced Trauma Life Support (ATLS) system.[15] The airway, breathing, and circulation (ABCs), with control of hemorrhage, are assessed in a quick primary survey. Following this, the resuscitation phase is started, and a secondary survey is performed. Intravenous access is established, appropriate antibiotics are given, initial laboratory tests are done, including typing and cross-matching of blood, nasogastric and bladder catheters are inserted, and chest and abdominal radiographs are performed. If the patient's vital signs are unstable, urgent laparotomy should be done.

Stab wounds to the abdomen in stable patients dictate a diagnostic work-up to (1) determine whether the peritoneum has been penetrated and (2) determine whether there is an abdominal injury that requires laparotomy. Because more than 25% of stab wounds fail to penetrate the peritoneal cavity,[16] selective management of stab wounds is practiced in many centers. This practice is further supported by complication rates of 8% to 41%[17, 18] for negative laparotomies or nontherapeutic laparotomies. As reported by Hasaniya and colleagues, the average hospital stay for uncomplicated nontherapeutic laparotomies is 5.1 days, and for patients with complications it is 11.9 days.[18] Reducing the incidence of unnecessary laparotomies promotes better use of allocated and scarce resources.

Diagnostic Modalities in Stab Wounds to the Abdomen

Physical Examination

In a classic study comprising over 2000 patients, Nance and colleagues advocated clinical observation with serial physical examinations in stable patients with stab wounds to the abdomen, proving that this method was safe and practical.[19] Using serial physical examinations in a series of 651 patients, Demetriades and Robinowitz reported a laparotomy rate of 53% and an observation rate of 47%. Only 2.9% of the observed patients required subsequent surgery. Their overall incidence of negative laparotomy was 5%.[20] In situations when it is not feasible to perform frequent serial examinations following the injury, the diagnostic work-up should be completed using other modalities.

Wound Exploration

The practice of wound exploration for anterior abdominal wounds (anterior is defined as the area bordered by the posterior axillary lines laterally, the nipple line superiorly, and the inguinal crease inferiorly) in the emergency room by the surgeon using local anesthesia to assess fascial penetration has been employed in many centers. Anterior abdominal and flank wounds should be explored locally because up to 35% of patients will be found not to have even fascial penetration. Further work-up is not necessary if the anterior fascia is intact. If penetration of the anterior fascia is present and this is used as the sole criterion for mandatory exploratory laparotomy, the nontherapeutic laparotomy rate will still be high. According to Feliciano and colleagues, in a series of 500 patients, even when the peritoneum has been penetrated, only 75% of the patients will have an injury to a viscus or vessel.[21] Consequently, additional diagnostic modalities have been investigated to better define true intraperitoneal injury, and these are discussed in the following sections.

Posterior stab wounds close to the midline are located over a thick muscular layer, making exploration difficult in these cases. Because of the central location, however, there is a risk of injury to major vessels as well as to the genitourinary system. A work-up with other modalities (see later section on computed tomography) should be undertaken if the injury is anything other than superficial.

Thoracoabdominal wounds carry the potential for injury to the diaphragm or thoracic or abdominal structures. In these situations, wound exploration is usually not helpful and may be risky. Even after thoracic penetration has been confirmed and a chest tube has been inserted, a coexisting intra-abdominal injury may be missed if the patient is not properly evaluated. Computed tomography has been notoriously inaccurate in diagnosing diaphragmatic lacerations. Diagnostic peritoneal lavage may be helpful, and in some cases, diagnostic laparoscopy (see later section on Laparoscopy) has been helpful in visualizing the diaphragm. Alternatively, diagnostic thoracoscopy has also been reported as a means of evaluating the diaphragm.[22]

Diagnostic Peritoneal Lavage

In 1965 Root and associates reported a new technique of paracentesis that involved a disposable catheter with multiple side-holes.[3] This technique allowed aspiration from the pelvis where blood is more likely to accumulate. If the aspirate is negative, peritoneal saline lavage is performed to increase the probability of retrieving a significant sample. It is important to understand that peritoneal lavage examines the presence of abnormal fluid only in the peritoneum and that retroperitoneal injury can escape detection by this technique.

Stab wounds to the abdomen cause intra-abdominal injury in 30% to 40% of cases.[23] Following the practice of selective management with serial physical examinations, patients are evaluated frequently, and if signs of peritoneal irritation develop, laparotomy is indicated. The rationale for diagnostic peritoneal lavage (DPL) is that it can quickly determine the presence of an intra-abdominal injury. A hemodynamically stable patient with an abdominal stab wound and a benign abdominal examination is evaluated next with local wound exploration. If anterior fascial penetration is found on local wound exploration, DPL is indicated, and DPL can be done using an open or closed technique. In the open technique the skin is incised and the abdomen is dissected to the peritoneum; then, under direct vision the peritoneum is incised and the catheter is inserted. The open technique should be used in patients with previous abdominal surgery to reduce the risk of puncturing bowel that is adherent to the anterior abdominal wall. It should also be done in patients with pelvic fractures and possible retroperitoneal hematomas because these hematomas can be so large that they are adjacent to the anterior abdominal wall, risking perforation and decompression of the hematoma. The closed technique requires a small skin incision and blind puncture of the fascial layers and peritoneum using a trocar-equipped catheter. This technique should be reserved for patients who are outside the above-mentioned categories and should only be done by physicians experienced in its use. As reported in a prospective study by Cue and colleagues,[24] the closed method is as safe and effective as the open technique in the hands of trauma surgeons. Regardless of the technique used, DPL has been extensively studied and has been shown to have an overall accuracy of 89% to 95%.[25-27]

Controversy exists about what red blood cell (RBC) count constitutes a "positive" lavage. Some centers have attempted to lower their missed injury rate by using lower RBC counts. The problem is that the incidence of nontherapeutic laparotomies will increase as the RBC count is lowered. Comparing the various reports may be confusing because different authors use different criteria to define a positive result. Oreskovich and Carrico reported the results for three lavage parameters.[26] DPL had the lowest sensitivity (59%) when a count of 100,000 RBC/mm³ was used; this increased to 100% when a figure of 1000 RBC/mm³ was used. Their overall accuracy rates were 78% and 77%, respectively. The specificity was 96.6%. They subsequently recommended using a 1000 RBC/mm³ threshold to maximize sensitivity.[26] Merlotti and associates, using 10,000 RBC/mm³ as a positive result, reported 87% sensitivity and an overall accuracy rate of 95%.[27] Henneman and colleagues suggested that Oreskovich and Carrico's recommendation would lead to an unnecessary laparotomy rate of 32%.[28] Feliciano and colleagues, with the largest series, used a figure of 100,000 RBC/mm³ and reported a sensitivity of 96% and an accuracy rate of 91%.[21] Adding to the confusion, many studies do not distinguish in their reports of true positives between an injury that requires intervention and one that does not (i.e., between therapeutic and nontherapeutic DPL). At the University of Miami, an RBC count of 20,000 cells/mm³ is used with an accuracy of 95% in stab wounds to the abdomen.

The white blood cell (WBC) count of the peritoneal lavage fluid is also used as an indicator of abdominal injury. It was noted by Root and colleagues that the peritoneum responds to abdominal trauma by increasing the protein content and the number of polymorphonuclear cells.[3] However, they also found that it takes 2 hours after injury for leukocytes to appear in the peritoneum; Feliciano and associates suggested an interval of 4 to 6 hours.[21] Other studies have suggested that the WBC count is unreliable and nonspecific for the diagnosis of intra-abdominal injury.[29, 30] The absence of leukocytes in the lavage fluid is therefore not significant unless at least 2, and possibly 4 to 6, hours have elapsed since the time of injury.

The amylase content of the lavage aspirate is also of questionable value. McAnena and colleagues examined peritoneal lavage enzyme determinations following blunt and penetrating abdominal trauma.[31] In addition to amylase, they also studied alkaline phosphatase. Of 1969 DPLs that were otherwise nondiagnostic, a lavage amylase value of greater than 200 IU/dl combined with a lavage alkaline phosphatase value of greater than 300 IU/dl was found to be 97% specific and 78% sensitive and had a positive predictive value of 88% for significant hollow visceral injury.[31] An elevated amylase content in the lavage fluid can occasionally identify a patient with significant intra-abdominal injury in the absence of an abnormal WBC or RBC count. There appears to be no delay after injury before the amylase count becomes elevated. It may be helpful in the assessment of small bowel injury.

In the end, the recommended values that define a positive peritoneal lavage evaluation following a stab wound to the abdomen are (1) RBC count of over 20,000 mm³, (2) WBC of over 500 mm³, and (3) bacteria, bile, or particulate matter suggesting bowel contents in the aspirate. Peritoneal amylase evaluation is not routinely done at many institutions (Table 10–1).

Computed Tomography

The use of computed tomography (CT) for diagnosis in patients with anterior abdominal stab wounds has been limited mainly because of the poor ability of CT to detect hollow organ injury. Marx and colleagues evaluated the use of CT in patients with anterior stab wounds and reported a sensitivity of only 14%, with a false-negative rate of 86%.[32] Rehm and colleagues studied the use of double-contrast CT in patients with penetrating abdominal injuries and concluded that it was unreliable in detecting bowel injury and did not reliably demonstrate diaphragmatic injury.[33] CT therefore appears to offer no advantage over DPL in patients with anterior abdominal stab wounds.

For patients with posterior stab wounds there is a lower incidence of bowel injury, and a selective approach is warranted.[34] The same structures that make injury less likely—namely, the paraspinal muscles and the vertebral column, can mask the signs and symptoms of an injury. This is especially true if the injury is limited to the retroperitoneum, in which case the result may be retroperitoneal abscess, arteriovenous fistula, or pseudoaneurysm. Double-contrast CT has been recommended by Meyer and colleagues, who reported an accuracy rate of 97% and a sensitivity of 89%.[35] Colon injuries are easily missed without contrast in the colon; hence, some authors have added rectal contrast. This has been called triple-contrast CT or CT enema. Himmelman and associates, for example, reported a prospective study of triple-contrast CT in 88 patients with stab wounds to the back or flank; they found that CT was effective in predicting the absence of significant retroperitoneal injuries. They concluded that the use of rectal contrast enhances the ability to diagnose colon injuries, and because it is not difficult to perform, is advocated.[36]

Diagnostic Laparoscopy

The use of diagnostic laparoscopy (DL) has been studied in trauma centers in asymptomatic or mildly symptomatic patients who have sustained penetrating abdominal trauma. In general, the accuracy of DL in detecting peritoneal penetration has been very promising. Ivatury and Simon[11, 12] used laparoscopy to evaluate patients with wounds to the lower chest and upper abdomen. Diagnostic laparoscopy was performed in 40 patients with penetrating thoracoabdominal wounds (34 stab wounds, 6 gunshot wounds) with the goal of lowering the number of negative laparotomies performed to rule out diaphrag-

Table 10–1. Suggested Parameters for Positive Results on Diagnostic Peritoneal Lavage

5 ml gross blood on aspiration	Bacteria (Gram's stain)
>20,000 RBC/mm³	Bile
>500 WBC/mm³	Food particles
>175 U amylase/100 ml	

matic injury. DL was negative in 50% of patients and therefore prevented laparotomies in these patients. Ten therapeutic laparotomies were performed after injuries were noted on DL. Finally, ten nontherapeutic laparotomies were performed after only hemoperitoneum was found on DL. These latter cases must be approached cautiously because the injury resulting in hemoperitoneum may be very difficult to identify on laparoscopy alone. Ivatury and Simon concluded that laparoscopy was a "superior method for the detection of diaphragmatic injuries." They cautioned, however, that "its role in diagnosing hollow organ injuries needs further study." Fabian and colleagues[37] performed DL in 182 patients (99 stab wounds, 66 gunshot wounds, and 17 blunt trauma injuries). In patients with stab wounds, DL demonstrated a lack of peritoneal penetration in 49%. These patients' average hospital stay was 1 day. In their study, 31% of patients underwent a therapeutic laparotomy, 13% had a negative laparotomy and 6% had a nontherapeutic laparotomy, for a combined unnecessary laparotomy rate of 19%. The average length of stay for those with an unnecessary laparotomy was 4.6 days. These authors also evaluated the cost of DL versus that of negative laparotomy and found the two to be very similar. They added that perhaps the use of nondisposable equipment could reduce the overall cost. Salvino and associates[38] reported on 16 patients with stab wounds in whom DL was performed in the emergency room under local anesthesia, eliminating some of the charges from the operating room. They found diaphragmatic lacerations in three patients who had insignificant RBC counts on DPL. At present, DL appears to have the highest value in the diagnosis of thoracoabdominal wounds to rule out diaphragmatic injuries.

In summary, DL can be very effectively used to rule out peritoneal penetration. The key point is that in patients without peritoneal violation, laparotomy can be avoided, thus reducing the attendant morbidity of hospital stays, days lost from work for recovery, and the potential for future small bowel obstruction. If the peritoneum has been violated, one should proceed with laparotomy except in select cases, for instance, a small nonbleeding laceration of the liver (which would be positive on DPL).

Ultrasonography

The use of ultrasonography (US) has been growing, particularly for evaluation of blunt abdominal trauma. However, experience with its use in penetrating abdominal trauma is limited. Rozycki and associates[39] reported on a series of patients evaluated with US after sustaining penetrating abdominal wounds. They reported a 14% (10 of 74 patients) false-negative rate and a 4% false-positive rate. They concluded that in patients with penetrating wounds the use of US is most valuable in those with multiple injuries or possibly suspected pericardial injuries when the cause of hypotension is obscure. At the current time, ultrasound probably has no role in the management of penetrating abdominal trauma.

GUNSHOT WOUNDS

Initial Management

As many as 96% to 98% of gunshot wounds (GSWs) that penetrate the peritoneum require an operation,[40] but the diagnostic considerations are similar to those with stab wounds in patients with equivocal findings. One must remember that bullets may follow an erratic course. Additionally, falls following gunshot injuries may lead to associated injuries. After the initial resuscitation has been completed and appropriate intravenous access has been established, a plain radiograph of the abdomen and chest is performed to look for the projectile and fragments, which may give a rough estimate of the potential for intra-abdominal injuries.

A detailed discussion of ballistics is beyond the scope of this chapter, but a basic knowledge of the pathophysiology of wound ballistics in general assists in understanding the potential for injury. Civilian gunshot wounds are generally caused by lower velocity handgun missiles, which have velocities of between 700 and 1500 feet/second, whereas military injuries generally result from higher velocity (around 3000 feet/second) rifle missiles (e.g., AK-47, M-16). The shotgun behaves like a high-velocity weapon at short range and like multiple low-velocity projectiles at more distant ranges.[41] Closer range shotgun injuries also concentrate the pellets in a smaller area, while longer range injury patterns are more diffuse and usually less severe. The tissue damaged is the tissue directly in the bullet's path that is crushed by the bullet. This is known as the permanent cavity. Therefore, the wider the bullet, the larger the permanent cavity and the more tissue that is damaged. For instance, a .22 caliber missile measures .22 inches in diameter, while a .45 caliber weapon is double that diameter (.45 inches). A hollow-point bullet expands on striking the target, thereby increasing its diameter. In addition to the permanent cavity, all missiles have associated temporary cavities of varying sizes. This expanding pressure wave in elastic tissue results in little permanent damage; however, the same pressure wave in the nonelastic liver will fracture the organ. High-velocity assault weapon missiles are usually significantly longer than they are wide and tumble (or "yaw") as they make their way through tissue, enlarging their permanent and temporary cavities. However, each type of missile begins this yaw at different depths and causes different injury patterns. For instance, an AK-47 begins its yaw at approximately 18 cm, whereas an AK-74 begins to yaw almost immediately. An AK-47 injury with an entry and exit less than 20 cm apart has only a small hole at both sites. However, a longer tissue path will probably have a small entry with a much larger exit hole.

Although the science of wound ballistics is interesting, the trauma surgeon treating a gunshot wound rarely knows what the offending weapon is, nor is it important. The goal is to repair what is injured or bleeding. Only obviously devitalized tissue should be debrided, and attempts to explore wound tracts should be avoided. Bullets generate friction heat but are not sterile when they strike tissue. Therefore, one or two doses of antibiotics should be considered.

Diagnostic Modalities in Gunshot Wounds to the Abdomen

Gunshot wounds to the abdomen generally require urgent exploration, but certain situations in stable patients may exist that warrant further diagnostic work-up before the decision is made to proceed to the operating room. It must be stated in no uncertain terms that urgent laparotomy is indicated in hemodynamically unstable patients, and no diagnostic modalities should delay such intervention. A preoperative x-ray to locate the bullet is helpful but can be obtained in the operating room as necessary.

Diagnostic Peritoneal Lavage

Diagnostic peritoneal lavage for the evaluation of GSWs is controversial. In a classic report evaluating DPL for GSWs of the lower chest and the abdomen, Thal and colleagues[42] sounded a cautionary note, stating that "patients who sustain gunshot wounds are best treated with exploratory celiotomy." Their report consisted of a prospective study of 168 stable patients with GSWs to the lower chest and abdomen. The patients first underwent clinical assessment with a reported 20.2% false-negative and 15.9% false-positive results for physical examination alone. Following DPL, 25.4% had false-negative results, and 6 of the 15 patients with a false-negative result had RBC counts of less than 1000/mm^3. These authors concluded that GSWs should not be treated using the same principles as those used for stab wounds and that these injuries differ from stab wounds in their unpredictable behavior. They went on to state that DPL cannot be relied on with the same degree of confidence as for stab wounds and blunt trauma. Some centers have used considerably lower red blood cell counts as criteria for a positive DPL result. Nagy and colleagues[87] have suggested that DPL can be an accurate test in this setting using a threshold of 10,000 RBC/mm^3.

Diagnostic Laparoscopy

Diagnostic laparoscopy has been studied for use in evaluating GSWs to the abdomen to rule out peritoneal penetration and for possible use therapeutically. Most series that report on DL group stab wounds with GSWs. A noteworthy study is one by Fabian and colleagues[37] in which 66 GSW victims underwent DL. Two thirds of GSWs in this series were in the upper torso. Peritoneal penetration was ruled out in 62%, 29% had a therapeutic exploratory laparotomy, 5% had a nontherapeutic laparotomy, and 4% had a negative exploratory laparotomy. Hospital stay was 4.3 days for patients with negative DL and associated injuries compared with 8.6 days for those requiring laparotomy. The remaining group of patients, with no associated injuries and negative DL, had an average hospital stay of 1.1 day.

Simon and Ivatury[12] reported six patients with GSWs.[12] Laparotomy was prevented in five patients with a negative DL, and therapeutic laparotomy was performed in one patient with a positive DL.

Sosa and colleagues[13] studied the impact of DL on the negative laparotomy rate. A retrospective review of 817 patients who underwent exploratory laparotomy for abdominal GSWs over a 4-year period showed a negative laparotomy rate of 12.4%. These patients had a reported 22% morbidity with an average length of hospital stay of 5.1 days. The authors then studied 85 patients with abdominal GSWs evaluated with DL. Negative results on DL were reported in 65%, with no missed injuries, and no patients required subsequent laparotomy. This group had a 3% morbidity rate (one patient had urinary retention), and the average hospital stay was 1.4 days. Of the 35% of patients with a positive DL (30 patients), 28 underwent exploratory laparotomy, of which 86% were therapeutic and 14% were nontherapeutic. The remaining two patients were observed with nonbleeding liver lacerations, and thus a nontherapeutic laparotomy was prevented in these patients. In another report by the same group at the University of Miami,[15] 121 patients with suspected tangential GSWs who were hemodynamically stable were prospectively studied by DL. A 65% negative DL rate was seen in the selected group. Of the 35% with a positive DL, 92.8% (39 patients) underwent exploratory laparotomy. In this group, 82% of the laparotomies were therapeutic (32 patients), 15.4% (six patients) were nontherapeutic, and 2.5% (one patient) had a negative laparotomy. There were no false-negative DL results and no delayed laparotomies, and the sensitivity for peritoneal penetration was 100%.

DL has emerged as a significant diagnostic and possibly therapeutic modality for managing abdominal GSWs. At present, cost effectiveness is still under study but it will likely improve with time.[38] DL should be considered in patients with abdominal GSWs who are stable and have equivocal evidence of peritoneal penetration. Since the ability of DL to detect hollow organ injury is limited, there should be a low threshold for performance of laparotomy.

Computed Tomography

In 1994, Renz and Feliciano[43] reported the nonsurgical management of 12 patients with GSWs to the right thoracoabdominal area based on CT evaluation. CT scanning detected injuries in all 12 patients—pulmonary contusions, hepatic lacerations, spinal cord transection, and renal lacerations. All patients were successfully managed nonoperatively. The authors concluded that hemodynamically stable patients with GSWs to the right thoracoabdominal region and with no evidence of peritonitis can be managed nonoperatively with a low incidence of minor intrathoracic complications. Furthermore, they concluded that CT scanning of right thoracoabdominal GSWs is a "comprehensive means" of evaluation and follow-up when nonsurgical management is chosen.

The report from Himmelman and colleagues[36] included 21 patients with GSWs to the back or flank and compared CT evaluation with serial physical examinations. From this report CT had no impact on the negative laparotomy rate compared to serial physical examinations.

Ginzburg and colleagues[85] demonstrated the safety and efficacy of abdominal CT in hemodynamically stable patients with suspected tangential GSWs. CT can therefore be used to delineate the missile tract in patients with suspected tangential wounds. If this tract remains clearly extraperitoneal, any operative procedure (laparotomy, laparoscopy) can be avoided. Its indication is similar to that used for laparoscopy, and further controlled trials are needed to establish superiority of one over the other. One potential advantage is that CT can provide additional information about injuries in the retroperitoneum and may dictate further work-up (e.g., arteriography).

GENERAL CONSIDERATIONS IN THE OPERATING ROOM

The Operation

Wide preparation of the patient is necessary to allow access to the chest and inguinal area. The most common incision used in patients with abdominal trauma is the midline incision from the xiphoid to the pubis. Inadequate exposure in the interest of cosmetics can be costly, limiting access to unknown and potentially lethal wounds. Quick and ample entrance to the abdomen should be the primary goal. Upon entry into the abdominal cavity all quadrants are packed with laparotomy pads to control any active bleeding. The pads are then systematically removed, and areas of active hemorrhage are controlled. Once hemorrhage is under control, perforations in the gastrointestinal tract are controlled by noncrushing clamps and the peritoneum is copiously irrigated with warm saline solution. Addition of antibiotics to the irrigating solution has not been shown to add any protection against infections.[44]

Prevention of Hypothermia

The presence of hypothermia contributes morbidity and mortality in addition to that caused by the injury itself.[45] It is important for the entire trauma team and the operating team to have an understanding of the principles that govern temperature regulation, since measures to prevent hypothermia should be taken from the moment rescue personnel meet the patient.[46] In the operating room these measures consist of keeping the operating room warm before the patient enters the room, preventing air currents by controlling personnel circulation, covering the patient with warm air convection blankets, employing warm lavage fluids, infusing warmed intravenous fluids and warmed blood products, and limiting the amount of time a surface area is exposed.[46] The high-flow infusion devices currently available help reduce the incidence of hypothermia and play a central role in actively rewarming patients.[47] Gentilello and his group have very eloquently reviewed the mechanisms and treatment of hypothermia, and his work is recommended reading.[46, 47]

Avoidance of Lengthy Operations

"Damage control" is a concept that has received emphasis in an effort to shorten operating times in massively injured, unstable patients. The previously mentioned problems that occur with hypothermia and the sometimes massive distention that occurs in the small bowel during rapid resuscitation with crystalloids are reasons why rapid, conservative methods are favored over involved, lengthy procedures. To this end, single-layer closures, delayed gastrointestinal reconstruction, diversion instead of resection, colon repair instead of colectomies or colostomies, and packing instead of prolonged and unsuccessful attempts at hemostasis should be considered.[48]

The "abdominal compartment syndrome"[49] has recently been addressed in many trauma centers by closing the abdomen at the skin level only or by using plastic silos to temporarily cover the abdomen. These techniques may allow unstable patients to reach the intensive care unit for resuscitation and have reduced the amount of time the patient spends in the operating room. Returning a warmed, noncoagulopathic, hemodynamically stable patient to the operating room in 2 to 3 days usually produces superior outcomes compared to making heroic, and probably unwise, attempts at the initial operation.

MANAGEMENT OF SPECIFIC INJURIES

Besides general surgical principles, specific considerations relating to specific injuries are helpful.

Stomach, Small Bowel, and Mesentery

Leakage of gastric contents results in peritonitis, although in patients with small perforations, the development of peritoneal signs may not be obvious initially. Bloody nasogastric drainage and the presence of pneumoperitoneum on x-ray of the abdomen or chest may be signs of gastric injury, but neither is specific or sensitive enough to be a reliable indicator of gastric injury.[50, 51] It must be kept in mind that the aorta and celiac trunk are immediately posterior to the gastroesophageal junction, and injuries to this area are occasionally missed. Also, when the stomach has been injured, the possibility of diaphragmatic injury must be considered. The association of gastric injury with diaphragmatic injuries is significant because of the potential for contamination of the thoracic cavity with stomach contents and subsequent empyema.[52]

The stomach must be visualized thoroughly. The triangular ligament is divided and the left lobe of the liver is retracted for visualization of injuries to the gastroesophageal junction. Care must be taken to protect the vagus nerve during incision of the gastrohepatic ligament located to the right of the stomach. The posterior wall is thoroughly evaluated by incising the gastrocolic ligament away from the gastroepiploic artery and entering the lesser sac. Unless there is extensive destruction of the stomach, in most circumstances debridement and primary repair suffice. This is possible because of the large lumen available and therefore the lower risk of narrowing. Also, the stomach has a generous and redundant blood supply. The pitfalls of gastric trauma occur with missed injuries. If in doubt, the stomach can be filled with diluted methylene-blue solution and the pyloric channel occluded to detect a leak.

The small intestine is the viscus most commonly injured in cases of penetrating abdominal trauma.[53] The morbidity resulting from contamination of the peritoneum varies and mostly depends on delay in diagnosis. However, injuries to the small bowel are usually not life-threatening if the diagnosis is made expeditiously and the patient is explored early.[20] Small bowel repairs should be done in a transverse fashion to prevent stricture formation. Adequate debridement of all nonviable tissue should be done, and adjacent perforations should be united and repaired as one unit. Resection of a segment with multiple perforations is preferable to making multiple repairs.

Associated mesenteric injuries, on the other hand, can sometimes produce life-threatening hemorrhage. Hematomas should be carefully explored through radial incisions, and hemostasis should be obtained. The superior mesenteric artery and vein should be repaired. Ligation of the superior mesenteric vein should be undertaken only when rapid hemostasis is needed to save the patient's life. When the viability of large segments of bowel is in question and the patient is not fully resuscitated, the surgeon may choose to leave the bowel in situ and reexplore the patient in 24 hours.[54] Inspection of the bowel with ultraviolet light (Wood's lamp) following intravenous injection of fluorescein can be useful in determining the viability of a region of bowel.[55]

Duodenum and Pancreas

The diagnosis of duodenal injury is based primarily on a high degree of suspicion on the part of the surgeon, since signs of retroperitoneal injury are often difficult to elicit and the diagnostic modalities currently available are notoriously deficient in diagnosing injury to the duodenum. The majority of duodenal injuries are the result of penetrating trauma. Fortunately, most duodenal injuries can be safely repaired primarily. Snyder and colleagues[56] reported on 247 patients with duodenal trauma and identified some factors that directly affect the morbidity and mortality of patients with duodenal injuries. Among these factors are the causative agent, its size and location, interval to repair, and associated adjacent injuries. Correspondingly, large injuries, injuries in the first and second portion, long elapsed time from injury to repair, and associated injury to the bile duct or pancreas are all associated with increased morbidity and mortality. The associated morbidity and mortality ranged from 6% to 16% each.

A multicenter review by Cogbill and colleagues of 164 patients with duodenal trauma[57] showed that primary repair was done in 71%. Of the 108 patients with Grade I or II injuries (see Chapter 18), 90 underwent primary repair. Of the 56 patients with Grade III to V injuries, 46% underwent more involved duodenal repairs, such as pyloric exclusion and pancreaticoduodenectomy. Injury to the duodenum in conjunction with an injury to the pancreas can present a difficult treatment decision. Combined duodenal and pancreatic injuries are very challenging and are associated with significant morbidity. Because of the intimate anatomic relationship of the duodenum and the pancreas and because of the digestive nature of their contents, these injuries need to be approached with caution. Only with this cautious attitude can the surgeon be prepared to deal with the morbidity associated with them. When a duodenal injury is suspected, mobilization should be done by performing a Kocher maneuver encompassing and mobilizing the ligament of Treitz. Minor duodenal injuries (stab wounds, injury less than 50% of the wall, injury of third portion of the duodenum, injury interval of less than 24 hours, and no associated biliary or pancreatic injuries) can usually be repaired primarily. Periduodenal drainage is recommended.

Duodenal injuries with an associated pancreatic injury have an increased rate of leakage, and diversion of the gastric contents may decrease this complication. Diversion can be accomplished by a "pyloric exclusion" procedure, which is less disruptive and less time consuming than a true duodenal diverticularization. The procedure involves closure of the pylorus from within the lumen of the stomach through a gastrotomy, after which a gastrojejunostomy is constructed. This operation in effect diverts the gastric contents away from the duodenal repair while it heals. The pylorus will usually reopen after 2 weeks and the gastrojejunostomy functionally closes.[58] Pyloric exclusion can also be accomplished by firing a staple line over the distal edge of the pylorus. The pylorus will reopen with time, and the procedure is quick and effective.

An alternative, or addition, to gastric diversion is duodenal decompression through a lateral duodenostomy or retrograde jejunostomy, as popularized by Stone and Fabian.[59] These involved techniques of dealing with the more complex duodenal injuries reflect the high potential for the development of fistulas and dehiscences, which can lead to sepsis and development of multisystem organ failure. Mortality directly related to duodenal injury ranges from 2% to 5%.[56, 57, 59-61] The Whipple procedure is rarely required unless there is combined severe duodenal, pancreatic, and distal common bile duct injury. Fortunately, few patients sustaining a traumatic injury require a procedure as extensive as a pancreaticoduodenectomy.

Injuries to the pancreas (see Chapter 18) are most often associated with vascular and other intra-abdominal injuries. In patients with penetrating trauma the diagnosis of pancreatic injury is usually made intraoperatively and is therefore straightforward. The single most important determinant of outcome following pancreatic injury is the status of the pancreatic duct. In evaluating the pancreas intraoperatively every effort should be made to evaluate the integrity of the duct.[62] Most injuries to the pancreatic duct generally result from penetrating missiles. Pancreatography in the setting of trauma can be very time consuming and difficult to perform, and at most, it only confirms the suspicion of ductal injury. Therefore, it is recommended that obvious distal ductal injuries be treated with a distal pancreatectomy and suspected injuries be treated with drainage alone.

Evaluation of the pancreas requires full visualization of the parenchyma. This is achieved by opening the lesser sac through the gastroepiploic omentum. Evaluation of the head and uncinate process is achieved by mobilizing the hepatic flexure of the colon and performing a Kocher maneuver; evaluation of the tail requires exposure of the splenic hilum.

Contusions and lacerations of the parenchyma without ductal injury require only hemostasis and external drainage with closed suction drains. No attempt should be made to repair the capsule. A controlled pancreatic fistula is usually self-limiting. Distal transections with duct disruption are best treated by distal pancreatectomy, with or without splenectomy, and suture closure of the transected duct. It must be emphasized that provision for early enteral feeding through a jejunal feeding tube will simplify the postoperative nutritional regimen in these patients. Combined pancreaticoduodenal injuries most often result from penetrating trauma. A review by Feliciano and colleagues of 129 cases of combined pancreaticoduodenal injuries showed that 29% were treated by simple repair and drainage, 50% were treated with repair and pyloric exclusion, and only 10% required a Whipple procedure.[63] Any patient with a combined pancreaticoduodenal injury requires a cholangiogram and evaluation of the ampulla.

Complications occur in 20% to 40% of patients treated surgically for pancreatic injuries and are particularly common in those with combined pancreatico-duodenal injuries.[64] Fistulas are the most common complication. Fortunately, most are self-limiting when external drainage has been provided. Abscess formation also occurs relatively frequently. Most abscesses are peripancreatic and are amenable to percutaneous drainage. The mortality rate for patients with abscesses remains at 25%.[65] A true pancreatic abscess results from inadequate debridement. Percutaneous drainage may not be adequate, and open surgical drainage may be required. Pancreatitis may be expected to occur in a significant number of patients and can be managed with bowel rest and nutritional support; it should resolve spontaneously.[66] Fortunately, only a small percentage of these patients progress to hemorrhagic pancreatitis, which has a mortality rate approaching 80% and for which there is no effective treatment.[64] Pseudocyst formation resolves with percutaneous drainage if the pancreatic duct is not stenosed or injured. Therefore, prior to embarking on drainage, endoscopic retrograde cholangiopancreatography (ERCP) should be performed to evaluate ductal integrity. Drainage of a cyst formed because of an injured duct will only convert it to an external pancreatic fistula. Exocrine and endocrine insufficiency rarely occur following a pancreatectomy of up to 80% to 90%.[66] Although the majority of complications related to pancreatic injuries are self-limiting, sepsis and multisystem organ failure cause a significant percentage of the deaths that result from pancreatic trauma.

Colon and Rectum

The majority of injuries to the colon result from penetrating trauma to the abdomen. Colonic injuries increase the overall mortality from associated injuries, and infectious complications are common, often requiring reoperation and percutaneous drainage of abscesses. Containing the amount of contamination resulting from fecal spillage is of primary importance following control of hemorrhage. To this end, copious irrigation is of utmost importance. The patient may be too unstable to perform definitive repair of the colonic injury; under these circumstances, isolation of the injured portion can be performed quickly by stapling both ends of the colon. Definitive repair and establishment of intestinal continuity can be performed after the patient has been stabilized (at the same or in a future operation). Injuries to the colon can be treated by primary repair, colostomy, or exteriorization of the repair, although the latter method is mostly of historic interest now. The management of colonic injuries has undergone considerable evolution, and at the present time, almost all patients with penetrating injuries to the colon can be managed by primary repair.[67–71] Most reports show excellent results when over 50% of the patients are treated with primary repair; one study[70] in particular reported an impressive 93% of cases who were repaired primarily. In series in which primary repair has been compared to colostomy, the wound infection rate and the rate of intra-abdominal abscess have consistently been significantly higher when colostomies were done.[70] Resections with anastomoses are also considered primary repairs. The report from Burch and colleagues[71] further differentiated ileocolostomy from colocolostomy. In their study, 36 ileocolostomies were reported with only one anastomotic leak (2.8%); in contrast, 3 of the 14 (21%) patients with colocolostomies developed anastomotic leaks.

Most injuries to the rectum result from penetrating trauma. In every patient with gunshot wounds to the torso, buttocks, and thighs a rectal injury must be suspected, and rectal examination should be done routinely. While blood in the rectum is neither specific nor sensitive for rectal injury, this finding should be followed by further evaluation and proctoscopic examination. Most rectal injuries continue to be managed by presacral drainage through the perineum with proximal colostomy for diversion and no attempt to repair the injury itself.[72] The need for presacral drainage is controversial and is presently under study. The timing of closure of the colostomy is related to the patient's overall condition and the resolution of any complications. Colostomy closure is generally performed 6 weeks after injury. Contrast enema studies are rarely indicated prior to closure and should be used only to rule out suspected stricture or pathologic lesion.

Spleen

The trend in managing injuries to the spleen is toward splenic salvage. This trend has been supported by a better understanding of the role played by the spleen in immunologic host defense and by the occurrence of postsplenectomy sepsis. Furthermore, advances in technology, surgical techniques, and resuscitation and postoperative management have contributed to support of the current concepts in treating injuries of the spleen.

Though nonoperative management of splenic injuries may be considered in stable patients sustaining blunt abdominal injuries, it is never an option in those with penetrating trauma. Any penetrating injury to the spleen carries a significant risk of injury to adjacent organs and must be explored. Low-grade (Grades I to III [see Chapter 18]) injuries to the spleen in hemodynamically stable patients can be repaired most of the time, and reoperation for bleeding after splenorrhaphy is infrequent.[73] Higher grade injuries, and splenic injuries in combination with multiple associated injuries, usually require splenectomy. Although reimplantation of slices of the spleen into the omentum was at one time a popular concept, it has never proved clinically effective and is not recommended. Methods of splenic salvage include electrocautery, argon beam coagulation, partial splenectomy, compression suture of the spleen, and wrapping the spleen in Gelfoam or Dexon mesh pockets. Patients who undergo splenorrhaphy should be monitored closely, undergoing serial hematocrit checks in the postoperative period.

Overwhelming postsplenectomy sepsis, which rapidly progresses to death in susceptible patients, occurs most commonly, but not exclusively, in children who have undergone splenectomy before the age of 2 years. The most common etiologic agent is *Streptococcus pneumoniae*, but other encapsulated bacteria have been implicated as well. A study by Singer of 684 patients who underwent splenectomy for trauma showed a rate of septic complications of 1.45% with a mortality of 0.58%.[74] Aggressive medical intervention can dramatically reduce the mortality. Pneumococcal vaccination is provided postoperatively. The duration of effective protection following vaccination is unknown (one study of marginal value suggested 10 years[75]). Current recommendations by the Centers for Disease Control and Prevention suggest a single revaccination at 3 years for children 10 years and younger, and at 5 years for those older than 10 years.

Liver and Biliary Tree

There has been a shift from hepatic resection and placement of deep liver sutures in the operative management of hepatic injuries to techniques favoring nonresectional procedures that rely on hepatotomy and direct vessel ligation,[76] selective hepatic artery ligation,[77] resectional debridement,[78] packing, and even nonoperative management. Nonoperative management of liver injuries secondary to penetrating trauma is possible in very selected cases. Criteria for nonoperative management include: (1) hemodynamic stability, (2) no associated injuries, (3) close monitoring in an intensive care unit, and (4) availability of an operating team at all times. CT scanning has allowed identification and follow-up of patients when nonsurgical management is chosen. Renz and Feliciano[43] and Ginzburg[85] have demonstrated the successful use of nonoperative management of abdominal GSWs when this was combined with CT scanning to demonstrate a bullet track either remaining extraperitoneal or damaging only the liver. Although these authors' patients overall recovered well, it must be cautioned that biliary-pleural fistulas have been seen when the injury was missed or the diaphragm was not repaired. Computed tomographic imaging would of course not demonstrate this injury initially. Nonoperative management of abdominal GSWs in general should be approached with great reluctance and should be reserved for surgeons and institutions experienced in trauma care.

Most liver lacerations have ceased bleeding by the time they are evaluated at laparotomy. For those that are still bleeding, a variety of techniques can be used to control the hemorrhage. Argon beam coagulation works especially well for hepatic lacerations that have failed to respond to ligation of obvious vessels, direct pressure, and electrocautery. The finger-fracture technique to expose damaged vessels is advocated by some but is only necessary infrequently. Chromic liver sutures on blunt needles can approximate the edges of a deep crack but should be used sparingly because they are associated with subsequent liver abscesses. Formal lobectomies are virtually never required, and for the most part should be limited to resectional debridement.

Hepatic vein and retrohepatic inferior vena caval (IVC) injuries challenge even the most experienced trauma surgeon and carry a very high mortality.[79] In rare instances, an atriocaval shunt can be placed to afford vascular isolation and direct repair of the injury. This technique requires exposure of the intrapericardial IVC, the right atrial appendage, and the infrahepatic IVC. To complete vascular isolation of the liver, the portal vein and common hepatic artery must be controlled.

When hemorrhage is not reasonably controlled, and when the patient is coagulopathic or hypothermic, liver packing is often the best option. The abdomen and liver are packed tightly with laparotomy pads, and the abdominal wall is reapproximated. The patient may be returned to the operating room in 1 or 2 days for unpacking. More often than not, bleeding will be found to have stopped without further intervention.

Lacerations, transections, or avulsions of the extrahepatic bile ducts are rare. The techniques of repair in stable patients depend on the extent of the ductal injury and range from simple repair to biliary enteric bypass. In general, a ductal laceration involving less than 50% of the bile duct wall may be repaired primarily. Lacerations of more than 50% of the circumference, complete disruption, and segmental loss require cholecysto-, choledocho-, or hepatico-jejunostomy. T-tubes and stents are frequently used.[80]

Retroperitoneal and Vascular Injuries

A quarter of patients with penetrating abdominal injuries have a major abdominal vascular injury as well.[81] Some may remain hemodynamically stable if the hematoma is contained within the retroperitoneum, but others may present with massive abdominal distention and hypotension. Preoperative diagnostic aortography is rarely used to diagnose intra-abdominal vascular injuries because these patients are usually not stable enough to undergo such procedures. Emergency room thoracotomy with cross-clamping of the descending thoracic aorta may be the only way to prevent exsanguination until laparotomy and vascular control can be performed. This can be achieved with vascular clamps or compression. Once vascular control has been obtained, spillage from associated gastrointestinal perforations should be contained to minimize further contamination. Vascular repair can then be performed with monofilament sutures and the use of autogenous vein graft, Dacron, or polytetrafluoroethylene (PTFE). PTFE grafts are the preferred grafts for vessels 6 mm in diameter or larger. Grafts smaller than 6 mm have an unacceptably high thrombosis rate; vessels smaller than 6 mm should be repaired with autogenous vein grafts. In patients with combined vascular and bowel injury with spillage, PTFE is the optimal material for vascular repair.[82, 83]

All retroperitoneal hematomas from penetrating injuries must be explored. Active hemorrhage encountered on entry into the abdomen should be controlled immediately by means of compression and minimal dissection in order to obtain proximal and distal control of the vessel. It is frequently advisable to gain proximal and distal control before entering a hematoma, if possible. Midline supramesocolic hematomas are usually approached by reflecting all left-sided intra-abdominal viscera to the midline to gain control of the aorta at the hiatus of the diaphragm.

If the aorta is injured, repair is performed based on the extent of the injury. Injuries to the left gastric or proximal splenic artery should be ligated. The common hepatic artery can be ligated as well but may be more amenable to repair. If the celiac axis is injured it is best to ligate all three vessels. Injuries to the superior mesenteric artery are difficult to manage because ligation usually compromises the viability of the midgut. Repair with vein or graft replacement should be attempted. Superior mesenteric vein injuries are sometimes amenable to repair; however, injuries to the proximal aspect of this vessel are difficult to handle. Ligation of the superior mesenteric vein, when followed by vigorous postoperative management, is associated with modest survival rates. With injuries to the inframesocolic midline area, injuries to the infrarenal aorta or inferior vena cava should be suspected. Exposure is usually obtained in the same fashion as that used for resection of an abdominal aortic aneurysm.

Injuries to the vena cava pose challenging problems in regard to exposure and repair. Care must be taken to avoid avulsing the branches while attempting to control and repair these injuries. In patients with exsanguination, ligation of the infrarenal cava is usually tolerated, necessitating specific postoperative management aimed at improving venous return from the lower extremities and preventing venous thrombosis. Ligation of the suprarenal and retrohepatic cava should be done when the patient appears to be in a terminal state but carries a very high morbidity and mortality.

Hematomas in the lateral retroperitoneum are usually associated with renal vessel injury or injury to the kidney itself. Renovascular injuries that are extensive and associated with instability are usually treated with nephrectomy. A preoperative one-shot intravenous pyelogram (IVP) to establish the presence of a contralateral functioning kidney may be helpful in these cases but is rarely warranted. Intraoperative IVP or palpation of a normal kidney on the opposite side is usually adequate. Exposure of the renal hilum is obtained by mobilizing the right colon and the duodenum on the right, or the base of the mesocolon at the midline on the left. The kidney is elevated by incising the retroperitoneum lateral to the kidney. Occasionally, direct repair of the renal artery is accomplished, but attempts to revascularize and salvage a kidney must be weighted against the potential for the development of thrombosis and subsequent complications. Most series agree that revascularization should be attempted only when less than 12 hours have elapsed since injury. Nephrectomy may be a better choice in patients with other intra-abdominal injuries or those with prolonged ischemia or hypotension. Renal vein injuries, if not repaired, should be treated with nephrectomy.

With a hematoma in the pelvis, injury to the iliac vessels should be suspected. Vascular control is achieved by incising the retroperitoneum at the midline at the aortic bifurcation. Ligation of the common iliac or external iliac artery carries a high rate of limb loss, and revascularization is therefore necessary. The internal iliac arteries can be ligated with impunity. Iliac vein injuries should be repaired if possible, however, ligation is well tolerated if postoperative management with elastic stockings is instituted. The challenge with the management of these injuries lies in obtaining adequate exposure for control and repair; in cases of exsanguination, packing of the pelvis should be considered early on. Lower extremity fasciotomies should be employed liberally with injuries that involve the iliac vessels, particularly the iliac veins.

Hematomas of the portal area are associated with injuries to the portal triad and to the liver itself; rarely are these injuries isolated to any single structure. Owing to the difficulty of obtaining adequate control and rapid exposure, these injuries are often lethal. The Pringle maneuver is performed by manually compressing the portal triad or by using clamps or tapes. Thereafter, maneuvers depend on the location along the portal area in which the injury is suspected. Repair can be done if adequate exposure can be obtained; other options include portosystemic shunting, transposition of the splenic and the superior mesenteric veins, and even ligation of the portal vein. In the latter case, a second-look operation 24 hours later should be performed to determine whether excessive venous engorgement of the small intestine has occurred and whether mesenteric venous thrombosis with bowel infarction is likely to develop. If this is the case, a portosystemic shunt should be considered at this time. As expected, these injuries have a high mortality and are followed by a high incidence of complications from hepatic necrosis, encephalopathy, or portal hypertension. Ligation of the hepatic artery appears to be tolerated and should be followed with cholecystectomy.

Diaphragm

Diaphragmatic injuries should be suspected in patients with penetrating thoracoabdominal trauma. Likewise, injuries in both the thoracic and abdominal compartments must be ruled out. Diagnostic laparoscopy has proved helpful in diagnosing diaphragmatic injuries in cases of isolated, stable penetrating thoracoabdominal trauma.

All injuries to the diaphragm should be repaired, with the possible exception of very small posterior lacerations to the right diaphragm in which post-traumatic diaphragmatic herniation is uncommon. Repair should be accomplished with tension-free nonabsorbable monofilament mattress sutures. Undiagnosed injuries, with delayed recognition in the form of incarcerated diaphragmatic hernias, have an associated mortality of 36%.[84]

References

1. Rosoff L, Cohen JL, Telfer N, et al: Injuries of the spleen. Surg Clin North Am 1972;52:667.
2. Shaftan GW: Indications for operation in abdominal trauma. Am J Surg 1960;99:657.
3. Root HD, Houser CW, McKinley CR, et al: Diagnostic peritoneal lavage. Surgery 1965;57:633.
4. Federle MP, Goldberg HI, Kaiser JA, et al: Evaluation of abdominal trauma by computed tomography. Radiology 1981;29:242.
5. Raptopoulos V: Abdominal trauma: Emphasis on computed tomography. Radiol Clin North Am 1994;32:696.
6. Gruessner R, Mentges B, Duber CH, et al: Sonography versus peritoneal lavage in blunt abdominal trauma. J Trauma 1989;29:242.
7. Tso P, Rodriguez Al, Cooper C, et al: Ultrasonography in blunt abdominal trauma: A preliminary progress report. J Trauma 1991;33:39.
8. Kimura A, Toshibum O: Emergency center ultrasonography in the evaluation of hemoperitoneum: a prospective study. J Trauma 1991;31:20.
9. Hoffmann R, Nerlich M, Muggia-Sullam M, et al: Blunt abdominal trauma in cases of multiple trauma evaluated by ultrasonography: A prospective analysis of 291 patients. J Trauma 1992;32:452.
10. McKenney M, Lentz K, Nunez D, et al: Can ultrasound replace diagnostic peritoneal lavage in blunt trauma. J Trauma 1994;37(3):439.
11. Ivatury RR, Simon R: The role of cavitary endoscopy in trauma. Surg Annu 1995;27:81.
12. Simon RJ, Ivatury RR: Current concepts in the use of cavitary endoscopy in the evaluation and treatment of blunt and penetrating trauma. Surg Clin North Am 1995;75(2):157.
13. Sosa JL, Baker M, Puente I, et al: Negative laparotomy in abdominal gunshot wounds: Potential impact of laparoscopy. J Trauma 1995;38(2):194.
14. Sosa JL, Arrillaga A, Puente I, et al: Laparoscopy in 121 consecutive patients with abdominal gunshot wounds. J Trauma 1995;39(3):501.
15. Subcommittee on ATLS of American College of Surgeons Committee on Trauma: Advanced Trauma Life Support. Chicago, American College of Surgeons, 1997.
16. Thal ER: Evaluation of peritoneal lavage and local wound exploration in lower chest and abdominal stab wounds. J Trauma 1977;17:642.
17. Renz BM, Feliciano DV: Unnecessary laparotomies for trauma: A prospective study of morbidity. J Trauma 1995;38:350.
18. Hasaniya N, Demetriades D, Stephens A, Dubrowskiz R, Berne T: Early morbidity and mortality of non-therapeutic operations for penetrating trauma. Am Surgeon 1994;60:744.

19. Nance FC, Wennar MH, Johnson LW, et al: Surgical judgment in the management of penetrating wounds to the abdomen: Experience with 2,212 patients. Ann Surg 1974;179:639.
20. Demetriades D, Rabinowitz B: Indications for operation in abdominal stab wounds—a prospective study of 651 patients. Ann Surg 1987;205:129.
21. Feliciano DV, Nitondo PA, Steed G, et al: Five hundred open taps or lavages in patients with abdominal stab wounds. Am J Surg 1984;148:772.
22. Ochsner MG, Rozycki GS: Prospective evaluation of thoracoscopy for diagnosing diaphragmatic injury in thoracoabdominal trauma: A preliminary report. J Trauma 1993;37:704.
23. Meyer AA, Crass RA: Abdominal trauma. Surg Clin North Am 1982;62:105.
24. Cue JI, Miller FB, Cryer HM, et al: A prospective, randomized comparison between open and closed peritoneal lavage techniques. J Trauma 1990;30(7):880.
25. Gruenberg JC, Brown RS: The diagnostic usefulness of peritoneal lavage in penetrating trauma: A prospective evaluation and comparison with blunt trauma. Am Surg 1982;48:402.
26. Oreskovich MR, Carrico CJ: Stab wounds of the anterior abdomen: Analysis of a management plan using local wound exploration and quantitative peritoneal lavage. Ann Surg 1983;198:411.
27. Merlotti GJ, Dillon BC, Lange DA, et al: Peritoneal lavage in penetrating thoracoabdominal trauma. J Trauma 1988;28(1):17.
28. Henneman PL, Marx JA, Moore EE, et al: Diagnostic peritoneal lavage: Accuracy in predicting necessary laparotomy following blunt and penetrating trauma. J Trauma 1990;30(11):1345.
29. Jacobs DG, Angus L, Rodriguez A, et al: Peritoneal lavage white count: A reassessment. J Trauma 1990;30(5):607.
30. D'Amelio LF, Rhodes M: A reassessment of the peritoneal lavage leukocyte count in blunt abdominal trauma. J Trauma 1990;30(10):1291.
31. McAnena OJ, Marx JA, Moore EE: Contribution of peritoneal lavage enzyme determination to the management of isolated hollow visceral abdominal injuries. Ann Emerg Med 1990;19:463.
32. Marx JA, Moore EE, Jorden RC, et al: Limitations of computed tomography in the evaluation of acute abdominal trauma: A prospective comparison with diagnostic peritoneal lavage. J Trauma 1985;25:933.
33. Rhem CG, Sherman R, Hinz TW: The role of CT scan in evaluation for laparotomy in patients with stab wounds of the abdomen. J Trauma 1989;29:446.
34. Demetriades D, Rabinowitz B, Sofianos C, et al: The management of penetrating injuries of the back—a prospective study of 230 patients. Ann Surg 1988;207:72.
35. Meyer DM, Thal RE, Weigelt JA, et al: The role of abdominal CT in the evaluation of stab wounds to the back. J Trauma 1989;29(9):1226.
36. Himmelman RG, Martin M, Gilkey S, et al: Triple contrast CT scans in penetrating back and flank trauma. J Trauma 1991;31(6):852.
37. Fabian TC, Croce MA, Stewart RM, et al: A prospective analysis of diagnostic laparoscopy in trauma. Ann Surg 1993;217:557.
38. Salvino CK, Esposito TJ, Marshall WJ, et al: The role of diagnostic laparoscopy in the management of trauma patients: A preliminary assessment. J Trauma 1993;34:506.
39. Rozycki GS, Ochsner MG, Jaffin JH, et al: Prospective evaluation of surgeon's use of ultrasound in the evaluation of trauma patients. J Trauma 1993;34:516.
40. Moore EE, Moore JB, Van Duzer-Moore S: Mandatory laparotomy for gunshot wounds penetrating the abdomen. Am J Surg 1980;25:522.
41. Ordog G, Wasserberger J, Balasubramabian S: Shotgun wound ballistics. J Trauma 1988;28:624.
42. Thal ER, May RA, Beesinger D: Peritoneal lavage its unreliability in gunshot wounds of the lower chest and abdomen. Arch Surg 1980;115:430.
43. Renz B, Feliciano DV: Gunshot wounds to the right thoracoabdomen: A prospective study of nonoperative management. J Trauma 1994;37(5):737.
44. Ablau CJ, Olen RN, Dobrin PB, et al: Efficacy of intraperitoneal antibiotics in the treatment of severe fecal peritonitis. Am J Surg 1991;162:453.
45. Jurkovich GJ, Greiser WB, Luterman A, et al: Hypothermia in trauma victims: An ominous predictor of survival. J Trauma 1987;27(9):1019.
46. Gentilello LM: Advances in the management of hypothermia. Surg Clin North Am 1995;75:243.
47. Gentilello LM, Cobean RA, Offner PJ, et al: Continuous arteriovenous rewarming: Rapid reversal of hypothermia in critically ill patients. J Trauma 1992;32(3):316.
48. Feliciano DV, Rozycki GS: The management of penetrating abdominal trauma. In Cameron JL (ed): Advances in Surgery. Chicago, Mosby–Year Book, 1995;28:1.

49. Schein M, Wittman D, Aprahamian CC, et al: The abdominal compartment syndrome: The physiologic and clinical consequences of elevated intra-abdominal pressure. J Am Coll Surg 1995;180:745.
50. Durham RM: Management of gastric injuries. Surg Clin North Am 1990;70:517.
51. Durham RM, Olsen S, Weigelt JA: Penetrating injuries to the stomach. Surg Gynecol Obstet 1991;172:298.
52. Madden MR, Paull DE, Finkelstein JL, et al: Occult diaphragmatic injury from stab wounds to the lower chest and abdomen. J Trauma 1989;29:292.
53. Moore EE, Dunn L, Moore JB, Thompson JS: Penetrating abdominal trauma index. J Trauma 1981;21:439.
54. Mullins RJ: Duodenum, small intestine, and colon. In Trunkey DD, Lewis FR (eds): Current Therapy of Trauma, 3rd ed. Chicago, Mosby-Year Book, 1991, p. 256.
55. Bukley GB, Zuidema GD, Hamilton SR, et al: Intraoperative determination of small intestinal viability following ischemic injury: A prospective, controlled trial of two methods (Doppler and fluorescein) compared with standard clinical judgment. Ann Surg 1981;193:168.
56. Snyder W, Weigelt J, Watkins W, et al: The surgical management of duodenal trauma. Arch Surg 1980;115:422.
57. Cogbill T, Moore EE, Feliciano DV, et al: Conservative management of duodenal trauma: A multicenter perspective. J Trauma 1990;30:1469.
58. Vaugham G, Grazier O, Graham D, et al: The use of pyloric exclusion in the management of severe duodenal injuries. Am J Surg 1977;134:785.
59. Stone H, Fabian T: Management of duodenal wounds. J Trauma 1979;19:334.
60. Flint L, McCoy M, Richardson J, et al: Duodenal injury: Analysis of common misconceptions in diagnosis and treatment. Ann Surg 1980;191:697.
61. Levison M, Peterson S, Sheldon G: Duodenal trauma: Experience of a trauma center. J Trauma 1984;24:475.
62. Smego D, Richarson J, Flint L: Determinants of outcome in pancreatic trauma. J Trauma 1985;25:771.
63. Felicano DV, Martin T, Cruse P, et al: Management of combined pancreatoduodenal injuries. Ann Surg 1987;205:673.
64. Jones R: Management of pancreatic trauma. Am J Surg 1985;150:698.
65. Sims E, Mandal A, Schlater T, et al: Factors affecting outcome in pancreatic trauma. J Trauma 1984;24:125.
66. Cogbill T, Moore EE, Morris JJ, et al: Distal pancreatectomy for trauma: A multicenter experience. J Trauma 1991;31:1600.
67. Chappuis CW, Frey DJ, Dietzen CD, et al: Management of penetrating colon injuries: A prospective randomized trial. Ann Surg 1991;213:492.
68. Adkins RB, Zirkle PK, Waterhouse G: Penetrating colon trauma. J Trauma 1984;24:491.
69. Shannon FL, Moore EE: Primary repair of the colon: When is it a safe alternative? Surgery 1985;98:851.
70. George SM, Fabian TC, Voeller GR, et al: Primary repair of the colon: A prospective trial in nonselected patients. Ann Surg 1989;209:728.
71. Burch JM, Martin RR, Richardson RJ, et al: Evolution of the treatment of injured colon in the 1980's. Arch Surg 1991;126:979.
72. Burch JA, Feliciano DV, Mattox KL: Colostomy and drainage for civilian rectal injuries: Is that all? Ann Surg 1989;209:600.
73. Feliciano DV, Spjut-Patrinely V, Burch JM, et al: Splenorrhaphy: the alternative. Ann Surg 1990;211:56.
74. Singer DB: Post splenectomy sepsis. In Rosenbur HS, Bolande RP (eds): Perspectives in Pediatric Pathology. Vol. 1. Chicago, Year Book, 1973, p. 285.
75. Konradsen HB, Nielsen JL, Pedersen HK, et al: Antibody persistence in splenectomized adults after pneumococcal vaccination. Scand J Infect Dis 1990;22:725.
76. Pachter HL, Spencer F, Hofsteter SR, et al: Experience with the finger fracture technique to achieve intrahepatic hemostasis in 75 patients with severe injuries to the liver. Ann Surg 1983;197:771.
77. Flint LM, Polk HC: Selective hepatic artery ligation: Limitations and failures. J Trauma 1979;19:319.
78. Feliciano DV, Mattox KL, Jordan GL Jr, et al: Management of 1000 consecutive cases of hepatic trauma. Ann Surg 1986;204:438.

79. Cogbill TH, Moore EE, Jurkovich GJ, et al: Severe hepatic trauma: A multi-center experience with 1,335 liver injuries. J Trauma 1988;28:1433.
80. Feliciano DV: Biliary injuries as a result of blunt and penetrating trauma. Surg Clin North Am 1994;74:897.
81. Feliciano DV, Burch JM, Spjut-Patrinely V, et al: Abdominal gunshot wounds: An urban trauma center's experience with 300 consecutive patients. Ann Surg 1988;208:362.
82. Feliciano DV: Abdominal vascular injuries. Surg Clin North Am 1988;68:741.
83. Smith SRG: Traumatic retroperitoneal venous haemorrhage. Br J Surg 1988;75:632.
84. Madden MR, Paull DE, Shires GT, et al: Occult diaphragmatic injury from stab wounds to the lower chest and abdomen. J Trauma 1989;29:292.
85. Ginzburg E, Carrillo ED, Kopelman T, McKenney MG, Kirton OC, Shatz DV, Sleeman D, Martin LC: The role of computed tomography in selective management of gunshot wounds to the abdomen and flank. J Trauma 1998;45:1005.
86. Grossman MD, May AK, Schwab CW, et al: Determining anatomic injury with computed tomography in selected torso gunshot wounds. J Trauma 1998;45:446.
87. Nagy KK, Krosner SM, Joseph KT, Roberts RR, Smith RF, Barrett J: A method of determining peritoneal penetration in gunshot wounds to the abdomen. J Trauma 1997;43:242.

Chapter *11*

Blunt Abdominal Trauma

Wide-impact blunt trauma (e.g., transportation accidents and falls from great heights) may cause limited or severe regional injury throughout the central and peripheral nervous system, thorax, abdomen, pelvis, and extremities. Early, comprehensive, precise, and nearly simultaneous diagnosis of all possible critical injuries is essential after the ABCs of trauma care triage have been addressed. The abdomen is a potential site of major blood loss. The mechanisms of blunt abdominal trauma include: direct impact, acceleration-deceleration forces, and shearing forces. One must always be aware that there is no correlation between the size of the contact area and the resultant injuries. Patients who have suffered blunt abdominal trauma and who present with peritonitis, progressive abdominal distention associated with hypovolemic shock, or both are best served by rapid resuscitation and prompt mandatory laparotomy.

Besides physical assessment, trauma evaluation includes laboratory and radiologic work-up. Hematocrit, white blood cell count, amylase determination, urine analysis, arterial blood gases, and blood type and cross-match are typically forwarded to the laboratory. The admission chest x-ray may reveal lower rib fractures, heralding associated hepatic or splenic trauma. Intrathoracic bowel gas or a displaced nasal or oral gastric tube is pathognomonic for a ruptured hemidiaphragm. Moreover, abdominal films may demonstrate free intraperitoneal or localized retroperitoneal air.

Volume resuscitation of the patient begins with isotonic crystalloid infusion via a large-bore intravenous catheter. A nasogastric tube is placed to decompress the stomach, and a Foley catheter is inserted to empty the bladder and allow monitoring of urine output. Antibiotics are given if celiotomy is planned. Greater judgment is required for patients in whom a satisfactory physical examination of the abdomen cannot be obtained because of coma, spinal cord or associated major thoracic or pelvic injuries, intoxication, or other degrees of mental obtundation.

DIAGNOSTIC APPROACH

Exploratory laparotomy is mandatory for overt peritonitis, progressive abdominal distention with unexplained hypotension, ruptured diaphragm, and free intraperitoneal or loculated retroperitoneal air on abdominal roentgenograms. However, the diagnosis of the hemodynamically stable patient with suspected intra-abdominal injury has steadily evolved during the past several decades. In this patient population, the approach of mandatory exploration for suspected abdominal injury has resulted in unacceptably high negative and nontherapeutic laparotomy rates, which are associated with 18% and 45% morbidity rates, respectively.[1] The management of blunt or penetrating abdominal trauma in the hemodynamically stable victim has evolved toward using diagnostic modalities that identify which patients do not require laparotomy, thus decreasing morbidity and overall hospital costs. In the hemodynamically stable victim of blunt abdominal trauma who has no signs of peritonitis, less invasive measures such as diagnostic peritoneal lavage, computed tomography, and ultrasonography have gained wide acceptance because they demonstrate a high degree of sensitivity, specificity, and diagnostic accuracy.[2-4]

The accuracy of diagnostic peritoneal lavage (DPL) approaches 95%.[2] However, although highly sensitive (its sensitivity approaches 100%), DPL lacks specificity (its specificity is approximately 85%) and is associated with a nontherapeutic laparotomy rate of 20%.[1, 5] Moreover, the clinician is unable to evaluate the retroperitoneum. DPL remains an appropriate diagnostic modality in the unstable patient when the source of blood loss is obscure and is also used in the hemodynamically stable patient with blunt abdominal trauma who is undergoing emergent general anesthesia for repair of associated injuries (e.g., orthopedic or maxillary facial injuries) (Table 11-1).

Abdominal ultrasound has demonstrated equivalence to DPL in these situations and in many centers has replaced DPL. Ultrasound can be used to evaluate the presence of free intraperitoneal fluid in both stable and unstable patients and has sensitivity, specificity, and accuracy rates of 90% to 92%, 88% to 90%, and 95% to 99%, respectively.[2-5] Unfortunately, like DPL it also lacks specificity in regard to the source of the fluid and does not evaluate the retroperitoneum. Another potential shortcoming is its inability to characterize the intraperitoneal fluid (i.e., to distinguish blood from bowel contents). Accordingly, an intestinal perforation may be missed (0.5% incidence).

Computed tomography (CT) offers a further refinement of diagnostic technique in the hemodynamically stable patient; not only can a diagnosis of hemoperitoneum be made, but the source of bleeding is often identified as well. Furthermore, it is the only imaging modality capable of evaluating the retroperitoneum, and the extent of organ-specific injury can be quantitated. The sensitivity, specificity, and accuracy rates of CT approach 97%, 95% and 96%, respectively.[2] The diagnostic accuracy of CT has greatly facilitated the nonoperative management of hepatic and splenic injuries in hemodynamically stable patients, reducing the incidence of nontherapeutic laparotomy.

Another situation in which computed tomography has proved useful is in the evaluation of patients who are hemodynamically stable when they arrive but then develop mild to moderate abdominal pain 12 to 48 hours after injury.

Table 11-1. Criteria for a Positive Diagnostic Peritoneal Lavage in Blunt Abdominal Trauma

Initial aspiration of blood (5 ml or greater)
Red blood cell count >100,000 mm^3
White blood cell count >500 mm^3
Presence of bile, bacteria, or food particles
Presence of lavage fluid via Foley or chest tube
Presence of pleural effusion on postlavage chest x-ray, suggesting an occult diaphragmatic rupture

Blunt Abdominal Trauma

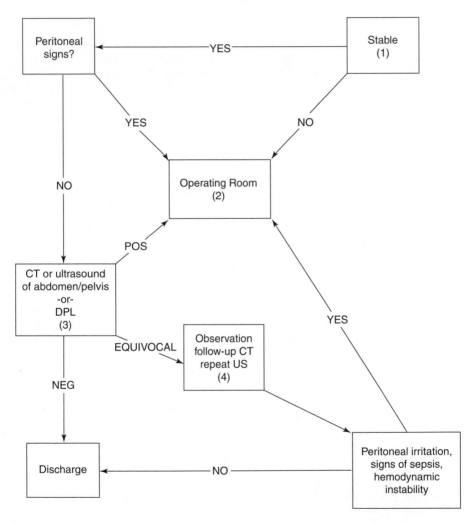

1. Basic evaluation for assessment of injury and stability should include a history and physical examination, determination of the mechanism of injury, vital signs, admission laboratory values (hematocrit, urinalysis, arterial blood gases, serum amylase, and toxicology), chest, cervical, and pelvic roentgenograms, insertion of large-bore intravenous catheters, central venous access if shock is present, Foley catheter insertion, and a nasogastric tube.
2. Mandatory exploratory laparotomy is indicated for shock in the presence of an expanding abdomen, pneumoperitoneum, or retroperitoneal air.
3. Indications for diagnostic peritoneal lavage (DPL), abdominal ultrasound, or computed tomography include the following:
   a. Unreliable or equivocal results of physical examination (e.g., altered mental status or pain perception associated with neurologic or musculoskeletal trauma) in a hemodynamically stable patient.
   b. Hypotension of uncertain etiology.
   c. Urgent or emergent need for general anesthesia and surgery for associated injuries precluding a "safe period" of observation (i.e., 24 hours).
   d. Unexplained blood loss.
   e. Associated major injuries (i.e., bilateral femoral fracture, multiple lower rib fractures, major pelvic fracture) suggesting a significant acceleration / deceleration mechanism in the presence of hemodynamic instability and requirement for extensive roentgenographic evaluation.
4. With equivocal findings on initial ultrasound (US), DPL, or CT, or in the face of clinical deterioration, follow-up studies should be done. Repeat ultrasound or CT may show development of a new or progression of a previously small or nonexistent hemorrhage.

Computed tomography is also used to evaluate patients with equivocal results on DPL or abdominal ultrasonography. The major limitation of CT is its relative inaccuracy in the identification of intestinal and mesenteric injuries. It is a costly examination and requires moving the acutely injured patient from the confines of a resuscitation unit to the relatively inaccessible scanning room. Therefore, *only* stable patients should be subjected to a CT scan.

Diagnostic laparoscopy for the evaluation of abdominal trauma was first introduced in the 1970s but failed to gain wide acceptance until the advent of videotechnology and improved instrumentation in the early 1990s. This technology is now used to evaluate blunt trauma in hemodynamically stable patients. Diagnostic video-assisted laparoscopy with direct visualization and evaluation of injuries has the potential to dramatically decrease the number of nontherapeutic laparotomies. However, its exact role continues to evolve.[5]

In summary, DPL and ultrasound can be used in the unstable victim of blunt trauma to perform a rapid assessment for intraperitoneal fluid. Both imaging modalities permit the prompt recognition and management of intra-peritoneal hemorrhage. In the stable patient requiring further evaluation, CT is appropriate. Use of diagnostic laparoscopy is limited to selected, hemodynamically stable patients. Like CT, it is appropriate for the evaluation of patients with multiple trauma and borderline DPL results (e.g., 80,000 to 120,000 RBC/high-power field) or in those who demonstrate intermittent mild hypotension or persistent tachycardia.[1–5]

BLUNT HEPATIC AND SPLENIC INJURIES

The liver and spleen are the two organs most commonly injured in blunt abdominal trauma.[6–9] In the hemodynamically unstable patient with suspected intra-abdominal hemorrhage, mandatory laparotomy is the rule. In hemody-namically stable patients, a selective nonoperative approach is now advocated and is substantiated by numerous clinical reports.[6–9] Early objections to nonop-erative management were based on the following concerns: (1) A rational decision was impossible without a visual assessment of the severity of injury, and (2) concomitant intra-abdominal injury could not be excluded.[6] The avail-ability of high-resolution CT has addressed these concerns by providing (1) pathologic accuracy, (2) grading of injury severity, (3) quantitation of the amount of hemoperitoneum, and (4) a highly reliable evaluation of the retro-peritoneum. However, all scans must be rapidly interpreted and classified to maximize treatment efficacy, and this requires the immediate availability of a radiologist or surgeon proficient in reading CT scans.

The overwhelming majority of hepatic injuries treated nonoperatively are classified as Grade I to III injuries (see Chapter 18); the overall success rate of such treatment is 94% in the hemodynamically stable patient. It is now well documented that approximately 20% of Grade IV and V hepatic injuries are also amenable to nonoperative management. However, the continued presence of hemodynamic stability, a stable hematocrit level, and observation in a critical care area is essential to success and patient safety.[6, 7] Complications include delayed hemorrhage as well as bile leaks, bilomas, and intra- and perihepatic abscesses, which are amenable to percutaneous drainage. Hemodynamically stable patients with evidence of ongoing bleeding may be candidates for angiographic embolization.

Nonoperative management of splenic injuries, first used by pediatric surgeons, has gained popularity in the adult population as well.[8] Hemodynamic stability is mandatory.[8, 9] Overall success rates are not as high as those for liver injuries, since splenic bleeding is likely to be due to arterial hemorrhaging at systemic pressures, whereas liver bleeding usually occurs in the venous system, which is under low pressure. Factors identified as predicting a successful outcome include hemodynamic stability, localized trauma to the flank or abdomen, age less than 60 years old, absence of associated injuries that preclude safe observation (associated major pelvic fracture, major closed head injury, and so on), and transfusion of less than 4 units of blood. Transfusion of any amount of blood, however, indicates a nonoperative failure; surgery should be considered long before blood loss is significant enough to require transfusion. Follow-up imaging studies (e.g., CT) showing early resolution of splenic defects are supportive of success. Grades I to III splenic injuries are most amenable to nonoperative management; Grades IV to V injuries almost invariably require operative intervention. Computed tomography offers accurate identification but does not always predict clinical outcome. The requirement for continuous clinical assessment and the ability to operate expeditiously in patients with delayed hemorrhage mandate the availability of surgical personnel and an operating room. Delayed hemorrhage after splenic injury that occurs hours to weeks after blunt trauma can occur; its incidence has been reported in several large series as 8% to 21% in adult patients.[8, 9] Delayed rupture is exceedingly rare in children.

BLUNT INJURY TO THE DIAPHRAGM

Diaphragmatic rupture can be silent, with few or no physical findings and hemodynamic stability, or it can be associated with significant hemodynamic and respiratory derangement secondary to tension pneumothoraces or displacement of mediastinal structures due to transdiaphragmatic herniation of gastrointestinal organs. Diaphragmatic rupture is estimated to occur in an average of 3% to 5% of all abdominal injuries.[10] Injury to the left hemidiaphragm occurs more frequently than that to the right. The rarity of right-sided blunt diaphragmatic injuries is attributed to the shock-absorbing effect of the liver on the right hemidiaphragm. The diagnosis of diaphragmatic rupture requires a high index of suspicion; therefore, the injury mechanism is of great importance (e.g., passenger compartment invasion, use and type of restraints, deformity of the steering wheel, need for extrication, fall from a great height [i.e., more than two stories]).

Radiographic findings can range from minimal to dramatic. Interestingly, the initial chest x-ray is not diagnostic in approximately 50% of patients with diaphragmatic rupture. Features associated with diaphragmatic rupture include prominence and immobility of the left hemithorax, obliteration of the left diaphragm on x-ray, elevation and irregularity of the costophrenic angle of the parietal pleura and diaphragm, pleural effusion, nasogastric tube in the chest, and presence of bowel sounds in the thorax. Diagnosis can be confirmed by gastrointestinal contrast studies such as upper gastrointestinal series and barium enema. CT and magnetic resonance imaging have proved to be valuable adjuncts but lack sensitivity. Minimally invasive technology (i.e., laparoscopy and thoracoscopy) have been used with success to confirm the diagnosis in a majority of cases.[5] Definitive management remains exploratory laparotomy and suture repair.

BLUNT INJURY TO THE DUODENUM AND PANCREAS

Pancreatic injury secondary to blunt abdominal trauma is relatively uncommon, representing 2% to 3% of all instances of significant abdominal trauma.[11, 12] Serum amylase abnormalities suggest injury to the pancreas or duodenum, but signs of pancreatoduodenal injury are often subtle. Obliteration of the right psoas muscle or retroperitoneal air on plain abdominal roentgenograms is suggestive. If there is any suspicion of such an injury, CT with oral and IV contrast is indicated and is often diagnostic. Diagnostic peritoneal lavage is unreliable in detecting isolated duodenal and pancreatic injuries.[12] At celiotomy, the finding of a central upper abdominal retroperitoneal hematoma, bile staining, or air, mandates visualization and thorough examination of the duodenum and pancreas. Eighty percent of duodenal lacerations can be repaired primarily by simple duodenorrhaphy (one or two layers). These represent Grade I and II injuries, which are characterized by injury to less than 50% of the bowel wall circumference with no associated pancreatic or biliary injury.[12, 13] Approximately 10% to 15% (Grade III to IV) of duodenal injuries require more complex procedures such as Roux-en-Y duodenojejunostomy, duodenal diverticularization, or pyloric exclusion.[12, 13] Pancreaticoduodenectomy (Whipple operation) is reserved for the rare occurrence of severe combined injuries to the pancreatic, duodenal, and distal common bile duct (Grade V injuries). Most patients who die from a pancreatic or duodenal injury do so within the first 48 hours; these injuries are often associated with exsanguinating vascular liver and splenic injuries.

Minor pancreatic contusions and capsular lacerations (Grade I to III) account for about 75% of all pancreatic injuries.[11] Time from injury to definitive treatment is an important factor in the development of late complications (e.g., pancreatic abscess, pseudocyst) and subsequent mortality. In the majority of cases (84%), the diagnosis of pancreatic injury is made at the time of laparotomy.[11] In the setting of blunt trauma, the CT scan may demonstrate a fractured or ischemic duodenal-pancreatic injury (Grade V), in which the duodenum is not reparable, and frequently the distal common bile duct cannot be reasonably repaired either. The guiding principles in management of pancreatic injuries include (1) hemorrhage control, (2) judicious debridement and resection, (3) wide drainage, and (4) limited use of pancreaticoenteric anastomoses. Distal pancreatic injuries (i.e., to the left of the mesenteric vessels) are often easily managed by resection of the distal pancreas or by closed suction drainage. If distal pancreatic resection is warranted and the patient is hemodynamically stable, consideration of splenic salvage is appropriate, albeit not mandatory. Complications include pancreatic fistula, pancreatic abscess, and pseudocyst;

all of these can be successfully managed with CT-guided drainage. Moreover, pancreatic fistulas, when well controlled by drainage, invariably close with time and adequate nutrition.

BLUNT INJURY TO THE STOMACH AND SMALL INTESTINE

Blunt injury to the stomach is rare. Most blunt gastric injuries occur on the anterior surface or greater curvature of the stomach. The lacerations caused by blunt injury are often large, are associated with significant intraperitoneal contamination, and associated injuries are almost universal. Blunt injury to the small bowel was relatively uncommon prior to the advent of high-speed motor vehicle traffic accidents.[14, 15] This injury is now often related to shoulder harness and lap belt devices. During rapid deceleration these harnesses and lap belts or the steering wheel can cause sudden deceleration and compression of the anterior abdomen. The small bowel, which is normally arranged in folds and convolutions, may become compressed by the steering wheel or seat belt or can twist to form a burst-type closed-loop obstruction. Stretching and traction of the small bowel is another mechanism of blunt intestinal injury. These shear-type blunt small bowel injuries occur at points of fixation (e.g., the ligament of Treitz and the retroperitoneal attachment to the ileocecal valve) or at fixed points secondary to adhesions caused by previous abdominal surgery. Significant blunt injury to the mesentery is also possible; this may range from very small tears in the overlying peritoneum to extensive avulsions with significant hemoperitoneum, consequent bowel ischemia, or even infarction. Mesenteric tears with small bowel devascularization account for approximately 25% of cases in which the small bowel requires operative intervention after blunt trauma. Traumatic injuries are common in 25% of patients with blunt intestinal injury, and not infrequently, there are multiple small bowel injuries, which emphasizes the need to fully inspect the entire length of the small bowel during abdominal exploration. The presence of a Chance fracture (i.e., a transverse fracture of the lower thoracic or lumbar vertebral body caused by flexion and distraction of the spinal column, usually involving a lap seat belt) raises the index of suspicion for possible injury to the small bowel and its mesentery.[14]

In patients with head injury, intoxication, or other conditions that make abdominal examination unreliable, DPL is sensitive for detecting blunt small bowel injuries that require operative intervention. However, DPL can be nondiagnostic for up to 6 to 8 hours after intestinal perforation. Moreover, peritonitis may not become manifest clinically until 6 to 12 hours following intestinal spillage. Laparoscopy can be used to detect staining with intestinal content. Alkaline phosphatase and amylase in the lavage fluid, as well as elevated serum levels, may be suggestive. Delayed perforation, although rare, does occur as a result of direct injury, transmural contusion, or ischemia from mesenteric vascular injury. If localized ischemia does result in full-thickness necrosis, stricture may occur, resulting in small bowel obstruction. Delayed perforation usually presents within days; delayed obstruction can present from weeks to months after injury.

INJURIES TO THE COLON AND RECTUM

Blunt colonic and rectal injuries are uncommon and therefore pose problems for diagnosis and treatment. Most blunt injuries to the colon occur in motor vehicle accidents and are evenly distributed throughout the colon. Implicated mechanisms include steering wheel compression of the abdomen as well as lap belt restraints.[15] The clinical presentation may include hemoperitoneum secondary to mesenteric vascular lacerations or peritonitis resulting from spillage of colonic contents. Definitive diagnosis is made at the time of surgery, which involves a thorough exploration. These injuries present either as large disruptions of the colonic wall or as avulsion injuries in which the mesentery is stripped from the colon. Occasionally, extensive disruptions of the serosa are encountered. Suture repair of small perforations is successfully employed for the majority of colon injuries. Mesenteric rents must be repaired to prevent internal small bowel herniation. When resection is required, treatment must be individualized, and an ostomy is created based on the patient's hemodynamic stability, degree of enteric contamination, and severity of associated injuries (e.g., pancreatic, renal). Resection of the right colon with ileocolostomy is ideally suited for injuries that require resection proximal to the right colonic artery. In the remainder of the colon, resection with colostomy is appropriate for injuries requiring resection. In the severely unstable patient, simple resection with staples can be done quickly; reanastomosis of the stapled bowel ends is performed in the next 1 to 2 days following stabilization of the patient.

The most common complication of colonic injury repair is an anastomotic leak, which can lead to subsequent fecal fistula. Fortunately, most colocutaneous fistulas close spontaneously after 2 to 3 weeks of bowel rest and parenteral nutrition.

References

1. Renz BM, Feliciano DV: Unnecessary laparotomies for trauma: A prospective study of morbidity. J Trauma 1995;38(3):350–356.
2. Liu M, Lee C-H, P'eng FK: Prospective comparison of diagnostic peritoneal lavage, computed tomographic scanning, and ultrasonography for the diagnosis of blunt abdominal trauma. J Trauma 1993;35(2):267–270.
3. Bode PJ, Niezen RA, van Vugt AB, et al: Abdominal ultrasound as a reliable indicator for conclusive laparotomy in blunt abdominal trauma. J Trauma 1993;34(1):27–31.
4. McKenney MG, Martin L, Lentz K, et al: 1,000 consecutive ultrasounds for blunt abdominal trauma. J Trauma 1996;40(4):607–612.
5. Sosa JL, Puente I: Laparoscopy in the evaluation and management of abdominal trauma. Int Surg 1994;79:307–313.
6. Pachter HL, Hofstetter SR: The correct status of non-operative management of adult blunt hepatic injuries. Am J Surg 1995;169:442–454.
7. Croce MA, Fabian TC, Menke PG, et al: Nonoperative management of blunt hepatic trauma is the treatment of choice for hemodynamically stable patients. Ann Surg 1995;21(6):744–754.
8. Powell M, Courcoulas A, Gardner M, et al: Management of blunt splenic trauma: Significant differences between adults and children. Surgery 1997;122:654–660.
9. Kohn JS, Clark DE, Isler RJ, et al: Is computed tomographic grading of splenic injury useful in the nonsurgical managment of blunt trauma? J Trauma 1994;36(3):385–389.
10. Brasel KJ, Borgstrom DC, Myer P, et al: Predictors of outcome in blunt diaphragm rupture. J Trauma 1996;41(3):484–487.

11. Patton JH, Lyden SP, Croce MA, et al: Pancreatic trauma: A simplified management guideline. J Trauma 1997;43(2):234–241.
12. Carrillo EH, Richardson JD, Miller FB: Evolution in the management of duodenal injuries. J Trauma 1996;40(6):1037–1046.
13. Ballard RB, Badellino MM, Eynon A, et al: Blunt duodenal rupture: A 6-year statewide experience. J Trauma 1997;43(2):229–233.
14. Wisner D, Chun Y, Blaisdell F: Blunt intestinal injury: Keys to diagnosis and management. Arch Surg 1990;125:1319–1323.
15. Carrillo EH, Somberg LB, Ceballos CE, et al: Blunt traumatic injuries to the colon and rectum. J Am Coll Surg 1996;183:548–552.

Chapter 12

Blunt Genitourinary Trauma

Blunt genitourinary trauma is often a covert entity associated with a wide spectrum of injuries. Approximately 3% to 10% of all injured patients have some manifestation of genitourinary involvement.[1] Genitourinary trauma is divided into upper tract injuries (renal or ureteral injuries) and lower tract injuries (bladder, urethra, and gonadal injuries). The kidney is most commonly injured, followed by the bladder, the urethra, and the ureter. Blunt trauma accounts for 85% to 94% of renal injuries, whereas penetrating trauma accounts for only 6% to 11% of renal injuries.[1-4] Eighty-five percent of these injuries are of limited severity and do not require exploration but can be treated conservatively with observation.[1, 2, 5] Five percent of these injuries consist of a shattered kidney or major collecting system disruption, and these injuries often require operation. The remaining 10% represent major parenchymal lacerations, for which management remains controversial, with opinions ranging from an operative approach (to avoid the late complications of urinoma, urosepsis, and hypertension) to expectant management (because of the availability of percutaneous and endourologic procedures).

Blunt injury to the genitourinary system is most commonly associated with motor vehicle accidents, sports injuries, occupational injuries, and assaults. The primary mechanisms include (1) a direct blow causing blunt parenchymal disruption by compression against an adjacent bony structures or surrounding muscle, (2) a direct blow with laceration caused by impaction on the bony edges of fractured ribs or vertebral transverse processes, and (3) a sudden deceleration force that induces a shearing laceration.[1, 2, 4, 5] Signs of flank trauma include lower rib fractures, fracture of the lumbar transverse processes, bruising of the flank, and flank tenderness.

Hematuria is the most common sign of renal trauma in all large series. Rarely, severe rhabdomyolysis produces large quantities of urine myoglobin which can be confused with gross hematuria. In rhabdomyolysis, urine analysis tests positive for blood, but red blood cells are absent, confirming myoglobinuria. It was previously taught that significant microscopic hematuria, or 50 or more red blood cells per high-power field, constituted an appropriate indication for urography. Currently, the only absolute indication for urologic radiologic evaluation is the presence of gross hematuria, blood at the urethral meatus, or microscopic hematuria with associated hypotension or shock (systolic blood pressure ≤90 mmHg).[1, 2, 5] Isolated microscopic hematuria is no longer considered adequate justification for urologic evaluation in the adult patient.[1, 2] Moreover, the degree of hematuria does not correlate with the severity of injury. Seven to fourteen percent of patients with major lacerations or renal vascular injury, and 6% to 10% of patients with minor lacerations do not present with hematuria.[2]

The guidelines for identifying adults at risk for significant renal injury do not pertain to children. Any child involved in a traumatic injury who demonstrates any degree of hematuria, microscopic or macroscopic, must have a complete urinary tract evaluation. Children may have congenital renal abnormalities (e.g., cyst and urethral pelvic junction obstruction) that predispose them to significant renal consequences with benign mechanisms of injury.[6, 7]

Owing to its frequent occurrence and subtle presentation, blunt genitourinary trauma is often overlooked in the initial evaluation of the trauma victim. Following the primary survey for life-threatening injuries, Foley catheter placement performed as part of the secondary survey may disclose the first sign of urinary tract injury. The urinary tract is unique in that diagnostic evaluation in the setting of blunt trauma is often performed in a retrograde fashion. Suspected urethral injury is evaluated before presumptive bladder injury, which is excluded before renal or ureteral disruption is sought. Adherence to this axiom permits discovery of virtually any important urinary tract injury, even during the resuscitation of critically injured patients.

Several authors recommend that a bolus intravenous urographic examination (intravenous pyelogram [IVP]) be performed in the hemodynamically unstable blunt trauma victim with gross hematuria who requires abdominal exploration.[1, 2] This is advocated because a normal IVP carries a very high positive predictive value for the absence of significant renal injury. Unilateral nonvisualization of the kidney suggests either a solitary kidney, a pedicle injury, a renal laceration, thrombosis, or spasm of the renal artery. Opponents of this approach argue that a "one-shot" IVP will not change the intraoperative management, especially if the surgeon adheres to the philosophy that no kidney should be removed unless it is unsalvageable and the patient's life is in jeopardy. Moreover, the limited roentgenogram is often indeterminant or nonconclusive in the hypotensive patient. And finally, an intraoperative "on-table" IVP can always be performed.[1]

Computed tomography with intravenous and oral contrast is considered the initial radiologic examination of choice in the hemodynamically stable patient with suspected blunt genitourinary trauma.[2, 3, 5] These studies identify 60% to 85% of renal injuries. Computed tomography is readily available and noninvasive, and it accurately documents the pattern and magnitude of renal injury and delineates the degree of parenchymal lacerations, the extent of extravasation, the amount of surrounding hemorrhage, and the presence of major renovascular injury (as manifested by the lack of renal enhancement, differential renal enhancement, or presence of a cortical rim sign, which suggests renal artery thrombosis). Moreover, CT can identify and stage nonrenal injuries.[2-5] Angiography is reserved for high-risk patients with indeterminate CT scans or for therapeutic embolization in hemodynamically stable patients.

BLUNT INJURY TO THE URETHRA

Three to twenty-five percent of patients sustaining a pelvic fracture suffer an injury to the posterior urethra.[1] Of these, approximately 65% experience

Blunt Genitourinary Trauma without Pelvic Fracture

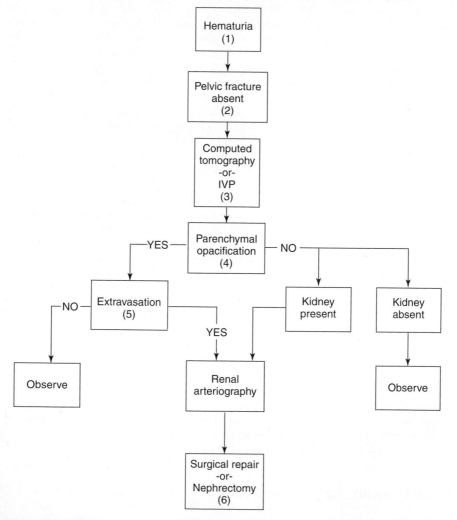

1. Traumatic hematuria is typically defined as either gross blood in the urine or greater than 50 red blood cells per high power field.

2. Hematuria in the presence of an anterior pelvic fracture mandates cystogram. Clinical suggestions of urethral injury (e.g., blood at the meatus, high-riding prostate gland, and/or a butterfly perineal ecchymotic pattern) mandate a retrograde urethrogram before placement of a Foley catheter. This avoids compounding the injury if the urethra is damaged.

3. In the acute setting, patients who are hemodynamically stable and have no clinical or radiologic evidence of lower or upper genitourinary tract injuries are best screened with computed, contrast-enhanced, tomography or excretory urography (intravenous pyelography [IVP]) to define the extent of renal function. Intravenous pyelography identifies abnormal findings in 85% to 97% of patients with Grade II to III renal injuries, although a normal study does not exclude the possibility of a major renal injury. Decreased renal perfusion, systemic hypotension, and technical factors are among the multiple factors that may preclude an adequate examination, resulting in poor visualization. Computed tomography has consistently demonstrated superior precision compared to either urography or sonography in determining the extent of injury and distinguishing between minor and major renal injuries. Computed tomography demonstrates perirenal collections, bilateral kidney function, and the integrity of other intra-abdominal organs.

4. If no function is demonstrable, renal arteriogram and/or celiotomy is mandatory. If renal arterial occlusion is evident, the chances of renal salvage depend on the time interval between the injury and the operative procedure (an interval of >6 hours carries a less than 5% chance of salvage). In the presence of signs of ongoing surgical bleeding (decreasing hematocrit, systemic hypoperfusion, or persistent gross hematuria), intervention is usually necessary, although angiographic embolization may occasionally be effective.

5. Extravasation of contrast from an injured but functioning kidney (indicating disruption to the collecting system) usually subsides within 72 hours, as determined by repeat IVP or CT scan. Delayed bleeding, urinary extravasation, hypertension, or perinephric infection are complications seen in 4% to 6% of all patients managed nonoperatively, and this figure may approach 40% in patients with major cortical or medullary lacerations or associated parenchymal fragmentation. Surgical exploration is required whenever urinary extravasation is extensive or when major vascular injury is associated with arterial occlusion or significant retroperitoneal bleeding. Angiography with embolization has a place. Renal exploration is rarely required for blunt renal injury. CT scans allow simultaneous assessment of the associated injury and accurate staging of the renal injury and result in less delay.

6. The transperitoneal approach facilitates renal exploration and allows early control of the pedicle as well as assessment of potential associated intra-abdominal injuries. In patients with severe trauma to the kidney, nephrectomy may be indicated to control hemorrhage. Partial nephrectomy may be possible in those with isolated injuries.

7. The posterior elements of the pelvis consist of the supporting ligaments (sacroiliac, sacrospinous, sacrotuberous, and iliolumbar) and bones (iliac wings and sacrum). Disruption of these structures is seen on plain films and CT scans as fractures of the bony elements and/or separation or malalignment of the sacroiliac joints (see Chapter 14).

8. The anterior pelvic ring includes the symphysis pubis, and bilateral inferior and superior pubic rami. Bone spicules from fractured rami can directly lacerate the bladder, and the force required to disrupt the anterior elements can be transmitted to, and result in, rupture of the full bladder.

9. When retrograde urethrography (RUG) shows extravasation with contrast medium in the bladder, a diagnosis of incomplete urethral separation is made. This injury commonly heals with 7 to 10 days of suprapubic catheter drainage and prophylactic antibiotics.

10. A normal antegrade urethrogram should precede removal of the catheter. Complete or suspected urethral disruption with extravasation and total absence of contrast medium reaching the bladder is generally treated with initial suprapubic catheter drainage and delayed urethroplasty 4 to 6 weeks after injury.

11. Intraperitoneal bladder rupture requires operative multi-layered repair and Foley or suprapubic catheter drainage.

Blunt Genitourinary Trauma with Pelvic Fracture

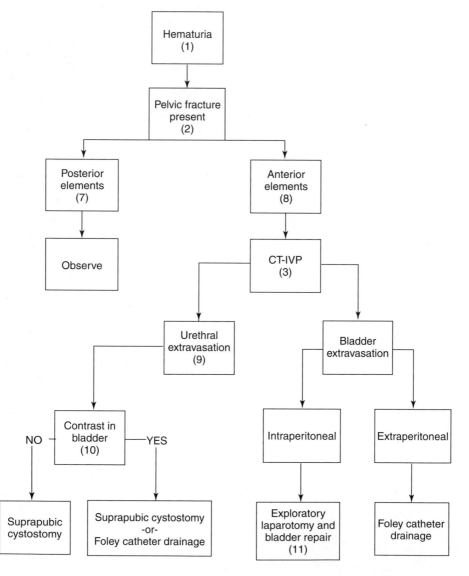

complete disruption, and 34% experience partial urethral disruption.[8, 9] Approximately 10% to 20% of patients with bladder rupture caused by pelvic trauma have concomitant urethral injury. Therefore, one must pay special attention to all patients who sustain pelvic trauma. Examination of the torso and pelvis during the secondary survey is the first step in evaluation. The likelihood of urethral disruption increases significantly in the presence of a pelvic fracture. In males, an anterior pelvic fracture may disrupt the pubic prostatic ligaments and injure the posterior positioned prostatic or membranous urethra, resulting in significant retropubic venous bleeding. This may produce a large pelvic hematoma that can displace the prostrate superiorly, an injury that is detected on rectal examination as a boggy, ill-defined mass.

Examination of the genitalia should be focused on evidence of hematoma or ecchymosis in the penile shaft, scrotal skin, or perineum. Blood at the male meatus is highly diagnostic of urethral injury and dictates the need for an early retrograde urethrogram. When emergent surgical exploration is required for life-threatening injuries, the retrograde urethrogram can be performed on the operating table or after the operative procedure. A Foley catheter should never be introduced when a urethral injury is suspected without first obtaining a retrograde urethrogram to ensure urethral integrity. However, in the absence of definitive signs and with a negative rectal examination, a gentle initial passage of the Foley catheter is acceptable. If any resistance is encountered, a urethrogram should be performed or a suprapubic cystostomy placed.[1, 4, 9]

The retrograde urethrogram is optimally performed under fluoroscopic control using retrograde injection, and can be performed in the emergency room or on the operating table using portable equipment. The patient is positioned in a 30- to 60- degree oblique angle and a 14- to 18-Fr Foley catheter is inserted 2 to 3 cm into the urethra. The balloon is then inflated with 25 to 30 ml of saline, and a water-soluble contrast agent is injected. If an injury is demonstrated, a suprapubic cystostomy with delayed urethral repair (urethroplasty) at 4 to 6 weeks is the consensus approach.[4, 8-10] Not repairing the urethra immediately does result in a primary stricture in nearly 100% of cases. However, the stricture is invariably amenable to urethroplasty. Moreover, this approach is associated with the lowest rate of impotence compared with the alternatives of either primary realignment or immediate suture repair.[8, 9]

Several situations exist in which suprapubic cystostomy and delayed urethral management are contraindicated and immediate repair should be considered. These include (1) associated bladder neck injury, (2) associated rectal injury, and (3) massive pelvic lacerations with extensive displacement of the proximal and distal urethral segments.[8, 9] Careful attention must always be paid to the female patient with a pelvic fracture. A thorough vaginal examination will detect vaginal lacerations or urethral disruption caused by displaced pelvic fragments. Early consultation with the gynecology service is important.

BLUNT INJURY TO THE BLADDER

Major bladder trauma is relatively uncommon. It accounts for less than 2% of abdominal injuries requiring surgical repair, and it occurs in only 5% to 10% of patients who sustain a fracture of the pelvis.[1] Moreover, bladder rupture rarely is an isolated injury and rarely presents without a fracture of the pelvis. The bladder is an extraperitoneal organ located in the space of Retzius posterior to the symphysis pubis. In children up to age 6, the bladder is an intraperitoneal organ. Blunt forces are directed to the dome of the bladder, where the urachus originates during embryonic life. Because of this developmental hiatus, the bladder dome is attenuated and represents the anatomic area most susceptible to rupture from blunt trauma.[10, 11]

Ninety to ninety-five percent of bladder ruptures present with gross hematuria. A plain film of the pelvis should be obtained prior to retrograde cystogram; accuracy approaches 85% to 100%. Three hundred and fifty to four hundred milliliters of a water-soluble contrast agent are instilled under gravity, and an anteroposterior roentgenogram is obtained. A drainage or post-void film is essential to identify extraperitoneal leakage that is not detected on the initial full-distention cystogram. Computed tomography with an on-table cystogram and a post-void scan have been demonstrated to have equivalent accuracy. Investigation of the bladder should never rely solely on an IVP, which can miss 15% of bladder injuries. Thirty-five to fifty percent of bladder injuries are contusions; diagnosis is by exclusion on cystogram.

Extraperitoneal injuries account for 66% to 75% of bladder ruptures. Expectant management with large-bore Foley catheter drainage and parenteral antibiotics is the standard of care for the patient with extraperitoneal bladder rupture. If the patient's urine is known or thought to be infected prior to the traumatic event, consideration must be given to both catheter drainage and surgical placement of drains in the perivesicular space to prevent the possibility of subsequent extraperitoneal infection. If urinary drainage is inadequate due to blood clot, a suprapubic cystostomy should be placed. Intraperitoneal bladder rupture causes extravasation of blood and urine into the peritoneal cavity and occurs in 17% to 30% of patients with bladder rupture. Combined intraperitoneal and extraperitoneal bladder rupture occurs in 5% to 10% of patients. The operation usually requires a two- to three-layer closure with chromic or polyglycolic acid sutures.[4, 10, 11]

BLUNT INJURY TO THE URETER

Blunt trauma does not commonly damage the ureter, owing to its protection by the latissimus dorsi and iliopsoas muscles. It is thought that violent torso hyperextension is capable of producing ureteral avulsion. Hematuria is characteristically microscopic. Missed ureteral injury ultimately is manifested by fever, flank mass, malaise, ileus, leukocytosis, or urinary fistulas. Avulsion of the ureter with development of urinoma increases the serum blood urea nitrogen level without causing a corresponding increase in serum creatinine, exaggerating the normal blood urea nitrogen-creatinine ratio. Ureteral injuries secondary to external trauma are relatively rare and are almost exclusively associated with penetrating trauma.[4]

Distal injuries should always be treated with a ureteroneocystostomy. Midureteral injuries require primary repair and should be spatulated. The outcome depends on the care taken in the initial mobilization of the ureter. The gonadal vessels and fat surrounding the ureter must be left attached to the injured segment to preserve as much collateral blood supply as possible.[4, 12] Primary repairs must always be stented and externally drained. If the repair is tenuous, a nephrostomy tube may be placed. Very close follow-up is required when stents are removed because of the high risk of delayed stricture. Delayed reconstruction with an interposed section of ileum is an option when a large segment of ureter is lost, making primary repair impossible. In these instances, ligation of the ureter and placement of a nephrostomy tube for drainage is the appropriate initial management; reconstruction is performed at 3 to 4 months. Also, in the unstable patient, the ureter can be divided and the proximal end brought up as a percutaneous nephrostomy.[10] Distal ureteral injuries are better managed by implantation (i.e., bladder hitch or a Boari flap).[1, 10]

BLUNT INJURY TO THE KIDNEY

Upper tract renal trauma secondary to blunt injury is rarely isolated and is often associated with disruption of other vital organs. However, the renal injury itself can be solely responsible for the observed morbidity and mortality and therefore demands immediate operative intervention. Blunt renal trauma is five times more common than penetrating trauma and accounts for 80% to 85% of all renal injuries. Approximately 20% of blunt renal injuries are associated with intraperitoneal injury, whereas 80% of penetrating trauma injuries are associated with intraperitoneal injury.

The American Association for the Surgery of Trauma has proposed a grading system to simplify the approach, evaluation, and management of renal injuries.[2] Grade I renal injuries are characterized as contusions or subcapsular hematomas without laceration; Grade II injuries are nonexpanding perirenal hematomas or cortical lacerations less than 1 cm deep without urinary extravasation; Grade III injuries are lacerations extending more than 1 cm into the cortex without urinary extravasation; Grade IV lacerations extend through the corticomedullary junction and into the collection system, or include a main renal artery or vein injury; and Grade V injuries include a shattered kidney or avulsion of the renal pedicle.

Treatment of minor renal injuries (Grades I and II) is observation. Patients with gross hematuria are admitted and placed on bed rest until the urine becomes clear. If hematuria persists, angiography and selected embolization should be performed.[1, 2] Management of major renal lacerations and pedicle injuries (Grades III to IV) in the hemodynamically stable patient continues to evolve. [2-4, 10] The literature increasingly points to a high success rate with nonoperative management in the majority of patients with Grade III to V injuries, and advancements in interventional angiography, endourologic and percutaneous techniques have lessened the morbidity of complications such as retroperitoneal urine collections, persistent urinary extravasation, and arteriovenous fistulas. Advocates of immediate surgical interventions for major lacerations (particularly injuries associated with urinary extravasation or devitalized segments) believe that debridement and repair maximize renal function and prevent the development of late complications. They believe that expectant management prolongs hospitalization and increases the rate of complications such as sepsis and post-traumatic hypertension. Those who fear nonoperative management believe that renal salvage is best maximized by observation, with surgery reserved for patients who develop complications amenable to angiography, endourology, or percutaneous drainage. They do not believe that delayed intervention is worse than the risk of a nephrectomy associated with immediate exploration.[2] Nonoperative management has been shown to be cost effective, and has the potential to maximize preservation of renal function. Specific indications for early surgical intervention include (1) an unconfined, expanding hematoma, (2) extensive, uncontrolled urinary extravasation, (3) large, nonviable renal fragments, and (4) uncomplete staging. However, the trauma victim who demonstrates persistent hemodynamic instability despite appropriate reconstruction requires prompt surgical intervention, and observation should not be attempted.

No accurate marker for renal injury exists, and the degree of renal trauma is not predicted by the degree of hematuria. Renal artery avulsions, intimal lacerations, and renal venous and pedicle injuries also are classified as significant injuries. In the stable patient, computed tomography with intravenous and oral contrast or an IVP represent an adequate initial work-up for upper tract injuries. Nonvisualization of the kidney requires angiography. Complete transection or thrombosis of the main renal artery can be repaired if it is detected early. Segmental renal artery injuries can be managed by ligation. The time period for functional recovery after renal artery repair is generally agreed to be 12 hours or less.[4, 10]

A midline transabdominal incision is recommended. This incision also allows assessment of other intra-abdominal organs. Vascular control of the renal vascular pedicle should be considered in all patients before Gerota's fascia is opened. Several studies show that nephrectomy is reduced with proper vascular control.[4, 5, 10] If medial vascular control cannot be performed safely, or if an extensive retroperitoneal hematoma extends to the midline, an expeditious lateral approach (without entering Gerota's fascia) can be performed with placement of noncrushing vascular clamps across the entire pedicle followed by selected vascular isolation. Nonviable tissue can be removed by means of a partial nephrectomy. Segmental vessels are ligated, and tears in the collecting system should be repaired with continuous 4–0 chromic or polyglycolic sutures.

Careful attention should be paid to obtaining a water-tight closure. Injection of methylene blue or indigo carmine should identify any collecting system leaks. If possible, the renal capsule should be reapproximated to provide hemostasis and promote healing. A pedicle of omentum can be used to cover the defect when the capsule has been destroyed or devitalized. Occasionally, deceleration may devascularize a large segment of the kidney. In these cases, partial nephrectomy is performed. Coverage of the partial nephrectomy surface is important and can be obtained using the remaining capsule, a pedicle of omentum, a synthetic bolster, or a mesh wrap (e.g., polypropylene and polyglycolic mesh). A closed suction drain is placed to control any consequent urinary leakage. The placement of a drain for bleeding or a hematoma is typically ineffective.[4, 5] Renal preservation is likely in 85% to 95% of patients who undergo exploration and reconstruction.

BLUNT TRAUMA TO THE EXTERNAL GENITALIA

Complete amputation of the penis rarely occurs; if it occurs it is often self-inflicted. The severed penis should be kept cool and moist, and the patient should be assessed for other injuries. If reimplantation is undertaken the first step is urethroplasty. No attempt is made to repair the tiny corporal arteries. Microsurgical anastomoses of one or both dorsal arteries, the main dorsal vein, and the nerves are performed.[4] Repair of the external genitalia in the unstable patient with multiple trauma can generally be managed by compression dressings for control of bleeding,[10] wound irrigation, and preservation of organ viability. Generally a tear or bleeding can be easily controlled by direct suturing or ligation while more critical injuries are addressed. Tissue desiccation and injudicious debridement of tissue that initially appears marginally perfused should be avoided, and the urology service members should be consulted for definitive treatment.

References

1. Carlin BI, Resnick MI: Indications and techniques for urologic evaluation of the trauma patient with suspected urologic injury. Semin Urol 1995;13(1):9–24.
2. Matthews LA, Spisnak JP: The non-operative approach to major blunt renal trauma. Semin Urol 1995;13(1):77–82.
3. Mirvis SE: Trauma. Radiol Clin North Am 1996;34(6):1225–1257.
4. Skinner EC, Parisky YR, Skinner DG: Management of complex urologic injuries. Surg Clin North Am 1996;76(4):861–878.
5. Nguyen HT, Carroll PR: Blunt renal trauma: Renal preservation through careful staging and selective surgery. Semin Urol 1995;13(1):83–89.
6. Kirton OC, Jacobs JP, Carrillo EH, et al: Incidental finding occult hydronephrosis after blunt abdominal trauma. Eur J Emerg Med 1994;1:139–144.
7. Medina J, Caldamone A. Pediatric renal trauma: Special considerations. Semin Urol 1995;13(1):73–76.
8. Griebling TL, Kreder KJ: Urethral reconstruction after pelvic fracture with urethral disruption: The gold standard. Semin Urol 1995;13(1):45–55.
9. Koraitim MM: Pelvic fracture urethral injuries: Evaluation of various methods of management. J Urol 1996;156:1288–1291.
10. Coburn M: Damage control for urologic injuries. Surg Clin North Am 1997;77(4):821–833.
11. Kotkin L, Koch MO: Morbidity associated with non-operative management of extraperitoneal bladder injuries. J Trauma 1995;38(6):895–898.
12. Rosen DM, Korda AR, Waugh RC: Ureteric injury at burch colposuspension. Aust N Z J Obstet Gynecol 1996;36(3):354–358.

Chapter 13

Rectal Trauma

The index of suspicion for a rectal injury is based on a knowledge of pelvic anatomy and the type of injury sustained. The most common traumatic injuries to the rectum result from penetrating gunshot wounds.[1-3] Other penetrating injuries occur with shotgun wounds, stab wounds, falls with impalement, sexual assaults or misadventures, and iatrogenic causes (endoscopic procedures, radiographic procedures, therapeutic manipulations, and enemas).[3-7] Blunt trauma is a less common cause of rectal injury but can occur with severe pelvic fractures and falls associated with perineal lacerations.[5-7]

ANATOMY

The rectum is approximately 15 cm in length in situ and is divided into the intraperitoneal and extraperitoneal segments. The intraperitoneal segment is 7 to 8 cm in length and extends from the rectosigmoid junction (the level of the sacral promontory) to the peritoneal reflection. The rectosigmoid junction can be recognized as the point where the three discrete taeniae coli diverge to form the outer longitudinal muscle layer. Other findings delineating the rectosigmoid junction include the termination of epiploic tags, sacculations, and obvious mesentery. The extraperitoneal segment begins at the level of the middle valve of Houston, which is approximately at the level of the anterior peritoneal reflection. This segment extends approximately 8 cm to the level of the anorectal ring formed by the pelvic floor muscles or the top of the anal canal (i.e., Alcock's canal). If the anorectal ring is divided, fecal incontinence usually occurs. Posteriorly, the rectum is related to the sacrum, coccyx, the levator ani muscles, the medial sacral vessels, and the root of the sacral nerve plexus.[8] Anteriorly, in men, the extraperitoneal rectum is related to the prostate, seminal vesicles, vas deferens, and bladder. In women, the extraperitoneal rectum lies behind the posterior vaginal wall.

The pelvic floor musculature is formed mostly by the levator ani muscle, which consists of three muscles: the iliococcygeus, the pubococcygeus, and the puborectalis. Potential spaces around the anorectal region are significant, especially if they are infected. Injuries below the peritoneal reflection may result in infections in these anatomic spaces. Posterior wall injuries usually develop infectious tracts that extend caudally in the retrorectal or supralevator spaces (presacral space); lateral wall injuries usually create infections that extend to the ischioanal (ischiorectal) and intersphincteric spaces. Anterior wall injuries usually are associated with adjacent organ injuries.[9, 10] Associated injuries that occur in the majority of patients include (in descending order of frequency) injuries of the bladder, small bowel, colon, pelvic fracture, pelvic arteries, and ureter.[3, 15, 16]

The arterial supply to the rectum is derived principally from the superior and inferior rectal arteries; the middle rectal artery has a variable contribution. The superior rectal artery is a continuation of the inferior mesenteric artery and bifurcates into left and right branches that ultimately anastomose with the middle rectal arteries. The inferior rectal arteries arise from the pudendal arteries, which themselves arise from the internal iliac artery, and supply the anal sphincters. The middle rectal arteries arise from the anterior divisions of the internal iliac arteries. There are no obvious anastomoses with the other rectal arteries, and they contribute insignificantly to the blood supply of the rectum.

The fascia propria (i.e., the pelvic fascia that covers the posterior part of the rectum that is devoid of peritoneum) envelops the rectal vessels. Below the anterior peritoneal reflection this fascia condenses on either side of the rectum to form the lateral ligaments (lateral stalks). These ligaments support the rectum, attaching it to the pelvic side wall (parietal pelvic fascia). The retrosacral fascia, known as Waldeyer's fascia, is a portion of the parietal pelvic fascia that runs from the level of the fourth sacral vertebral segment and attaches to the fascia propria at the anorectal junction. Anteriorly, the extraperitoneal rectum is covered with a visceral pelvic fascia known as Denonvilliers' fascia. This fascia extends from the anterior peritoneal reflection to the urogenital diaphragm. It separates the rectum from the prostate gland and seminal vesicles or vagina.

ADVANCED TRAUMA LIFE SUPPORT PROTOCOL

Routine Advanced Trauma Life Support (ATLS) protocols should be followed in all patients who sustain penetrating or blunt trauma.[11] A primary survey (assessment) of the *airway, breathing, circulation, and disability* is necessary. The patient should then be completely exposed to allow the detailed secondary survey. A complete abdominal examination is performed as well as genital, perineal, and digital rectal examinations. The examiner should be concerned about microscopic or macroscopic evidence of blood on the digital rectal examination. After the rectal examination, a urinary drainage catheter is passed to allow inspection of the urine; if found, hematuria is an indication that the urinary system (bladder or other retroperitoneal structure) has sustained an injury as well. Levine and colleagues demonstrated the inadequacies of fecal guaiac testing in identifying rectal injuries.[12] They found that guaiac testing associated with rectal injuries had a 69% sensitivity and 33% specificity rate. A negative test result does not mean that the diagnosis of a rectal injury should not be pursued if the index of suspicion is high. Gross blood or blood mixed with stool and/or a positive sigmoidoscopic examination (for blood) is a positive predictor of rectal injury in 80% to 96% of cases.[13–17] Burch and colleagues[3] from Baylor found that a heme positive rectal examination had an 80% positive predictive value for rectal injury. Blood was noted in 88% of patients undergoing protoscopy when blood was present on digital rectal examination and in 38% when *no* blood was present on digital rectal examination.[3]

The mechanism of injury must be identified, and other related factors (e.g.,

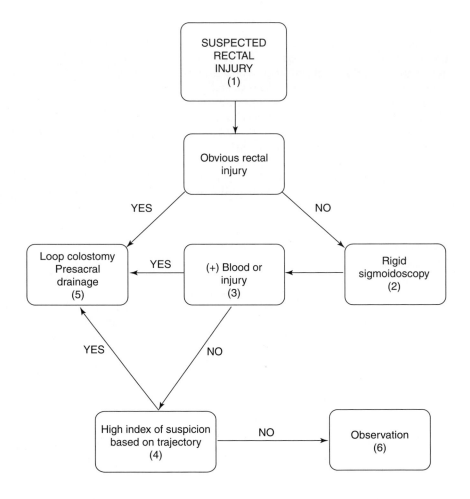

1. A rectal injury is suspected based on the history and physical examination, including a digital rectal examination and, if necessary (based on suspicion), rigid sigmoidoscopy. If an abdominal, pelvic, gluteal, perineal, or proximal thigh wound is encountered, a rectal injury must be suspected and evaluated.
2. When the examination indicates an acute abdomen and an urgent laparotomy is imminent but a rectal wound is suspected, the surgeon must plan to perform rigid sigmoidoscopy before the end of the case. This simple procedure *must* be performed because a positive finding requires a change in operative management. Preferably, if the circumstances allow, sigmoidoscopy should be performed at the end of the secondary survey to look for an injury or, more commonly, evidence of blood.
3. Patients with rectal blood or an injury identified during the physical examination or secondary survey require operative intervention. Gross blood or blood mixed with stool and/or positive results on a sigmoidoscopic examination (for blood) are positive predictors of rectal injury in 80% to 96% of cases.
4. During the secondary survey, all entrance and possible exit wounds must be identified to allow trajectory mapping. Projection of the trajectory of the gunshot is most important to assess potential injuries adequately. Suspicion of an injury based on the trajectory of a bullet constitutes sufficient evidence to treat the patient for a rectal injury.
5. Diversion is accomplished by performing a sigmoid loop colostomy. This procedure does not require a formal laparotomy if the injury is limited to the extraperitoneal rectum and there is no other indication for an exploratory laparotomy. A "mini" laparotomy is sufficient if there are no other indications for a formal exploratory laparotomy. A laparoscopic assisted loop colostomy is another option. Presacral or transperineal drainage should *always* be employed for management of rectal injuries. One or two 3- to 4-cm curvilinear incisions are made outside the lateral margin of the anal sphincters, and these are extended through the endopelvic fascia into the presacral space (Fig. 13–1). One or two 1-inch Penrose drains should be placed adjacent to the rectal injury or injuries and sutured to the perineal skin.
6. Patients who are admitted for observation *must* undergo serial abdominal examinations. If the condition of the patient deteriorates or if peritonitis develops, operative intervention is warranted. Missed isolated extraperitoneal rectal injuries may become manifest as new-onset fever or as rectal or perineal pain; reevaluation is then mandatory.

combined blunt and penetrating injuries, multiple penetrating injuries, type and caliber of weapon) must be elucidated. The trajectory of gunshot wounds must be mapped, noting the entrance and exit wounds. For patients with multiple penetrating gunshot injuries, a simple rule is that the number of entrance and exit wounds *plus* the number of bullets (visible on radiographs) should be an even number. If this equation produces an odd number, either a wound or a bullet is missing, and the secondary survey should be repeated. In the series reported by DiGiacomo and associates[14] from the University of Pennsylvania, the wound trajectory correctly predicted the presence or absence of injuries requiring surgical intervention in 93% of their patients.[14] Radiographic procedures are indicated if improved trajectory mapping is necessary and to look for associated injuries and retained foreign bodies.

INTERVENTIONS

There are case reports of nonoperative management of rectal gunshot wounds.[5] As stated by Burch and colleagues, "Certainly some of these injuries will heal satisfactorily without surgery; however, selecting the appropriate patients must be difficult and the consequences of failure may be severe. This approach is not recommended."[3] Other less severe rectal injuries (i.e., iatrogenic incomplete perforations) can be treated without surgery. In these patients, admission with actual not just intended serial abdominal examinations is warranted. If the condition of the patient deteriorates or if other signs and symptoms of peritonitis or rectal injury become evident, an operation is performed.

Operative intervention is performed when (1) rectal injury is obvious, (2) blood is found on rigid sigmoidoscopy with or without evidence of an injury, and, (3) injury is suspected based on physical evidence or the trajectory of the penetrating object.[3, 14, 15, 18] Parenteral antibiotics that cover the lower intestinal flora (aerobes and anaerobes) should be used. The first dose should be given prior to laparotomy, and the antibiotics should be continued for 24 hours.[19, 27]

The goals of laparotomy are to control hemorrhage from intra-abdominal (intraperitoneal) injuries, contain enteric spillage and contamination, and evaluate and manage associated injuries. Most intraperitoneal rectal injuries can be repaired primarily.[20, 21] Those that are associated with extensive soft tissue trauma will probably require resection with primary reanastomosis.

Extraperitoneal rectal injuries are usually not repaired unless they are visualized during exposure of other closely associated structures (e.g., iliac vessels, bladder, and vagina. The techniques needed to manage extraperitoneal rectal injuries are diversion of the fecal stream and presacral drainage.[3, 5, 15, 16, 24, 25]

Diversion is accomplished by performing a sigmoid loop colostomy. This procedure does not require a formal laparotomy if the injury is limited to the extraperitoneal rectum and there is no other indication for an exploratory laparotomy. Methods of forming the loop sigmoid colostomy include the laparoscopic assisted technique and the limited laparotomy. The "bridge" (a device used to support the loop at or above the skin level) should elevate the central portion of the loop well above the skin level so that spillover is unlikely and the colostomy diverts the fecal stream completely. Maturation of the colostomy is recommended at the time of operation; this is achieved by suturing the mucosa of the colon to the skin. The bridge or supporting rod is removed on postoperative day 7. That loop colostomy is sufficient for complete diversion was demonstrated by Rombeau and associates[22] in a prospective study that made use of barium meals; the loop colostomy completely diverted the fecal stream even though the loop was not divided. Advantages of the loop colostomy are ease of construction and a simpler reconstruction at the time of closure. In a controlled, prospective, randomized trial, Velmahos and colleagues[23] compared early colostomy closure (performed within the first 15 postoperative days) with late colostomy closure (after postoperative day 90, performed in a second admission).[23] The operating time was shorter and there was less intraoperative blood loss in the early colostomy closure group. These authors also found that reconstruction of a loop colostomy was associated with decreased operative time and less blood loss than reconstruction of a divided colostomy. They identified nonhealing distal bowel, persistent wound sepsis, and persistent postoperative instability as contraindications to early closure.

Presacral and transperineal drainage should be employed for management of rectal injuries. This remains an issue of controversy and one that has not yet been resolved by a randomized prospective trial; therefore, we continue to advocate its use in all cases. An undrained injury dramatically increases the incidence of associated infection and morbidity.[24] This may be explained by the high proportion of fat in the retrorectal area, its relative avascularity, and fecal contamination of traumatized tissues.[6, 25] The drain or drains should be placed adjacent to the site of injury. One or two 3- to 4-cm curvilinear incisions are made outside the lateral margin of the anal sphincters and extended through the endopelvic fascia into the presacral space (see Fig. 13–1). A 1-inch Penrose drain is typically used. It is advanced with a finger or instrument to a position adjacent to the rectal injury and is then sutured to the perineal skin. This procedure is done after the abdominal wound has been closed and a dressing has been applied. These drains are removed in 5 to 7 days unless purulent or fecal drainage persists.

Irrigation of the distal rectum may be used at the discretion of the surgeon. There are conflicting reports about this in the literature. Support (decreased morbidity) for distal rectal washout was derived from wartime experience.[26] Because the procedure is time consuming and cumbersome, it could be reserved for patients with large extraperitoneal rectal wounds or high-velocity gunshot injuries. The benefit of distal rectal washout has not been confirmed in patients with the typical civilian low-velocity gunshot wound to the extraperitoneal rectum.[3, 15] If distal rectal washout is used, the technique is as follows: Sterile normal saline is introduced into the distal loop of the colostomy while continuous manual anal dilatation is maintained. The saline bag is elevated 2 to 3 feet above the level of the patient, and the infusion is performed using gravity (not pressure). The contaminated irrigation may go through the injured rectum into the perirectal space; hence, adequate presacral drainage is still needed, even after irrigation.

COMPLICATIONS

The potential for complications is usually associated with the degree of injury. Fistulas can occur from the site of injury to the presacral drain tract or to adjacent organs. Inadequate or incomplete drainage can lead to abscess formation (pelvic sepsis) in one or more of the perirectal spaces previously described. Armstrong and colleagues demonstrated a more than 50% reduction in the incidence of pelvic infections with the use of presacral drains.[23] Missile tract infections as well as wound infections do occur. The use (preoperatively and perioperatively) of appropriate antibiotics that cover aeorbic (especially enterococcus) and anaerobic organisms can reduce the overall infection rate.[27]

SUMMARY

Based on present knowledge, recommendations for the diagnosis and treatment of rectal injures are as follows: (1) Digital examination *and* rigid sigmoidoscopy should be performed, but false-negative results may occur in up to 5% of cases. (2) Projection of the trajectory of the missile is useful in identifying rectal injury in up to 93% of cases. (3) Operation should be performed if an injury even is *suspected*. (4) Descending loop colostomy and transperineal presacral drainage are considered appropriate operative treatment by most authors today.

References

1. Abcarian H: Rectal trauma. Gastroenterol Clin North Am 1987;16:115–123.
2. Lung JA, Turk RP, Miller RE, et al: Wounds of the rectum. Ann Surg 1970;172:985–990.
3. Burch JM, Feliciano, DV, Mattox KL: Colostomy and drainage for civilian rectal injuries: Is that all? Ann Surg 1989;209:600–611.
4. Bousamra M, Guisto DF, Gervin AS: Rectal impalement. Surg Rounds 1990; Dec, 55–59.
5. Haas PA, Fox TA: Civilian injuries of the rectum and anus. Dis Colon Rectum 1979;22:17–23.
6. Marcet JE, Gottesman L: Anorectal trauma and necrotizing infections. *In* Beck DE, Wexner SD (eds): Fundamentals of Anorectal Surgery. New York, McGraw-Hill, 1992, pp. 440–452.
7. Smith L: Traumatic injuries. *In* Gordon PH, Nivatvongs S (eds): Principles and Practice of Surgery for the Colon, Rectum, and Anus. St. Louis, Quality Medical Publishing, 1992, pp. 957–980.
8. Pemberton JH: Anatomy and physiology of the anus and rectum. *In* Shackelford's Surgery of the Alimentary Tract, 3rd ed. Philadelphia, WB Saunders, 1991, p. 243.
9. Nivatvongs S, Gordon, PH: Surgical anatomy. *In* Gordon PH, Nivatvongs S (eds): Principles and Practice of Surgery for the Colon, Rectum, and Anus. St. Louis, Quality Medical Publishing, 1992, pp. 4–37.
10. Pemberton JH: Anatomy and physiology of the anus and rectum. *In* Beck DE, Wexner SD (eds): Fundamentals of Anorectal Surgery. New York, McGraw-Hill, 1992, pp. 1–24.
11. American College of Surgeons, Committee on Trauma: Advanced Trauma Life Support. Chicago, American College of Surgeons, 1997.
12. Levine H, Simon RJ, Smith TR, et al: Guaiac testing in the diagnosis of rectal trauma: What is the value? J Trauma 1992;32:210.
13. Mangiante EC, Graham AD, Fabian TC: Rectal gunshot wounds. Am Surg 1986;52:37.
14. DiGiacomo JC, Schwab CW, Rotondo MF, et al: Gluteal gunshot wounds: Who warrants exploration? J Trauma 1994;37:622–628.
15. Levy RD, Strauss P, Aladgem D, et al: Extraperitoneal rectal gunshot injuries. J Trauma 1995;38:273–277.
16. Tuggle D, Huber PJ: Management of rectal trauma. Am J Surg 1984;148:806–808.
17. Fallon WF, Reyna TM, Brunner RG, et al: Penetrating trauma to the buttock. South Med J 1988;81:1236–1238.
18. Duncan AO, Phillips TF, Scalea TM, et al: Management of transpelvic gunshot wounds. J Trauma 1989;29:1335–1340.

19. Fabian TC, Croce MA, Payne LW, et al: Duration of antibiotic therapy for penetrating abdominal trauma: A prospective trial. Surgery 1992;112:788–795.
20. Stone HH, Fabian TC: Management of penetrating colon trauma: Randomization between primary closure and exteriorization. Ann Surg 1979;190:430–436.
21. George SM, Fabian TC, Voeller GR, et al: Primary repair of colon wounds. Ann Surg 1989;209:728–734.
22. Rombeau JL, Wilk PJ, Turnbull RB, Fazio VW: Total fecal diversion by the temporary skin-level loop transverse colostomy. Dis Colon Rectum 1978;21:223–226.
23. Velmahos GC, Degiannis E, Wells M, et al: Early closure of colostomies in trauma patients—A prospective randomized trial. Surgery 1995;118:815–820.
24. Armstrong RG, Schmitt HJ, Jr, Patterson LT: Combat wounds of the extraperitoneal rectum. Surgery 1973;74:570–583.
25. Trunkey D, Hays RJ, Shires GT: Management of rectal trauma. J Trauma 1973;13:411–415.
26. Laverson GJ, Cohen A: Management of rectal injuries. Am J Surg 1971;122:515.
27. Weigelt JA, Easley SM, Thal ER, et al: Abdominal surgical wound infection is lowered with improved perioperative *Enterococcus* and *Bacteroides* therapy. J Trauma 1993;34:579–585.

Chapter 14

Pelvic Fractures

Mortality from pelvic fractures remains as high as 60%, with major hemorrhage accounting for as many as 65% of the deaths. Associated injuries found in victims with significant pelvic fractures may account for a large proportion of these deaths.[1] Emergent treatment of the fracture and hemorrhage may include application of military antishock trousers (MAST), external skeletal fixation, and arterial embolization, the chosen therapy being at least partially dictated by the stability of the fracture. Though orthopedic consultation is required in most instances, an understanding of pelvic fractures by the trauma surgeon aids in producing an optimal therapeutic decision in this potentially lethal injury.

Ligamentous support of the pelvis includes contributions from the sacroiliac (SI), sacrospinous (SS), and sacrotuberous (ST) ligaments posteriorly and from the symphysis pubis and anterior sacroiliac ligaments anteriorly. Posterior vertically positioned ligaments (long posterior sacroiliac ligaments, sacrotuberous and lateral lumbosacral ligaments) provide vertical stability. Damage to the transverse ligaments (short posterior sacroiliac, anterior sacroiliac, iliolumbar, and sacrospinous ligaments) results in rotational instability. Fractures through the iliac wing simulate ligamentous disruption, which shows the same instability patterns.

Various classification systems of pelvic fractures can be found in the literature, but the underlying theme of these systems is an attempt to define stability.[2-4] Singular fractures (pelvic ring, rami, acetabulum) have traditionally been classified as stable, but isotope scanning has proved the invariable presence of a second injury in pelvic ring fractures, some of which lead to significant instability. Young and colleagues[2] and Young and Resnick[4] defined a system based on directional forces of injury, and Tile developed a system based both on directional forces and on stability.[3] Although the Tile system groups injuries by stability, the Young-Burgess system also defines injuries by stability and is perhaps easier to use. Injuries are classified into one of three categories: lateral compression, anterior-posterior compression, or vertical shear (Fig. 14–1). Knowledge of vector forces, fracture pattern, and ligamentous anatomy allows a clinical assessment of stability and the requirements for therapy.

Force applied from the side results in a lateral compression fracture. Force applied to the posterior aspect of the lateral surface thrusts the ilium onto the sacrum, resulting in a stable impaction fracture that produces no significant physiologic or ligamentous damage (Type I fracture). Forces applied anteriorly rotate the fracture segment inward, disrupting the posterior SI joint (Type II) and fracturing the pubic rami horizontally. If this force is stronger, it is transmitted to the contralateral hemipelvis, disrupting the anterior SI joint and the SS and ST ligaments and rotating the contralateral hemipelvis externally

172

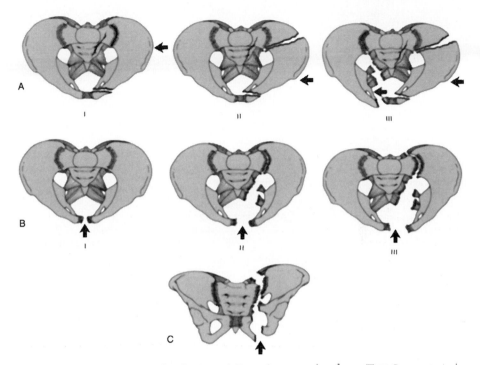

Figure 14–1. Young Burgess classification. *A*, Lateral compression force. Type I: a posteriorly directed force causing a sacral crush and horizontal pubic rami fractures ipsilaterally. This is a stable injury. Type II: a more anteriorly directed force causing horizontal pubic rami fractures with an anterior sacral crush and disruption of either the posterior sacroiliac joints or fractures through the iliac wing. This is an ipsilateral injury. Type III: an anteriorly directed force that is continued, leading to a type I or type II ipsilateral fracture with an external rotation component to the contralateral side, opening the sacroiliac joint posteriorly and disrupting the sacrotuberous and spinous ligaments. *B*, Anteroposterior compression fractures. Type I: an anteroposterior-directed force opening the pelvis but with the posterior ligamentous structures intact. This is stable. Type II: continuation of a type I fracture with disruption of the sacrospinous and potentially the sacrotuberous ligaments and an anterior sacroiliac joint opening. This is rotationally unstable. Type III: a completely unstable or a vertical instability pattern with complete disruption of all ligamentous supporting structures. *C*, A vertically directed force or forces at right angles to the supporting structures of the pelvis leading to vertical fractures in the rami and disruption of all the ligamentous structures. This is equivalent to an anteroposterior type III or a completely unstable and rotationally unstable fracture. (Redrawn with permission from Young JWR, Burgess AR: Radiologic Management of Pelvic Ring Fractures. Baltimore-Munich, Urban & Schwarzenberg, 1987.)

while internally rotating the ipsilateral side. This Type III injury is completely unstable and is associated with significant brain and abdominal visceral injury.

Anterior-posterior compression injuries are also subdivided into three categories, which also progress to complete instability in Type III fractures. In Type I injuries the anterior pelvis is disrupted by a fracture of the pelvic rami (vertically) or a rupture of the ligaments of the symphysis pubis. Diastasis of less than 2.5 cm defines a Type I injury, which is not associated with posterior ligamentous damage. A stronger force splays the pelvis open further, and causes

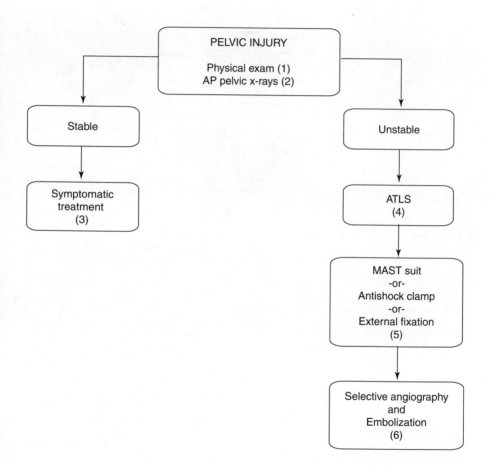

1. Tests for pelvic stability on physical examination include the use of lateral and anterior-posterior compression. Fractures of the pelvic rami can be detected by exerting pressure over the pubic symphysis, eliciting pain or movement. Posterior pressure with the examiner's hands placed over the anterior superior iliac spines and medial pressure with the hands over the lateral iliac crests tests for fractues of the pelvic ring and rotational instability. Acetabular, femoral neck, and vertical shear fractures may be manifest with a foreshortened ipsilateral lower extremity.
2. Anteroposterior (AP) pelvic radiographs should be obtained in all patients with blunt trauma of the torso. The need for pelvic films in the patient with a penetrating injury is determined by the location of the wound and the type of weapon used (e.g., a gunshot wound of the chest might require radiographs to locate the bullet, whereas a stab wound would not). Displacement of the pubic symphysis and sacroiliac joint and fractures of the bony structures of the pelvic ring can be evaluated with a single AP radiograph. Specialized views (inlet, outlet, and so on) should be ordered by the orthopedic surgeon as needed. Computed tomograms of the pelvis are essential for evaluation of the posterior elements.
3. The hemodynamically stable patient who has a stable pelvic fracture should be evaluated for 24 hours in an intensive care unit setting to monitor hematocrit values. Mobilization of the patient over the ensuing days is dictated by the nature of the fracture. Pelvic fractures, regardless of their extent, are painful. Pain control, usually achieved with narcotics, is important to ensure a functional return to activity. Physical therapy is usually helpful and should be instituted early in the course of treatment of the injury and rehabilitation. Consultation with the orthopedic surgery service should be obtained to determine the degree of weight bearing allowable for each individual fracture.
4. Persistent hypotension and/or tachycardia in the presence of a falling hematocrit must be treated with aggressive fluid resuscitation, which may include blood transfusions. Advanced Trauma Life Support (ATLS) protocols should be followed closely. Although significant hemorrhage may result from a fractured pelvis, hemodynamic instability is multifactorial, and aggressive and prompt evaluation of the chest and abdomen must be carried out. Hemothoraces or pneumothoraces should be quickly decompressed with tube thoracostomy. Intra-abdominal injuries should be evaluated with diagnostic peritoneal lavage (DPL) or ultrasonography in unstable patients or with computed tomography (if necessary) in stable patients, and exploratory laparotomy should be performed as needed.
5. Control of bleeding in the fractured pelvis is of paramount importance to prevent excessive transfusion requirements and the potential severe complications of adult respiratory distress syndrome (ARDS), sepsis, multiple organ system failure (MOSF), and death. Initial management measures include use of the MAST suit, which must be inflated to 40 mmHg, or, when available and applicable, the pelvic antishock clamp. Both can be applied quickly and easily in the trauma resuscitation room or emergency room and can close down the pelvic ring, favoring tamponade and slowing or halting ongoing hemorrhage. *Note:* A MAST suit applied at 40 mmHg of pressure may cause respiratory compromise and may require intubation and assisted ventilation of the patient. External fixation is also an alternative to achieve pelvic stabilization but requires an orthopedic surgeon, and usually an operating room and therefore necessitates some delay. Emergent reduction may be accomplished with the MAST suit or pelvic antishock clamp, with definitive reduction by external fixation scheduled some hours later.
6. Patients with ongoing pelvic hemorrhage despite use of the previously outlined measures and correction of coagulopathy should undergo prompt selective angiography. Delay in definitive therapy only increases transfusion requirements and prolongs the coagulopathy. Evidence of extravasation of contrast on pelvic CT scans indicates vessel damage with ongoing hemorrhage and warrants immediate angiographic embolization. Although pelvic bleeding is most often venous in nature, such bleeding ought to tamponade early and should not be a source of instability. Selective angiography and embolization, usually with Gelfoam, is frequently effective in controlling arterial hemorrhage.

progressively more severe disruption of the ligamentous support; the pelvis remains hinged at the posterior aspects of the SI joints. The SS and ST ligaments are damaged in Type II injuries, which lead to rotational instability. When all sacroiliac ligaments are disrupted (Type III injuries), rotational and vertical instability results.

Vertical shear fractures, typified by the Malgaigne fracture, usually result from a fall in which the person lands on the lower extremities. A vertically oriented fracture through the anterior and posterior pelvis occurs, and the fracture segments are superiorly displaced. Pelvic disruption is complete and leads to a completely unstable hemipelvis. These injuries, like Type III anterior-posterior compression injuries, usually include a significant amount of abdominal visceral and pelvic vascular damage and are associated with potentially lethal retroperitoneal hemorrhage, shock, sepsis, and death.

Acetabular fractures are often associated with pelvic ring fractures.[6] Fractures through the posterior rim and posterior column are often accompanied by an anterior-posterior compression fracture, as are fractures of the anterior column. Lateral compressive forces may fracture the acetabular wall, and vertical shear injuries fracture the roof of the acetabulum.

Among the complications resulting from pelvic fractures are immobility with fat embolism and respiratory insufficiency, genitourinary trauma, and long-term disability in the form of chronic back pain and gait abnormalities. Perhaps the most significant acute complication is that due to hemorrhage. Bleeding due to venous injury is typically limited because tamponade occurs in the intact retroperitoneal space. However, this space may accumulate up to 4000 ml of blood before tamponade occurs. Using geometric principles, a 3-cm diastasis of the pubic symphysis increases the radius of the pelvis and doubles the normal volume.[4] Patients with posterior instability may require as much as 10 units more blood than those without. Cadaver studies have shown that a disrupted pelvis without prior reduction and stabilization increases in volume up to 26% when it is further destabilized by a laparotomy incision, and the pubic diastasis increases nearly threefold.[5] Bleeding in such injuries results from laceration of the superior gluteal artery, anterior branches of the internal iliac artery, the sacral venous plexus, or the fractured bony surfaces.

Therepeutic decision-making in patients with pelvic fractures is based on (1) the mechanism of injury, (2) the stability of the pelvic ring, and (3) the hemodynamic stability. Baseline hemoglobin and hematocrit levels should be obtained, along with anteroposterior pelvic bone x-rays. Additional views of the pelvis (Judet's view, inlet-outlet view, and so on) should be reserved for special request by the orthopedic service. Computed tomography is mandatory for the evaluation of posterior sacral element injuries and is helpful in evaluating the acetabulum. If blood is present at the urethral meatus, urethral injury should be suspected, and insertion of a urinary catheter should be delayed until a retrograde urethrogram (RUG) is performed. The same applies to male patients with a high-riding or boggy prostate.

If diagnostic peritoneal lavage (DPL) is used to evaluate the patient for abdominal injury, the procedure should be performed early before extensive dissection of the hematoma occurs, increasing the possibility of false-positive DPL results, and it should be performed using the open technique, which decreases the risk of entering the expanded retroperitoneal space. Although a reluctance to proceed with laparotomy, which thereby releases the tamponade, is justifiable, penetrating trauma resulting in a pelvic fracture and/or retroperitoneal hematoma must be addressed like any other penetrating abdominal injury. Any patient who sustains blunt trauma and has a positive result on DPL should similarly undergo laparotomy. If the result of lavage is negative or equivocal, or if CT examination shows a hematoma contained within the retroperitoneal space, the hemodynamically unstable patient should be immediately placed in a MAST suit inflated to 40 mmHg, and simultaneous consultation with the orthopedic service should be sought for evaluation of the patient for external fixation.[6] Prophylactic intubation should be considered early when the MAST suit is applied because 40 mmHg pressure is difficult to tolerate, even in the nontraumatized person.

External fixation in hemodynamically unstable patients with an unstable pelvis should be considered for several reasons. First, immobilization of the bone fragments will prevent further disruption of the affected vascular beds and any formed clot. In addition, as mentioned previously, reduction of the pelvic radius to normal will decrease the volume of the pelvis, thereby reducing the hemorrhage required before tamponade occurs. For patients undergoing laparotomy, external fixation should be considered preoperatively.

The antishock pelvic clamp, first reported in the American literature in 1991,[7] has been described as an alternative to the formal external fixator, which requires an orthopedic surgeon and usually an operating room to apply. The antishock pelvic clamp can be applied in the emergency room by personnel other than orthopedic surgeons if they have been properly trained. However, this clamp should be considered only as temporary fixation and used only in patients with life-threatening hemorrhage from pelvic fractures.

All patients with significant pelvic fractures or physiologic alterations resulting from such fractures should be monitored closely in the intensive care unit for ongoing blood loss as well as respiratory compromise due to decreased functional residual capacity (FRC) secondary to the MAST suit or retroperitoneal hematoma. Temperature and coagulation parameters should be normalized as quickly as possible. If bleeding continues despite all measures taken, arteriography with transcatheter embolization of damaged arteries should be performed. An interventional radiologist with experience and adherence to strict criteria are vital for effective use of the arteriography-embolization technique. Because most bleeding resulting from pelvic fractures is venous, spontaneous tamponade in the retroperitoneal space is the rule. However, if arterial injury is present, as evidenced by persistent hypotension despite crystalloid challenges, large blood transfusion requirements (four or more units in the first 24 hours), or a large expanding pelvic hematoma at laparotomy or on CT, and if an intraperitoneal source has been excluded, patients should be considered for angiography and transcatheter embolization.[8]

References

1. Poole GV, Ward EF, Muakkassa RR, et al: Pelvic fracture from major blunt trauma: outcome is determined by associated injuries. Ann Surg 1991;213(6):534.
2. Young JWR, Burgess AR, Brumbach RJ, et al: Pelvic fractures: Value of plain radiography in early assessment and management. Radiology 1986;160:445.

3. Kellman JF, Browner BD: Fractures of the pelvic ring. *In* Browner BD, Jupiter JB, Levine AM, Trafton PG (eds): Skeletal Trauma, Vol I. Philadelphia, WB Saunders, 1992, pp. 859–860.
4. Young JWR, Resnick CS: Fracture of the pelvis: Current concepts of classification. AJR Am J Roentgenol 1990;155:1169.
5. Ghanayen AJ, Wilber JH, Lieberman JM, et al: The effect of laparotomy and external fixator stabilization on pelvic volume in an unstable pelvic injury. J Trauma 1995;38(3):396.
6. Latenser BA, Gentilello LM, Tarver AA, et al: Improved outcome with early fixation of skeletally unstable pelvic fractures. J Trauma 1991;31:20.
7. Ganz R, Krushell RJ, Jakob RP, et al: The antishock pelvic clamp. Clin Orthop 1991; 267:71.
8. Panetta T, Sclafani SJ, Goldstein AS, et al: Percutaneous transcatheter embolization for massive bleeding from pelvic fractures. J Trauma 1985;25(11):1021.

Chapter 15

Penetrating Trauma of the Extremity

Penetrating trauma of the extremity runs the gamut from minor injury to life-threatening injuries in which quick action can save the victim's life and ensure a rapid return to normal activity. Just a few inches difference in the trajectory of a gunshot wound of an extremity makes the difference between an injury that requires only a few hours observation and a critical life-threatening injury of a major artery. With modern techniques (rapid evacuation, shortened ischemia time, aggressive debridement, and appropriate use of fasciotomy), the incidence of amputation following penetrating trauma to the extremities is less than 10%.[1-5] Thus, the physician who treats trauma patients must be conversant with the care required by these injuries, from resuscitation of the profoundly hypotensive patient to definitive care of complex vascular, soft tissue, and bony injuries.

ANATOMY OF THE LOWER LIMB

The lower limb is divided into six segments: hip, thigh, knee, leg, ankle, and foot. The hip is connected to the bones of the pelvic girdle and forms the uppermost aspect of the lower limb. Penetrating injuries to the superiormost aspect of the leg may involve the pelvic structures. Bleeding within the pelvis is sometimes not clinically evident, and a high degree of suspicion of pelvic pathology must be maintained.

The femur is the longest and generally the strongest bone in the human body. The upper end consists of the head, neck, and greater and lesser trochanters. The shaft separates the upper femur from the distal end, which consists of the lateral and medial epicondyle, the adductor tubercle, and the condylar surface of the knee joint. The patella is a sesamoid bone located within the quadriceps femoris tendon.

The bones of the leg are the tibia and the fibula. The tibia is the larger of the two and supports the weight of the body during ambulation. The fibula is important as a site of muscle attachment (peroneus brevis and longus, soleus, extensor digitorum longus, peroneus tertius, and extensor hallucis longus) and because it provides stability to the ankle joint by forming the lateral malleolus. The bones of the foot include the talus, calcaneus, navicular, cuboid, cuneiforms, metatarsals, and phalanges.

The arterial supply to the lower limb comprises the common femoral artery, which is a continuation of the external iliac artery after it passes under the inguinal ligament. The common femoral artery gives off the profunda femoris artery and then continues distally as the superficial femoral artery. The pro-

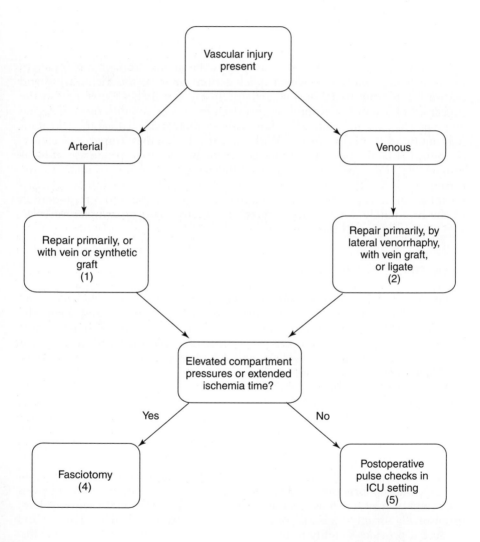

1. Repair of arterial injuries depends largely on the degree of destruction of the native vessel. A partial clean laceration of the vessel, such as that caused by a knife, may be reparable using simple suture closure. Caution is in order, however, because such a repair should not be done at the expense of the luminal diameter. If the lumen will be narrowed significantly by such a repair the vessel may be mobilized proximally and distally to effect primary and end-to-end anastomosis without the need for a graft. If this is not possible, some form of graft is used to bridge the gap between the noninjured vessel ends. Reverse saphenous vein graft is usually quite adequate and should be used preferentially in certain circumstances, for example, for vessels smaller than 6 mm or for vessels that extend across the knee joint. Synthetic grafts such as polytetrafluoroethylene (PTFE) are manufactured in a variety of sizes and are convenient and easy to use. Even in contaminated fields, these grafts do well, and they eliminate the extra time required to harvest and prepare a vein graft. Synthetic grafts less than 6 mm in diameter should be avoided to prevent thrombosis in the future. Vascular injuries can be bypassed by means of a temporary shunt in patients who are too unstable to tolerate extended operative time. When they are stable, these patients can be returned to the OR for definitive repair.

2. Venous injuries can be a challenging endeavor for the trauma surgeon because these vessels are thin walled and tear easily. As with arterial injuries, a clean partial laceration can be repaired by performing lateral venorrhaphy. A venous injury that is repaired with a vein graft frequently fails but such repairs should be attempted in locations where the vessel is the major or sole conduit (e.g., the axillary vein). The question of ligation versus repair continues to be a controversial one. Most studies indicate that thrombosis is likely in even well-repaired veins in the postoperative period, but advocates of repair believe that this period of time allows for collateralization of adjacent vessels. Venous ligation of major veins should be reserved for patients who are in an unstable condition.

3. Warm ischemia that lasts for more than 6 hours is likely to result in necrotic tissue distal to the site of injury. However, extensive data are available on the mechanism and effects of ischemia/reperfusion and the cell-damaging effects of the products of ischemia. Locally, ischemia results in interstitial edema; within nonexpansile fascial compartments, the small vessels (e.g., vasonevorum) collapse, resulting in ischemia of nerves and small vessels and ultimately ending in massive muscle necrosis.

4. The potential need for fasciotomy must be remembered at all times, and this procedure should be used liberally if the situation is at all questionable. Compartment pressures that exceed 15 mmHg are abnormal but do not necessarily require surgical intervention. Patients in whom elevated compartment pressures may develop should be examined frequently for subtle changes related to increasing pressure. Certainly any compartment should be opened with fasciotomy if the pressure rises above 40 to 50 mmHg. Compartment syndrome can occur any tissue space enveloped in a nonyielding fascia, including the abdomen. The key therapeutic maneuver is to release the constriction. Most compartment syndromes, and therefore most fasciotomies, involve the lower leg. Specifically, the lower leg has four fascial compartments, each of which must be opened to allow proper decompression. As the patient recovers and edema lessens, fasciotomy sites can be closed primarily or with skin grafts.

5. All patients undergoing vascular reconstruction should be monitored closely during the postoperative period (24 hours) for any alteration in pulse characteristics and sensorimotor function. Acute changes demand prompt evaluation, with possible return to the operating room for repair.

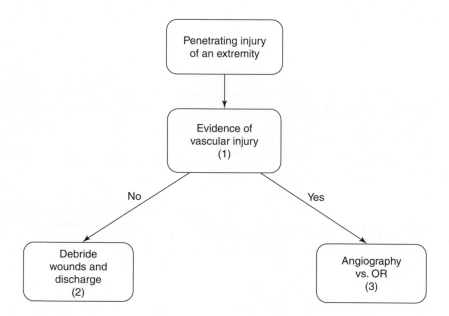

1. Hard signs of an arterial injury include the presence of an expanding hematoma, a pulsatile mass or pulsatile blood flow from the wound, lack of distal pulses on the affected side, pallor, and paresthesias. Proximity of the bullet path to a vessel does not constitute an indication for radiologic or surgical examination. Although approximately 20% of patients with pulses are found to have a vascular injury on angiography, in fact, all but about 20% of these are small intimal disruptions that will heal spontaneously and therefore do not require surgical intervention. For patients with subtle pulse changes, ankle-brachial indices or simply Doppler blood pressure measurements can be compared bilaterally. Most patients with arterial injury on physical examination do not require an angiogram because the level of injury is obvious. However, patients who have sustained shotgun blasts, those at risk of peripheral vascular occlusive disease, and those who have sustained a longitudinal gunshot wound in which the segment of vessel damaged is unclear warrant preoperative or intraoperative angiography. The fine quality of the study is not important; one is only attempting to define the level of injury.
2. If no vascular injury is suspected, entry and exit wounds should be debrided of any necrotic tissue. No attempt should be made to remove the bullet unless it is easily palpable. If the bullet is removed, handle it delicately to avoid altering the rifling (the bullet's fingerprint) and save it for forensics or law-enforcement officials. Do not close entry or exit wounds. Remember, bullets may be hot, but they are not sterile, nor is the necrotic tissue in the track of the wound.

funda femoris artery gives off many muscular branches including the medial and lateral circumflex femoral arteries, which supply the thigh. It is the rich anastomoses between these vessels with branches of the inferior gluteal artery that may allow palpable pulses in patients with penetrating injuries of the common femoral artery. The distal profunda femoris artery terminates just above the knee. The profunda femoris artery may be ligated distally because the rich collaterals about the knee from the superficial femoral artery provide adequate vascular supply in this location. The superficial femoral artery continues distally to form the popliteal artery at the adductor hiatus. Another rich anastomosis consisting of the genicular arteries and the tibial recurrent branches forms around the knee. Although these collaterals allow limb preservation if the popliteal artery is occluded during chronic atheromatous processes, they are generally not sufficient to allow limb preservation during acute trauma. Thus, an injured popliteal artery requires not only rapid diagnosis but expedient repair as well.

The popliteal artery divides into the anterior and posterior tibial arteries at the popliteus muscle, the posterior tibial being the larger branch. The posterior tibial gives off the peroneal artery deep to the soleus muscle. The anterior tibial artery continues distally to the foot, where it is known as the dorsalis pedis, while the peroneal artery also continues to the foot, where the two then form the arcuate artery. The posterior tibial artery terminates as the medial and lateral plantar arteries, which anastomose with the arcuate artery through perforating arteries. The superficial nature of the posterior tibial artery in the posteromedial leg subjects it to injury relatively easily. Anastomoses between the posterior tibial artery and the peroneal artery usually allow one of the two to be ligated without causing permanent injury to the foot.

Venous return in the lower extremity parallels arterial supply with the exception of the superficial saphenous system. The more superficial system should be well known to the surgeon because of its use as a bypass conduit and because of its propensity to form pathologic varices that require either ligation or excision. The saphenous vein should be preserved whenever possible because it may be needed for arterial repair. The saphenous vein is found distally on the anteromedial thigh and may be cannulated by way of a cutdown technique to achieve emergent venous access.

Innervation to the lower limb occurs via the sciatic and femoral nerves. The femoral nerve is formed from segments L2 to L4 of the lumbar plexus. It descends lateral to and outside of the femoral sheath. It supplies motor function to the muscles of the anterior thigh (sartorius, pectineus, and quadriceps femoris) and sensation to the anteromedial thigh, hip, and knee. The saphenous nerve is the longest branch of the femoral nerve and supplies sensation to the medial leg and foot. The obturator nerve is formed from the lumbar plexus and exits the pelvis through the obturator foramen; it supplies sensation to the superior medial thigh and adduction of the leg through the adductor magnus, brevis, and longus as well as the gracilis and obturator externus muscles.

The sciatic nerve is the largest peripheral nerve in the body. It comprises the tibial and common peroneal nerves and is made up of nerve segments from L4 to S3. It leaves the pelvis through the sciatic foramen and generally passes inferior to the piriformis muscle. The common peroneal may divide before it leaves the pelvis and passes either through or superior to the piriformis, making it more likely to be injured. This nerve supplies the hamstring group of muscles including the semitendinosus, semimembranosus, and biceps femoris. The tibial nerve, the largest branch of the sciatic nerve, innervates the gastroc-nemius, soleus, plantaris, and popliteus muscles. The tibial nerve gives rise to the sural nerve, which supplies sensation to the lateral leg and foot. The peroneal nerve runs posterior to the fibula before it winds around the fibula and runs with the peroneus longus muscle. Injury to this nerve results in foot-drop due to lack of innervation of the foot dorsiflexors as well as loss of sensation to the lateral leg and dorsum of the foot. Injury to the tibial nerve results in loss of sensation to the sole of the foot and decreased flexor activity of the foot.

ANATOMY OF THE UPPER LIMB

The upper limb may be divided into the shoulder, arm, elbow, forearm, wrist, and hand. Bony support for the upper arm consists of the clavicle, scapula, humerus, radius, ulna, carpals, metacarpals, and phalanges. The clavi-cle extends from the manubrium to the acromion of the scapula. The scapula is a triangular bone with many muscular attachments including the supraspinatus, infraspinatus, rhomboid major, levator scapulae, trapezius, deltoid, and teres major and minor muscles.

The humerus connects the glenoid cavity of the scapula to the elbow. It consists of a head and greater and lesser tubercles connected to the body. The surgical neck is immediately distal to the head of the humerus and is the most common site of fractures. The distal humerus consists of the medial and lateral epicondyles, the capitellum, and the trochlea. The coronoid and olecranon fossae articulate with the corresponding processes of the proximal ulna. The capitellum connects to the radius, which consists of a head, neck, radial tuberosity, body, and styloid. The ulna, the longer of the two bones of the forearm, consists of the olecranon, tubercle, coronoid process, body, and styloid process. The bones of the wrist comprise the scaphoid, lunate, triquetrum, hamate, capitate, trapezoid, and trapezium. The hand contains the metacarpal and phalangeal bones.

The arterial supply of the upper limb consists proximally of the axillary artery, which begins as a continuation of the subclavian artery after crossing under the first rib. The axillary artery is divided into three parts based on the pectoralis minor muscle. The first portion has a single branch, the superior thoracic artery. The second portion lies behind the pectoralis minor and is intimately associated with the brachial plexus. Two branches exit from this portion, the thoracoacromial and the lateral thoracic arteries. The third seg-ment extends from the distal segment of the pectoralis minor muscle to the teres major muscle. It has three branches: the subscapular artery and the anterior and posterior circumflex humeral arteries. Beyond these branches the size of the axillary artery decreases substantially.

The brachial artery, which lies medial and then anterior to the humerus, begins as a continuation of the axillary artery beyond the teres minor. Because of the smaller size of the brachial artery compared with the axillary, repairs of the brachial artery usually require saphenous vein segments to ensure long-term patency, whereas the axillary artery can usually be safely repaired with synthetic materials such as polytetrafluoroethylene (PTFE). Just beyond the epicondyles the brachial artery bifurcates into the radial and ulnar arteries. It gives off many muscular branches including the profunda brachii and superior and inferior ulnar collateral arteries. As in the knee, there is a rich anastomotic arterial supply about the elbow, including the above mentioned arteries and the ulnar recurrent arteries. The radial artery extends laterally across the forearm deep to the brachioradialis muscle. Its branches include the recurrent radial artery, muscular branches, a palmar carpal branch, a superficial palmar branch, and a dorsal carpal branch. The ulnar artery extends across the forearm in a medial position. It passes inferiorly to the pronator teres between the heads of the flexor digitorum superficialis and superior to the flexor digitorum profundus. Its branches include the previously mentioned anterior and posterior ulnar recurrent arteries, the common interosseous artery, and the palmar carpal branch.

The venous drainage of the upper limb is complex. The arteries of the hand are accompanied by superficial and deep venous arches that drain into a dorsal venous network and from there into the cephalic vein. There is a rich venous network about the forearm with numerous communications between the basilic and cephalic veins. The cephalic vein may be used as an alternate arterial substitute if other options are not available. The basilic vein becomes the axillary vein at the inferior border of teres major. The cephalic vein also drains into the axillary vein. The axillary vein ends at the outer border of the first rib, where it becomes the subclavian vein. Unlike injuries of the veins of the arm or forearm, penetrating wounds of the axillary vein should be repaired if possible. Significant pulmonary emboli from this location are rare but do occur.

An understanding of the complex innervation of the upper limb is necessary for proper repair of penetrating injuries to this region of the body. The brachial plexus is formed by nerve roots spanning C5 to T1. These form three trunks: superior (C5 to C6), middle (C7), and inferior (C8 to T1). The lower trunk is immediately behind the subclavian artery. Each trunk has an anterior and a posterior division. The three posterior divisions supply the extensor muscle groups and form the posterior cord. The upper and middle trunks form the lateral cord, while the inferior trunk continues as the medial cord. Each cord then bifurcates into two segments. The posterior cord forms the axillary and the radial nerves. Both the medial and lateral cords contribute to the median nerve. The medial cord also gives rise to the ulnar nerve, and the lateral cord gives rise to the musculocutaneous nerve.

The supraclavicular branches of the brachial plexus are as follows:

1. Dorsal scapular nerve.
2. Long thoracic nerve.
3. Nerve to subclavius.
4. Suprascapular nerve.

The infraclavicular branches of the cords of the brachial plexus are:

1. Lateral pectoral nerve.
2. Musculocutaneous nerve.
3. Lateral root of the median nerve.

The medial cord has the following branches:

1. Medial pectoral nerve.
2. Medial brachial cutaneous nerve.
3. Medial antebrachial cutaneous nerve.
4. Ulnar nerve.
5. Medial root of the median nerve.

The posterior cord also has five branches:

1. Upper subscapular nerve.
2. Thoracodorsal nerve.
3. Lower subscapular nerve.
4. Axillary nerve.
5. Radial nerve.

Four of these nerves progress distally into the arm: the median, radial, ulnar, and musculocutaneous. The median nerve has no branches in the arm but passes into the forearm to supply the flexors of the forearm and both muscular and sensory function in the hand. The ulnar nerve also passes through the arm into the forearm around the medial epicondyle of the humerus and the olecranon. The radial nerve provides muscular control of the triceps, brachioradialis, supinators, and extensors of the hand. In addition, it provides sensation to the dorsum of the hand. The musculocutaneous nerve provides innervation to the biceps, brachialis, and brachioradialis muscles. It later becomes the lateral antebrachial cutaneous nerve and supplies sensation to the lateral forearm.

Three nerves pass through the forearm: the median, ulnar, and radial nerves. The median nerve has the following branches: nerves to the pronator teres, the pronator quadratus, and all flexors except the flexor carpi ulnaris and half of the flexor digitorum profundus (which is supplied by the ulnar nerve), the anterior interosseous nerve, which supplies articular branches to the wrist, and the palmar cutaneous branch, which supplies sensation to the palm. The ulnar nerve supplies fibers to the flexor carpi ulnaris and the medial half of the flexor digitorum profundus, the palmar cutaneous branch, which supplies sensation to the medial palm, and the dorsal cutaneous branch, which supplies the medial portion of the dorsum of the hand. The radial nerve has two main branches: the superficial and deep radial nerves. The deep radial nerve supplies the extensor muscles of the forearm, including the extensor carpi radialis brevis, the supinator, and the remaining extensors of the forearm. The superficial radial nerve passes to the hand under the brachioradialis to supply the dorsum of the hand, wrist, thumb, and lateral two fingers.

RESUSCITATION

Resuscitation of the patient with isolated trauma to the extremity begins with airway control and establishment of adequate respiratory effort according to the Advanced Trauma Life Support (ATLS) guidelines. Next, an attempt is made to control bleeding and establish adequate intravenous lines to permit rapid restoration of adequate circulating volume. In the patient with multiple injuries including trauma to the extremity, other areas of the body such as the

Table 15–1. Signs of Arterial Injury

Hard Signs
Absent or diminished pulses
Active hemorrhage
Large, expanding, or pulsatile hematoma
Bruit or thrill
Distal ischemia (pain, pallor, paralysis, paresthesias, coolness)

Soft Signs
Small, stable hematoma
Injury to anatomically related nerve
Unexplained hypotension
History of hemorrhage no longer present
Proximity of injury to a major vessel

neck, thorax, and abdomen take precedence. Bleeding must be controlled as soon as possible, and perfusion must be maintained to permit later reconstruction of a viable, functional extremity. For obvious reasons, the injured extremity is not the preferred site of placement of intravenous lines, especially when venous trauma is suspected. In the multiply injured patient, choices may be limited, and venous access may be placed in an injured extremity proximal to the site of injury. In the absence of "hard signs" of arterial injury (Table 15–1), two large-bore peripheral intravenous catheters may be adequate for fluid resuscitation. Although it is somewhat controversial, large-bore central venous access lines may be placed once the patient has been initially resuscitated to facilitate further resuscitation and aid in the replacement of intravascular volume that may be lost during intraoperative arterial repair. In patients who require operative repair of their injuries a urinary catheter and nasogastric tube are also placed.

Intravenous (IV) antibiotics and tetanus prophylaxis should be given during the early resuscitation phase. During the initial physical examination the patient should be assessed for arterial supply, sensory and motor function, viability of muscle and integument, and the possible presence of a compartment syndrome. Auscultation near the site of a penetrating injury may detect the presence of a bruit, which is indicative of an arteriovenous communication. Pulses can be ascertained only after the patient has been appropriately resuscitated, and all extremity pulses should be examined by the same physician.[6, 7] Roentgenographic studies should also be performed to rule out the presence of a bony fracture and delineate the trajectory of a bullet as closely as possible. Any bony fracture caused by penetrating trauma is by definition an open fracture. These fractures may require antibiotic therapy and early irrigation and debridement as permitted by the patient's condition. In addition, compartment syndrome should be suspected and appropriately treated in any extremity in which a long bone fracture occurs following penetrating trauma. Treatment of a suspected or confirmed compartment syndrome should be performed in the operating room, with the patient appropriately anesthetized and positioned for immediate exposure of the major arteries of that extremity. Decompression of extremity compartments, via fasciotomy, may result in an unsuspected arterial hemorrhage that had temporarily stopped owing to a tamponade effect.

BALLISTICS

Bullet types in civilian use of which the surgeon should be aware include those with a full metal jacket, the "glaser," and the "talon" type. The full metal jacketed round bullet is commonly used in civilian handguns because of its ease in firing in semiautomatic handguns. These bullets occasionally fragment when they hit bone but generally remain intact during their passage through the tissues. They may exit the intended target with enough velocity to injure a second victim. The hollow-pointed bullet is commonly available and is used by police forces and private citizens. This bullet expands or "mushrooms" while passing through tissue, thereby increasing the cross-sectional area of injury and thus the tissue crushed in its path. On hitting bone, these rounds often fragment, but the inner core of soft lead metallic fragments generally poses no danger to the treating surgeon. Talon bullets, marketed as the Winchester SXT, Speer Gold Dot, and Remington Golden Saber, are hollow-pointed round bullets with a jacket that is designed to peel back, exposing metallic talons as the bullet passes through tissue. This design maximizes the amount of tissue lacerated by the spinning bullet. This bullet has the additional side effect of leaving sharp fragments in the tissues of the victim that may cause serious damage to the gloves and/or hands of the unwary trauma surgeon. The surgeon's best defense is to discover a history of a talon type bullet or to identify these bullets on plain x-rays. Glaser bullets contain many small metal spheres inside a metal jacket and are designed to fragment on hitting a target. Once inside the tissues, these multiple projectiles act like a shotgun round at close range, creating maximum probability of damage to a vital structure. As with shotgun injuries, angiographic study of an extremity injured by a bullet of this type may be warranted solely by the proximity of an artery to the injury.

Shotgun injuries remain a difficult problem because of the large amount of tissue involved and the complexity of the repair process. Bony fractures may have to be repaired, usually with external fixation. Angiography may be necessary to localize the site of vascular injury, even though long segments of injured artery may exist. Vascular repair may proceed with PTFE or saphenous vein interposition grafts as necessary. Porcine skin grafts have been used as a temporary method of coverage until skin grafting is appropriate. Soft tissue defects may be filled with free flaps. The primary amputation rate following shotgun wounds to the extremities has been reported to be as high as 17%.[8] Meyer and colleagues have reported a lower rate, although with the amputation rate of 4% an additional 8% of patients had an unacceptable outcome.[9]

MANGLED EXTREMITY

The mangled extremity can be thought of as an extremity that has sustained extensive damage to the vascular, bony, nervous, and soft tissues. Although these injuries have traditionally been described after blunt trauma, they can also occur after high-velocity assault rifle gunshot wounds and shotgun injuries at close range. Salvage of the extremity depends on the ability of the reconstructive team to create a sensate extremity of normal length. Thus, the crucial factors involved are the degree of bone and nerve injury.[10, 11] Plain roentgenographic studies can usually determine whether adequate bone remains for satisfactory repair. Determination of the total extent of nerve tissue damage requires operative exploration and consideration of sural nerve grafting. Although from a technical standpoint, primary nerve grafting may be performed, the patient may not be stable for an extended procedure, and nerve grafting may be safely performed at a later date. Loss of soft tissue can generally be compensated for by surgical tissue transfer, but adequate muscle mass must remain for mobility of the injured extremity. Most tissue flaps are performed after the first 48 hours following the injury, but before the first 2 weeks have elapsed. The latissimus dorsi free flap, the most commonly used free flap, associated with a 92% to 96% success rate in centers specializing in this operation.[12]

The decision between attempted salvage and early amputation is never an easy one and requires input from both the general surgeon and the orthopedic surgeon. In centers where special services exist, consultation with plastic surgery and hand specialists in appropriate cases is also of great value. Concomitant injuries must also be considered when deciding between salvage and early amputation, with co-morbid conditions pushing the decision toward amputation.

There are several scoring systems that attempt to predict which injuries are salvageable. The most commonly used is the MESS, or mangled extremity severity score, which incorporates four criteria in a scoring system that tries to predict salvage or loss of a mangled lower extremity. The four criteria are (1) type of skeletal or soft tissue injury, (2) length and degree of limb ischemia, (3) presence and severity of shock, and (4) patient age (Table 15–2).[13] This

Table 15–2. Mangled Extremity Severity Score (MESS) Variables and Scoring

	Points
Skeletal/Soft Tissue Injury	
Low-energy (stab, simple fracture, low velocity gunshot wounds)	1
Medium-energy (open or multiple fractures, dislocation)	2
High-energy (close range shotgun, high-velocity gunshot wound, crush injury)	3
Very high-energy (plus gross contamination or soft tissue avulsion)	4
Limb Ischemia	
Pulse reduced or absent but perfusion normal	1
Pulseless; paresthesias, diminished capillary refill	2
Cool, paralyzed, insensate, numb	3
(Score doubled for ischemia >6 hours)	
Shock	
Systolic blood pressure always >90 mmHg	0
Transient hypotension	1
Persistent hypotension	2
Age (years)	
<30	0
30–50	1
>50	2

A score of 7 or greater was associated with a 100% amputation rate when the scoring system was studied retrospectively and prospectively, whereas a score of 6 or less was associated with a 100% limb salvage rate.[13]

scoring system must be used in addition to clinical judgment to decide which limbs should undergo a salvage effort. The cost of delayed amputation has also been studied. These costs, both monetary and psychological, are significant. It is thus even more incumbent on the trauma team to determine which limbs deserve an attempt at salvage and which require early amputation.[14] Because neural function is critical for the proper rehabilitation of a mangled extremity, the diagnosis of compartment syndrome must be made expeditiously and treated without delay.[7, 15, 16] Compartment pressures are useful in making this diagnosis, but clinical evidence of compartment syndrome (pain and paresthesias without other cause), even in the presence of so-called normal compartment pressures (less than 40 mmHg pressure), must lead to a fasciotomy with documented reduction of pressure and resolution of symptoms.

ORTHOPEDIC INJURY

As stated earlier, fractures associated with penetrating trauma are considered open fractures. Intravenous antibiotics are begun in the resuscitation area. Fractures caused by gunshot wounds can be incomplete or complete fractures of a long bone. The three types of incomplete fractures are "drill-hole" through-and-through fractures, "divot" fractures in which a portion of bone, usually cortical but occasionally medullary, is damaged, and the "chip" fracture, which may also be seen with stab wounds.[17] Patients with "divot" and "chip" fractures may be treated with oral antibiotics. The length of treatment depends on the severity of the fractures.

Repair of fractures associated with penetrating trauma may consist of cast immobilization, external fixation, or open reduction with internal fixation (ORIF). Chip and divot fractures may be treated with splinting and limited weight bearing, while drill-hole fractures usually require a cast and nonweight-bearing therapy. Comminuted fractures require greater stabilization, either with an external fixation device or with ORIF. Generally, vascular repairs are performed first unless rapid (less than 6 hours from injury) external fixation can be accomplished. Occasionally, vascular shunts must be placed to achieve perfusion, and definitive repair must await orthopedic fixation. ORIF should be used when little soft tissue injury exists and the potential for infection is low. Immediate ORIF is preferred in stable patients. In severely injured patients, ORIF can be delayed up to 1 week after injury, when the potential for infection is better known and the patient's condition has stabilized.

VASCULAR INJURY

The primary survey of the injured patient with extremity trauma must include a physical examination to detect penetrating trauma. Several obvious signs of arterial trauma may be present on examination. The generally accepted "hard signs" of arterial injury are absent or diminished pulses, distal ischemia, active arterial hemorrhage, a large, expanding or pulsatile hematoma, and bruit or thrill. One or more of these signs is usually present on physical examination if arterial injury is present.[18] These so-called hard signs should alert the physician to the presence of arterial injury, which should be treated expeditiously. The site of arterial injury is usually obvious, but occasionally there may be multiple projectiles or a trajectory that is so unusual that an angiogram is necessary to allow proper surgical planning and exposure. In these cases, an angiogram may be performed in the emergency department, in the operating room, or in the angiography suite. Injuries to the shoulder girdle and pelvic region may require angiographic localization because of the potential need for thoracotomy or laparotomy. Elderly patients with known or suspected atherosclerotic disease may need preoperative angiography to properly place the distal limb of a bypass or interposition graft to achieve adequate distal runoff.

In the absence of the hard signs of penetrating arterial trauma, an attempt is made to find other signs on physical examination that may indicate a need for further radiologic or surgical work-up. These "soft signs" include a stable hematoma, injury to an anatomically related nerve, unexplained hypotension, hemorrhage no longer present, and proximity to a major vessel.[19] Controversy exists about the treatment of these wounds. The older literature suggests that patients with any of these wounds should undergo angiographic exploration, even if the physical examination is normal.[20-24] This practice, however, yields a negative angiographic exam rate that is as high as 95%. Given that angiography is invasive, time consuming, and costly, some have questioned this approach.[25-29] One alternative modality is that of screening Doppler pressure measurements, also known as ankle-arm indices or ankle-brachial indices (AAI or ABI). This method is cheap, noninvasive, and technically easy to perform. However, lesions that may not cause a pressure drop, such as a developing intimal flap or a false aneurysm, will be missed by this technique.[30] Another noninvasive method of screening patients for asymptomatic injuries in proximity to a major artery is ultrasound. This method is highly operator dependent and may suffer from low sensitivity. At present, positive findings on ultrasound are usually followed up with an angiographic study.[31-36] Enthusiasm now exists for reliance on physical examination alone. Patients with the hard signs of arterial trauma require surgical and/or arteriographic exploration. Patients with injuries far from the major vessels and normal findings on physical examination can be safely watched with sequential physical examinations. The position advocated by some is that sequential careful physical examinations over a 24-hour period are reliable in excluding penetrating arterial trauma in proximity to a major extremity artery.[37-42]

Repair of arterial trauma is generally surgical, although there is evidence that radiographically placed transluminal stents may have a role in the treatment of pseudoaneurysms and arteriovenous fistulas.[43] The preferred method of repair of an arterial injury is resection of the injured segment and primary end-to-end anastomosis. Vein patch angioplasty also has an acceptable patency rate. If primary repair techniques are not possible, larger arteries (axillary, common iliac, external iliac, common femoral, superficial femoral) are generally repaired with PTFE grafts, whereas the smaller arteries (brachial, popliteal, tibial) or arteries crossing joints generally require a saphenous vein interposition graft (Table 15-3).[44, 45] PTFE can be used in contaminated fields.[46-48] In unstable patients in whom the time needed for dissection of saphenous vein and performance of anastomoses is prohibitive, a temporary shunt can be placed to

Table 15–3. Polytetrafluoroethylene (PTFE) Graft Sizes

Arteries	Size (mm)	Veins	Size (mm)
Subclavian	8	Inferior vena cava	14–24
Axillary	6	Iliac	10–12
Brachial	5–6	Common femoral	10–12
Iliac	6–8	Superficial femoral	8–10
Common femoral	6–8	Popliteal	8–10
Superficial femoral	6		
Popliteal	6		

Externally supported grafts may be indicated for venous interpositions. Use of PTFE grafts at the brachial and popliteal artery locations should be limited to situations where saphenous or cephalic vein is unavailable or its use would be inappropriate. PTFE grafts of 4 mm or smaller are associated with an unacceptably high thrombosis rate.

restore perfusion to distal tissue. Patients are then returned to the OR when stability has been achieved, and definitive repair of the vessel or vessels is performed.

Venous injuries are generally found during exploration of proximate arterial injuries or as part of a Doppler examination. In the unstable patient, venous ligation is acceptable, while reconstruction should be attempted in the stable patient or the patient at risk for compartment syndrome.[49, 50] Early partial thrombosis of a venous repair is common, but recanalization appears to occur frequently with long-term follow-up.[51] Pulmonary embolism is an often cited concern but has been only rarely reported after failed venous repair.

References

1. Shah DM, Naraynsingh V, Leather RP, et al: Advances in the management of acute popliteal vascular blunt injuries. J Trauma 1985;25:793.
2. Pasch AR, Bishara RA, Lim LT, et al: Optimal limb salvage in penetrating civilian vascular trauma. J Vasc Surg 1986;3:189.
3. Lim LT, Michuda MS, Flanigan DP, et al: Popliteal artery trauma. Arch Surg 1980;115:1307.
4. Menzoian JO, Doyle JE, Cantelmo NL, et al: A comprehensie approach to extremity vascular trauma. Arch Surg 1985;120:801.
5. Feliciano DV, Herskowitz K, O'Gorman RB, et al: Management of vascular injuries in the lower extremities. J Trauma 1988;28:319.
6. Drapanas T, Hewitt RL, Weichert RF III, et al: Civilian vascular injuries: A critical appraisal of three decades of management. Ann Surg 1970;172:351.
7. Morris GC, Beall AC, Roof WR, et al: Surgical experience with 220 acute arterial injuries in civilian practice. Am J Surg 1960;99:775.
8. Stewart MPM, Kinninmonth A: Shotgun wounds of the limbs. Injury 1993;24:667.
9. Meyer JP, Lim LT, Schuler JJ, et al: Peripheral vascular trauma from close-range shotgun injuries. Arch Surg 1985;120(10):126.
10. Lange RH, Bach AW, Hansen ST, et al: Open tibial fractures with associated vascular injuries: Prognosis for limb salvage. J Trauma 1985;25:203.
11. Gregory RT, Gould RJ, Pecler M, et al: The mangled extremity syndrome (M.E.S.): A severity grading system for multisystem injury of the extremity. J Trauma 1985;25:1147.
12. Khouri RK, Shaw WM: Reconstruction of the lower extremity with microvascular free flaps: A 10-year experience with 304 consecutive cases. J Trauma 1989;29:1086.
13. Johansen K, Daises M, Howey T, et al: Objective criteria accurately predict amputation following lower extremity trauma. J Trauma 1990;30:568.

14. Bondurant EJ, Cotler HB, Buckle R, et al: The medical and economic impact of severely injured lower extremities. J Trauma 1988;28:1270.
15. Feliciano DV, Cruse PA, Patrinely VS, et al: Fasciotomy after trauma to the extremities. Am J Surg 1988;156:533.
16. Perry MO, Thal ER, Shires GT: Management of arterial injuries. Ann Surg 1971;173:403.
17. Billings JB, Zimmerman MC, Aurori B, et al: Gunshot wounds to the extremities: Experience of a level I trauma center. Orthop Rev 1991;20:519.
18. Rutherford RB: Diagnostic evaluation of extremity vascular injuries. Surg Clin North Am 1988;68:683.
19. Frykberg ER: Advances in the diagnosis and treatment of extremity vascular trauma. Surg Clin North Am 1995;75:207.
20. Geuder GA, Kreis DJ, Ratner L et al: The role of contrast arteriography in suspected arterial injuries of the extremities. Am Surg 1985;51:89.
21. Menzoian JO, Doyle JE, Cantelmo NL, et al: A comprehensive approach to extremity vascular trauma. Arch Surg 1985;120:801.
22. Rose SC, Moore EE: Trauma angiography: The use of clinical findings to improve patient selection and case preparation. J Trauma 1988;28:240.
23. Sirinek LR, Levine BA, Gaskell HV, et al: Reassessment of the role of routine operative exploration in vascular trauma. J Trauma 1981;21:329.
24. Snyder WH, Watkins WL, Whiddon LL, et al: Civilian popliteal artery trauma. An eleven-year experience with 83 injuries. Surgery 1979;85:101.
25. Dennis JW, Frykberg ER, Crump JM, et al: New perspectives on the management of penetrating trauma in proximity to major limb arteries. J Vasc Surg 1990;11:84.
26. Francis H, Thal ER, Weigdt JA, et al: Vascular proximity: Is it a valid indication for arteriography in asymptomatic patients. J Trauma 1991;31:512.
27. McDonald EJ, Goodman PC, Winestock DP: The clinical indications for arteriography in trauma to the extremity. A review of 114 cases. Radiology 1975;116(1):45.
28. Reid JDS, Weigdt JA, Thal ER, et al: Assessment of proximity of a wound to major vascular structures as an indication for arteriography. Arch Surg 1988;123:942.
29. Rose SC, Moore EE: Trauma angiography. The use of clinical findings to improve patient selection and case preparation. J Trauma 1988;28:240.
30. Lynch K, Johansen K: Can doppler pressure measurement replace "exclusion arteriography" in the diagnosis of occult extremity arterial trauma. Ann Surg 1988;214:737.
31. Anderson RJ, Hobson RW, Lee BC, et al: Reduced dependency on arteriography for penetrating extremity trauma: Influence of wound location and noninvasive vascular studies. J Trauma 1990;30:1059.
32. Bergstein JM, Blair J-F, Edwards J, et al: Pitfalls in the use of color-flow duplex ultrasound for screening of suspected arterial injuries in penetrated extremities. J Trauma 1992;33:395.
33. Bynoe RP, Miles WS, Bell RM, et al: Noninvasive diagnosis of vascular trauma by duplex ultrasonography. J Vasc Surg 1991;14:346.
34. Knudson MM, Lewis FR, Atkinson K, et al: The role of duplex ultrasound arterial imaging in patients with penetrating extremity trauma. Arch Surg 1993;128:1033.
35. Meissner M, Paun M, Johansen K: Duplex scanning for arterial trauma. Am J Surg 1991;161:551.
36. Schwartz M, Weaver F, Yellin A, et al: The utility of color flow Doppler examination in penetrating extremity arterial trauma. Am Surg 1993;59:375.
37. Frykberg ER, Crump JM, Dennis JW, et al: Nonoperative observation of clinically occult arterial injuries: A prospective evaluation. Surg 1991;109:85.
38. Frykberg ER, Crump JM, Vines PS, et al: A reassessment of the role of arteriography in penetrating proximity extremity trauma: A prospective study: J Trauma 1989;29:1041.
39. Frykberg ER, Dennis JW, Bishop K, et al: The reliability of physical examination in the evaluation of penetrating extremity trauma for vascular injury: Results at one year. J Trauma 1991;31(4):502.
40. Frykberg ER, Feliciano DV: Arteriography of the injured extremity: Are we in proximity to an answer? J Trauma 1992;32:551.
41. Frykberg ER, Vines PS, Alexander RH: The natural history of clinically occult arterial injuries: A prospective evaluation. J Trauma 1989;29:577.
42. Gomez GA, Kreis DJ, Ratner L, et al: Suspected vascular trauma of the extremities. The role of arteriography in proximity injuries. J Trauma 1986;26:1005.

43. Marin ML, Veith FJ, Panetta TF, et al: Transluminally placed endovascular stented graft repair for arterial trauma. J Vasc Surg 1994;20:466.
44. Martin LC, McKenney MG, Sosa JL, et al: Management of lower extremity arterial trauma. J Trauma 1994;37:591.
45. Cargile JS, Hunt JL, Purdue GF, et al: Acute trauma of the femoral artery and vein. J Trauma 1992;32:364.
46. Shah PM, Ito K, Clauss RH, et al: Expanded microporous polytetrafluoroethylene (PTFE) grafts in contaminated wounds. Experimental and clinical study. J Trauma 1983;23:1030.
47. Stone KS, Walshaw R, Sugiyama GT, et al: Polytetrafluoroethylene versus autogenous vein grafts for vascular reconstruction in contaminated wounds. Am J Surg 1984;147:692.
48. Ward RE, Hudson M, Flynn TC: Gram-negative infections of arterial substitutes. J Surg Res 1982;33:510.
49. Timberlake GA, Kerstein MD: Venous injury: To repair or ligate, the dilemma revisited. Am Surg 1995;61:139.
50. Nypaver TJ, Schuler JJ, McDonnell P, et al: Long-term results of venous reconstruction after vascular trauma in civilian practice. J Vasc Surg 1992;16:762.
51. Feliciano DV, Mattos KI, Graham JM, et al: Five-year experience with PTFE grafts in vascular wounds. J Trauma 1985;25:71.

Chapter 16
Crush Injuries

Injury resulting from entrapment of the body, usually an extremity, was first noted in 1909 after the earthquake of Messina and was described by German authors in 1916. Early descriptions focused on the tissue damage at the site of the crushing object, and distant renal impairment was not recognized until 1923.[1] Bywaters, in his War Medicine Series lecture in 1942, provides an insightful description of crush injuries and their treatment, based on his experience with bombing victims in the 1940 London air raids. It is somewhat disturbing that Bywaters' suggestion to give fluids "rapidly at the earliest possible moment . . . [preferably] while the patient is still trapped under the wreckage" was not followed until 50 years later with the formation of the Federal Emergency Management Agency's Urban Search and Rescue program.[2, 3] With the institution of the Urban Search and Rescue Task Forces, protocol now dictates early aggressive fluid and drug therapy in victims trapped in collapsed structures. This suggestion should be expanded in paramedic protocols to include victims involved in prolonged extrications in such situations as motor vehicle accidents.

The crush syndrome, of which crush injury is a component, is the systemic manifestation that occurs following reperfusion of the crushed tissue. The characteristic triad of the syndrome includes rhabdomyolysis, hyperkalemia, and myoglobinuria. The basis for the initiation of the entire syndrome is the restoration of blood flow to a previously ischemic area, usually an extremity. With the interruption of blood flow, conversion to anaerobic metabolism results not only in inefficient energy metabolism and lactic acidosis, but also in conversion of xanthine dehydrogenase to xanthine oxidase and the subsequent initiation of reperfusion injury via production of hydroxyl ions and superoxide radicals. These latter substances are in large part the cause of distant systemic third space fluid loss and multiple organ damage.

Measures that block the far-reaching effects of the products of reperfusion injury should begin as early as is physically possible.[4] Measures that prevent the production of oxygen free-radicals are the ideal option and should be initiated immediately along with fluid resuscitation. Allopurinol has been shown to block xanthine oxidase activity but is currently available in intravenous form on an experimental basis only. However, folate is actually more effective than allopurinol and is readily available.

Once produced, oxygen free-radicals can be inactivated with scavengers. Two commonly available substances, mannitol and albumin, are effective free-radical scavengers.[4] Besides its scavenging effects, mannitol may also assist in volume expansion and in creating the necessary diuresis to reduce the risks of myoglobin-induced renal failure. Although albumin should not be considered a volume expansion agent, its activity as a free-radical scavenger as well as its

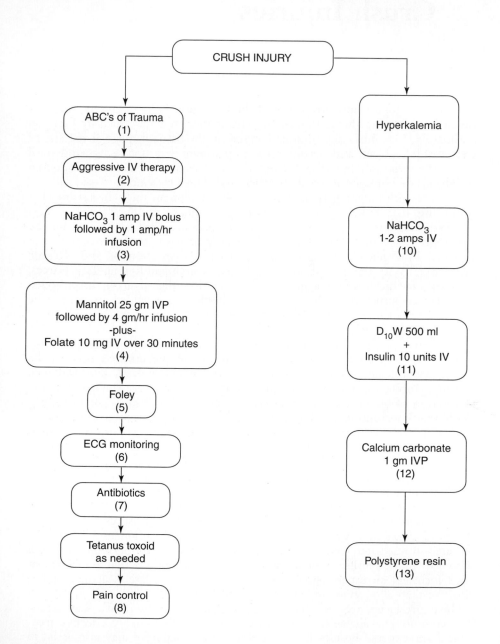

1. As with any trauma victim, airway, breathing, and circulation must take priority before any other therapy is initiated.
2. Depending on the duration of the crush injury, patients may be dehydrated and may need aggressive hydration *before* attempts at extrication are made. It should be remembered that volume replacement must account for not only the absence of fluid intake since the injury but also the volume of fluid that has extravasated into the reperfused tissue. Normal saline or lactated Ringers' solution are acceptable. Colloid solutions should not be used.
3. Alkalinization of the urine may increase myoglobin solubility, as documented in vitro, but there is no in vivo proof of benefit. Caution: The sodium load that accompanies sodium bicarbonate may be excessive. Metabolic acidosis resulting from reperfusion should be treated with volume expansion.
4. Mannitol is given simultaneously with aggressive volume replacement to improve renal perfusion and decrease the risk of myoglobinuria, as well as to gain its effect as a free-radical scavenger. Other free-radical scavengers such as albumin can be given, as well as inhibitors of xanthine oxidase production (e.g., folate).[4]
5. Urine output should be abundant (300 ml/hour) to promote clearing of myoglobin from the renal tubules.
6. Reperfusion of injured tissue results in systemic distribution of the products of rhabdomyolysis, including potassium. The cardiac effects of hyperkalemia must be monitored by electrocardiography.
7. The presence or absence and mechanism of open soft tissue injury will dictate the need for and type of antibiotics given. Victims caught in a collapsed building will need staphylococcal and streptococcal coverage as well as antipseudomonal agents.
8. Victims of a building collapse with crush injuries are often reached several days after the injury. These patients have sustained not only a significant physical injury but also a tremendous psychological challenge. All efforts should be made to relieve their physical *and* mental discomfort.
9. Hyperkalemia results when tissue damaged by both a direct crush injury and an indirect ischemia or reperfusion injury releases its intracellular contents. The acidotic environment created by anaerobic metabolism in the nonperfused tissue increases the hyperkalemia as the H^+ ion entering the cell forces the similarly charged K^+ ion into the extracellular space. Elevated systemic concentrations of potassium can cause refractive and lethal cardiac dysrhythmias, and should be treated promptly. Although laboratory values may not be available, the electrocardiogram should be monitored closely for changes in T wave morphology (peaked T waves), and therapy should be instituted immediately if such changes occur.
10. One goal of treating extracellular hyperkalemia is to drive the H^+ ions back into the intracellular space. Alkalinization with sodium bicarbonate, which creates a temporary alkaline extracellular environment, accomplishes this.
11. Insulin also reverses the extracellular migration of K^+ ions but must be given with dextrose to prevent systemic hypoglycemia.
12. Although sodium bicarbonate and insulin act directly on elevated potassium levels, calcium acts to stabilize the cardiac membranes and raises the dysrhythmia threshold, thereby decreasing the adverse cardiac risks of hyperkalemia.
13. Polystyrene resins are administered via the gastrointestinal tract to absorb potassium. They are not useful for the immediate life-threatening aspects of hyperkalemia but may be given to control elevated potassium levels during the ensuing days.

volume expanding capabilities may make it an agent to be considered for patients with the crush syndrome.

Beside lethal dysrhythmias resulting from hyperkalemia and renal failure secondary to rhabdomyolysis, hypotension is a major and immediate cause of death in patients with the crush syndrome. A tremendous amount of plasma volume is lost at the site of the injury and also systemically when the products of anaerobic metabolism wash out with reperfusion, initiating third space fluid loss through capillary leak. With the loss of circulating plasma volume to the interstitium, hypotension and hemoconcentration appear. Hemoconcentration is rarely if ever of clinical concern, but hypotension must be aggressively reversed with volume replacement. Both lactated Ringer's and normal saline are acceptable solutions for volume replacement, but both have disadvantages. The potassium in lactated Ringer's solution (4 mEq/L) may be of some concern in patients who are already faced with hyperkalemia resulting from the initial injury and the potential ensuing acute renal failure. However, unless a tremendous volume of fluid is needed, the potassium content should present few problems, and in fact, the subsequent hepatic conversion of lactate to bicarbonate may assist in treating the metabolic acidosis and myoglobinuria seen in these patients. The high sodium and chloride content of normal saline may be beneficial in the initial fluid resuscitation phase but may also exacerbate the metabolic acidosis of anaerobic metabolism and renal failure by adding a hyperchloremic component. Ultimately, either crystalloid solution is acceptable, the key point being aggressive, adequate fluid resuscitation.

Rhabdomyolysis associated with the crush syndrome unleashes several metabolic alterations. Skeletal muscle contains approximately 100 mEq K^+/kg of tissue, and as cells are lysed, systemic hyperkalemia results. This may lead to lethal arrhythmias in the first 1 to 3 days after injury. Calcium is deposited in damaged muscle, leading to hypocalcemia. This condition should not be treated with exogenous calcium because the extra calcium may activate further enzyme degradation of the muscle. Overproduction of purines and a decreased ability to excrete them lead to increased uric acid formation. The resultant hyperuricemia, however, does not require treatment. Systemic metabolic acidosis follows reperfusion of the ischemic limb, and as such, is a lactic acidosis. This acidosis may be exacerbated if the patient is underresuscitated at the time of reperfusion, leading to global hypotension. Acute renal failure appearing within the first few days also perpetrates the acidosis. The underlying cause must be corrected, but correction of the acidosis with sodium bicarbonate should be reserved only for patients with a significantly low pH (<7.00). Damaged muscle also leaks phosphates (approximately 2.25 g/kg of tissue), leading to hyperphosphatemia; this can be corrected with phosphate-binding antacids.

Creatine is a storage form of high-energy phosphate, its degradation product being creatinine. In crushed tissue, production of creatine exceeds filtration, resulting in an increase in creatinine relative to blood urea nitrogen (BUN) and a narrowing of the BUN-creatinine ratio. Also released in high concentration from damaged muscle is creatinine phosphokinase (CPK), which usually peaks in 24 hours and is degraded by 50% every 48 hours. A secondary delayed increase may indicate ongoing ischemia. In muscle cells, myoglobin binds oxygen, which then transports it across the cell membrane and delivers it to

Table 16–1. Solubility of Myoglobin Based on Urine pH

Urine pH	% Precipitated
8.5–7.5	0
6.5	4
5.5	23
5.0	46
<5.0	73

the mitochondria. Myoglobin is concentrated in muscle at a rate of approximately 2.5 g/kg and is released with injury. At or below a pH of 5.6, myoglobin degrades into hematin and the globin moiety. Hematin has a direct toxic effect on tubular cells, whereas the globin molecule precipitates and can obstruct the renal tubules. Although benefit has been demonstrated in vitro, alkalization of the urine in vivo has not proved to be clinically beneficial. Based on a knowledge of the solubility of myoglobin (Table 16–1) and the fact that most crush injury patients are acidotic, the judicious administration of sodium bicarbonate seems appropriate, because of the sodium load that accompanies bicarbonate. In addition to maintenance of circulating volume (and therefore renal perfusion) and alkalization of the urine, forced diuresis may lessen or prevent myoglobin-induced acute renal failure. Although furosemide is effective, mannitol may provide not only an osmotic diuresis but also its effects as a free-radical scavenger. Because renal tubular sodium resorption is an energy-requiring process, increased tubular flow may also decrease oxygen and substrate requirements and decrease the potential for anoxic renal injury.

Ultimately, it must not be forgotten that in victims with crush injuries due to a structure collapse, "pain must be relieved and steps taken to see that the patient is comfortable in body and mind. We are treating not only an injured limb, but a human being who has passed through an exhausting and terrifying ordeal."

References

1. Bywaters EGL: Crush Injury. Br Med J 1942;2:643.
2. Barbera JA, Lozano M: Urban search and rescue medical teams: FEMA task force system. Prehosp Disaster Med 1993;8(4):349.
3. Federal Emergency Management Agency, Task Force Medical Procedures: Federal Emergency Management Agency urban search and rescue response system: A component of the federal response plan under emergency support function 9. Washington, DC, Federal Emergency Management Agency, 1991, Appendix J.
4. Kirton OC, Civetta JM: Ischemia-reperfusion injury in the critically ill: A progenitor of multiple organ failure. New Horiz 1999;7:87.

Chapter 17

Resuscitation of the Burn Patient

General principles of burn care include adequate fluid resuscitation, burn wound coverage and healing, and rehabilitation to achieve the best functional and cosmetic outcome. The functions of the skin, including fluid balance, protection, immunity, reception, thermoregulation, and metabolism, are most often appreciated only when skin integrity is compromised. While the physical evidence of the burn often appears to be the compelling issue, it must be remembered that *the patient with burns is a trauma patient*: The issues extend well beyond wound care. Resuscitation is best performed within the familiar framework of the Advanced Trauma Life Support protocol, which maintains the focus on ensuring adequate tissue perfusion while preventing further injury. In the burn patient, this protocol sustains life while preventing further extension of the burn injury (and conversion to a deeper burn). Care is directed through the phases of primary survey, resuscitation, and secondary survey, on the way to definitive care. This discussion emphasizes aspects of the management of patients with major burns as integrated within these phases. Patients with minor burns move very quickly through, or do not require, resuscitation care.

HISTORY

As the primary survey is initiated, the mechanism of injury and patient characteristics must be fully ascertained (Table 17–1).

PRIMARY SURVEY

Patients should be approached in full mask/gown/glove regalia consistent with universal precautions to minimize the risk of patient contamination. Handwashing and strict attention to detail in infection control processes must be emphasized throughout the course of care of burn patients.

Airway. Inhalation injury results from heat and chemical (smoke) burns and is suspected from signs of stridor, carbonaceous sputum, singed nasal hair, hoarseness, mechanism of injury, and deep facial burns. Because the upper airway can be rapidly compromised by evolving edema, it is essential to anticipate the need for early intubation.

Breathing. Chemical burns caused by inhalation of smoke into the lower airway and alveoli can result in progressive respiratory compromise. Monitoring via pulse oximetry for early detection of hypoxia and assessment of the need for intubation are essential.

Table 17–1. Primary Survey of the Burn Patient

Question	Considerations
What kind of burn injury is present?	Flame, flash, contact, electrical, liquid, chemical, or tar
When did the injury occur?	Time of burn is the starting point for resuscitation
Where and how did the injury occur?	Note suspicious circumstances indicative of child abuse
Is there potential for inhalation injury?	Enclosed space
What is the general extent of the burn?	Major: >20% body surface area (BSA)
	Burns of face, hands, feet, genitals
	Minor: <10% BSA with combined second- and third-degree burns
	<2% BSA with third-degree burns
	No other injuries
Was there other mechanical trauma coincident with the burn?	Explosion
What is the patient's age?	Higher morbidity and mortality at extremes of age
What are the patient's co-morbid conditions?	Preburn pathophysiology affects resuscitation (e.g., heart disease, diabetes, asthma)

The history can also lead to a suspicion of carbon monoxide poisoning, which can be further diagnosed by measuring carboxyhemoglobin levels; it is treated by administering 100% oxygen. Cyanide toxicity can occur with inhalation of smoke from burning synthetics; it is treated with hydration, followed by 15 ml of 3% sodium nitrate and then 50 ml of 25% sodium thiosulfate.

Circulation. Loss of the skin covering causes massive salt and fluid loss through tissue leak and evaporation. This loss is most impressive within the first 48 hours after the burn and requires significant volume replacement and close monitoring of tissue perfusion.

Disability. Coincident mechanical trauma can result in a closed head injury, but the most common causes of altered mental status in trauma and thus burn patients are hypoxia and hypovolemia.

Exposure. First, the burning process must be stopped quickly by removing clothing that can retain heat and chemicals (dry powder chemicals should be lightly brushed away, and then the skin is copiously irrigated; neutralizing agents are not used because the heat generated causes more damage). Second, the extent of the burns can be determined only by a complete examination of the patient, which requires removal of all clothes. Third, because the skin is an important organ in thermoregulation, its loss can lead to "exposure," or hypothermia. Thus, the room must be kept warm, and wounds must be covered promptly. Fourth, all potential "tourniquets" must be removed, including rings and bracelets.

RESUSCITATION

Resuscitation is timed from the onset of the burn. Each problem uncovered in the primary survey is corrected in sequence.[1–3]

Intubation for management of the airway and initiation of ventilatory support

Burn Patient Resuscitation

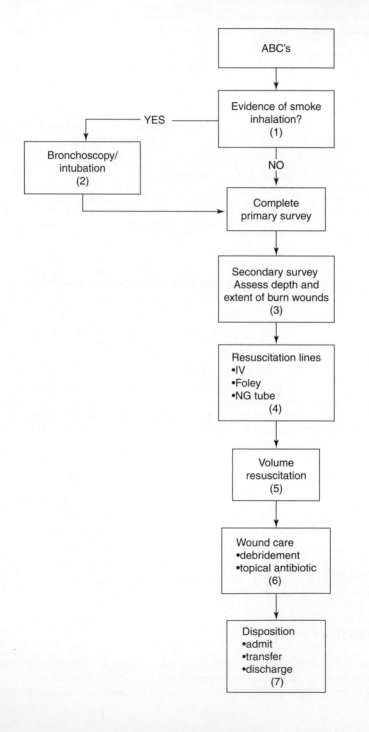

1. Smoke inhalation injury is a thermal injury only when super-heated steam is the cause of the burn. In all other cases, the oropharynx and upper airway regulate the temperature of inhaled gases and prevent thermal injury. In the majority of cases, smoke inhalation injury results from inhalation of the noxious products of combustion, which induce erythema and edema of the airway. Smoke inhalation should be suspected in patients who have been burned in an enclosed space, where the products of combustion are trapped and concentrated. Soot in the mouth and on the tongue, as well as edema of the oral cavity and carbonaceous sputum are all strong indicators of smoke inhalation.
2. If inhalation injury is suspected, patients should undergo bronchoscopy to evaluate the trachea and upper airway. Any evidence of injury should lead to prompt intubation. Patients can always be extubated at a later time, but if edema is allowed to progress to the point of obstruction and no airway has been established, the patient will die. An easy method that can be employed during bronchoscopy is to thread the bronchoscope through an endotracheal tube. If intubation is necessary, the endotracheal tube can simply be slid down over the bronchoscope and into the trachea.
3. The extent of the burn is estimated by determining the amount of body surface area burned (total body surface area = TBSA). This can be done using the rule of nines (Fig. 17–2), the 1% rule (the patient's hand equals 1% of the TBSA), or a Lunden-Browder chart. Burn wounds are charted by depth as first degree, second degree, third degree, or fourth degree.
4. All patients with extensive burns require aggressive volume resuscitation. Adequate intravenous access demands at least two large-bore peripheral intravenous (IV) lines or a central venous line. Urine output must be monitored to guide volume replacement and requires a Foley catheter for accurate measurement. Large burns induce gastrointestinal ileus; these patients require nasogastric decompression with a nasogastric tube. Mechanical trauma must be diagnosed and treated aggressively.
5. Several formulas can be used to guide the fluid resuscitation of the burn patient. Probably the most frequently used is the Parkland formula: $4 \times$ (TBSA) $\times$ (weight in kilograms) = milliliters of fluid to be given over a 24-hour period. The first half of the calculated volume is given in the first 8 hours, and the remaining half is given over the next 16 hours. Time starts at the time of the injury, not the time of evaluation. One must remember that these formulas are only a guide; true volume requirements should be based on patient response. The best measure is urine output, which should be monitored every 15 to 30 minutes, and IV rates should be adjusted accordingly to produce a urine output in the range of 0.5 ml/kg/hr in the adult. Lactated Ringer's solution is the agent of choice for volume replacement.
6. Wound care is critical in burn patients to control pain and to avoid complications such as burn wound (and systemic) infection and extension of the burn injury. Burn wounds should be debrided soon after admission to the hospital; this step requires only removal of blisters and cleansing of the burned areas. Tangential excision of deep wounds is usually undertaken in the ensuing days. Systemic prophylactic antibiotics are contraindicated, but topical antimicrobial agents such as silver sulfadiazine should be applied to all burned surfaces. Because silver sulfadiazine is water soluble, and because burn wounds weep fluid extensively, burns to the face may be better treated with a cream such as bacitracin. Also, because silver sulfadiazine does not penetrate burn eschar well, and because cartilage has a poor blood supply, cartilaginous structures such as the ear and nose may be better treated with agents such as sulfamyalon, which does penetrate eschar well. More extensive use of sulfamyalon can cause acid-base disturbances because of its capacity to inhibit carbonic anhydrase.
7. Following evaluation and initial treatment of the burns, a decision about disposition must be made. Patients with complicated burns, by virtue of depth, size, or location (see text), should be admitted to the hospital. Surgeons with burn experience as well as the services of support staff, including practitioners in physical therapy, nursing, dietary, rehabilitation, and psychology, are needed to properly treat these patients. If these facilities are not available, these patients must be transferred to a recognized burn center. For optimal outcome, even small burns should be treated by a surgeon with significant experience in treating burns.

for compromised breathing are guided by the same indications used for any trauma patient. The key is to recognize the *potential* for airway compromise and the development of pulmonary compromise *early*. Bronchoscopy is important to evaluate the upper airway for injury. It is far better to intubate the patient based on the potential for airway compromise than to confront an occluded airway because of the rapid progression of upper airway edema. Radiographic evidence of alveolar injury lags behind the clinical picture by several days, and thus a normal chest radiograph provides little reassurance. Once the spine has been cleared (clinically or radiographically, depending on the mechanisms of injury), the head of the bed should be elevated to 30 degrees to prevent edema.

Vascular access is best obtained through large-bore peripheral intravenous (IV) lines placed through nonburned tissue. Introducer central lines are the second choice and again should be placed through nonburned tissue if possible. However, if there are no burn-free sites, IV lines can be placed through burn eschar.

Administered fluids should be warmed. Fluid management in the first 24 hours is guided by a variety of formulas, of which the most commonly used is:

24-hour volume = (% body surface area burned) ×
(uninjured body weight in kg) × (4 ml lactated Ringer's/kg)

Half of this amount is administered in the first 8 hours after the burn (*not* the first 8 hours since presentation), and the remaining half is given during the subsequent 16 hours. Lactated Ringer's is chosen because it is a balanced salt solution that provides isotonic replacement. In adults, glucose is not added at this time because it promotes an osmotic diuresis during the initial state of "glucose intolerance" and thus exacerbates hypovolemia. However, infants and children require glucose (5% dextrose) because of low glycogen stores and higher basal metabolism characteristic of growth.

Hypertonic saline is another option for fluid replacement and highlights the importance of Na^+ loss through the fluid leak and the need for its extracellular replacement in burn resuscitation. Both the isotonic and hypertonic methods use sodium as the volume expander and deliver the same amount of sodium in the first 24 hours; the difference between them is that the volume administered with hypertonic saline is significantly less. Hypertonic saline can be made by adding 100 mEq of sodium acetate to lactated Ringer's solution and is administered at a rate that provides

$(0.52$ mEq $Na^+) \times$ (% body surface area burned) × (weight in kg)

over 24 hours. Hypertonic saline resuscitation requires experience and close electrolyte monitoring; it should be discontinued when the serum sodium concentration exceeds 148 mEq/L.

Colloid is not administered during the initial resuscitation period because the capillary leak generated by the burn pathophysiology leads to protein retention in interstitial tissues and tenacious edema. Blood is generally not needed (prior to burn excision) and is transfused in accordance with standard guidelines.

The success of fluid resuscitation is monitored clinically using evidence of end-organ perfusion, the most important and accessible of which is the urine output. Placement of an indwelling bladder catheter facilitates this monitoring. For adults, the targeted urine output is 0.5 ml/kg/hour; in children, it is 1 ml/kg/hour. The fluid resuscitation formula serves as a guideline, which may overestimate or underestimate the volume needed; contributing factors include preburn volume status, inaccurate estimation of burn size and/or depth, and the presence of inhalation injury, which increases the requirement. *Fluid volume is adjusted based on the response of the patient.* During the resuscitation period, return of the concentrated hematocrit to normal indicates that resuscitation is moving in the right direction, but this value should not be considered an endpoint for resuscitation.

The importance of completing a flow sheet of the care rendered merits comment. Not only does such a flow sheet guide care during the initial evaluation, it also provides a link to care rendered elsewhere. Proper fluid management can be rendered only with a knowledge of what has been done already and is being done now.

Baseline laboratory studies (complete blood count, electrolytes, blood urea nitrogen, creatinine, glucose, liver chemistries, and urinalysis), a chest radiograph, and 12-lead electrocardiogram (in patients over age 40) are obtained for later comparison.

Patients with electrical burns usually have extensive soft tissue damage underlying what can be a small surface burn, which represents the entrance or exit of the electrical current. The burn represents the tip of the iceberg of the total body injury. Muscle cell lysis causes myoglobinemia and consequent myoglobinuria, which may induce renal failure. Volume resuscitation and alkalinization of the urine (using two ampules of sodium bicarbonate per liter of lactated Ringer's) diminish this threat.

SECONDARY SURVEY

Coincident trauma must be aggressively diagnosed and treated in the secondary survey. During the course of the secondary survey, the burns are further characterized by more precise determination of their size (as a percentage of body surface area) and depth.[4] The four burn degrees are (Fig. 17–1):

First degree: epidermal injury, such as a sunburn—red, painful, no blisters.

Second degree: injury through the epidermis to the dermis—mottled and red, painful (even air motion across the skin hurts), and swelling with blisters; these burns are further characterized as superficial and deep.

Third degree: full-thickness burn extending to the subcutaneous fat or deeper—dry, leathery, and waxen, with no blanching and no pain (the nerve endings are dead); the skin does not hold hair (which is easily pulled out with forceps) and is dead.

Fourth degree: full-thickness skin and hypodermis extending to muscle, tendon, or bone—black, no pain, dry, gangrenous; necrosis typically involves an appendage.

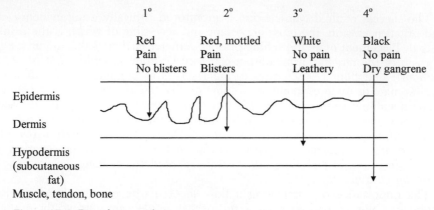

1°	2°	3°	4°
Red	Red, mottled	White	Black
Pain	Pain	No pain	No pain
No blisters	Blisters	Leathery	Dry gangrene

Epidermis

Dermis

Hypodermis
(subcutaneous
fat)
Muscle, tendon, bone

Figure 17–1. Burn degree and appearance.

The burns are mapped over the body by degree. The "rule of nines" correlates specific body areas with percentage of body surface area. In an alternative method the patient's hand is used as an approximate measure of 1% of the body surface area. Separate diagrams are used for adults and children (Fig. 17–2). The total percentage of body surface area burned is the sum of the second- and third-degree burn areas over the body and indicates the

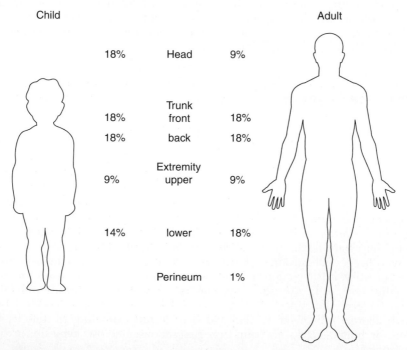

Child		Adult
18%	Head	9%
18%	Trunk front	18%
18%	back	18%
9%	Extremity upper	9%
14%	lower	18%
	Perineum	1%

Figure 17–2. Rule of nines.

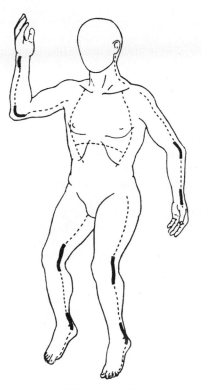

Figure 17–3. Escarotomy incisions. Parallel and medial/lateral incisions for extremities and digits; bilateral/lateral incisions for chest.

severity of the burn (major vs. minor). This is the percentage used in the calculation of fluid resuscitation (first-degree burns are mapped but not included in this calculation).

A resuscitative intervention that is performed based on the findings of the secondary survey is the escharotomy.[5] Circumferential third-degree burns of the extremities (including the digits) and chest can apply tourniquet-type pressure, compromising blood flow and chest wall compliance, respectively. The solution is to perform "tourniquet" release by cutting through the eschar along parallel lines (Fig. 17–3).[6] The incisions are carried only through the eschar and not to the fascia. Electrocautery is particularly useful for this purpose and anticipates the need to stop potential subcutaneous bleeding. Burned extremities should be elevated to reduce the development of edema. Fasciotomy is indicated for intramuscular compartment pressures greater than 30 torr but is *not* a part of escharotomy.

Tetanus status is determined, and tetanus toxoid is administered as necessary. Patients without a current tetanus immunization series must receive tetanus immunoglobulin in addition to the complete series given over the ensuing several months. Prophylactic antibiotics are not recommended; they do not prevent infection, and they promote colonization of the wounds by resistant organisms.

Pain management is essential, and morphine is administered liberally for patient comfort, particularly during the initial dressing application and changes.

Initial wound debridement is limited. Only blisters that compromise function (e.g., over joints) are unroofed. Wounds are dressed using silver sulfadiazine cream and gauze. Silver sulfadiazine has moderate wound penetration and an acceptable antibacterial coverage (it is less effective against *Staphylococcus*). It prevents burn wound infection, and the gauze provides coverage and absorption. It is helpful to place a single-sheet gauze layer on the wound as a lattice to hold the silver sulfadiazine cream. The dressings help to decrease pain, heat, and fluid loss. Definitive wound management involves tangential or full excision of burned tissue followed by skin grafting.

Early nutrition affects the long-term outcome. A nasogastric tube is placed during the first 24 to 48 hours to decompress the stomach in the presence of burn ileus mediated by catecholamines and the edema of fluid resuscitation. Enteral feeds are then started, preferably using a nasoduodenal feeding tube. Nutritional support and prevention of infection are key elements in managing the burn hypermetabolism that is generated 5 to 7 days after the burn by the needs of burn wound healing and inflammation.

Resuscitation and surveys continue from the initial point of patient care to the critical care area and typically last 24 to 36 hours, depending on the severity of the burn, coincident trauma, and underlying co-morbidities. Capillary integrity is usually reestablished at 24 hours, at which time free water and colloid replacement can be started. Amounts used are based on a calculation of deficits.

Rehabilitation is integrated into care from the moment the patient enters the system. Form, represented by a healed patient with closed wounds, is quite distinct from function. Early range of motion exercises, both passive and active, are critical for long-term function.

As resuscitation progresses, a decision must be made about the best place for the patient to receive comprehensive burn care. Criteria for patient transfer to a burn center include:

>20% body surface area with second- and third-degree burns
>10% body surface area with second- and third-degree burns at the extremes of age (<10 and >50 years of age)
>5% body surface area with third-degree burns
All patients with burns of the face, hands, feet, genitalia, perineum, or major joints
Electrical (and lightning) injuries
Inhalation injury
Any percentage of second- and third-degree burns with preexisting co-morbidity or coincident mechanical trauma that complicates management

Complete patient healing requires normalization of the physiology, coverage of the wounds, and rehabilitation sufficient to return the patient as close as possible to his or her pre-burn functional level. Multidisciplinary care is the best way to accomplish these goals.

References

1. Demling RH: Burn care in the immediate resuscitation period. *In* Wilmore D (ed): Care of the Surgical Patient, 3rd ed, Vol. I. New York, Scientific American, 1995.

2. Morehouse JD, Finkelstein JL, Marano MA, Madden MR, Goodwin CW: Resuscitation of the thermally injured patient. Crit Care Clin 1989;8(2):355–365.
3. Warden GD: Burn shock resuscitation. World J Surg 1992;16:16–23.
4. Demling RH: Burn care in the early postresuscitation period. *In* Wilmore D (ed): Care of the Surgical Patient, 3rd ed, Vol. 2. New York, Scientific American, 1995.
5. Hammond JS, Ward CG: Complications of the burn injury. Crit Care Clin 1982;1(1):175–187.
6. Zawacki BE: Burns. *In* Donavan AJ (ed): Trauma Surgery: Techniques in Thoracic, Abdominal, and Vascular Surgery. St. Louis, Mosby-Year Book, 1994, p. 263.

Chapter 18

Organ Injury Scoring Systems

Proper documentation is necessary not only from a medicolegal point-of-view but also because it is crucial for valid clinical research. Unfortunately, the International Classification of Disease (ICD-9) does not provide detailed categories for most injuries, thereby limiting the validity of most retrospective studies. In 1989, a committee of the American Association for the Surgery of Trauma (AAST) began to develop injury scoring systems for various organs. Each level of injury of every organ or organ system also includes the ICD-9 codes representing the specific injury. If injuries are described according to these nationally accepted scoring systems, future research efforts will be not only far easier but also far more accurate. To that end, this chapter describes all of the AAST scoring systems available. The use of these grading systems should be encouraged both in dictated operative reports and in general discussion.

The Abbreviated Injury Scale—1990 Revision (AIS-90) for each injury is included in the tables.

Table 18–1. Splenic Injury Scale

Grade*	Type	Injury Description†	ICD-9	AIS-90
I.	Hematoma:	Subcapsular, <10% surface area	865.01 865.11	2
	Laceration:	Capsular tear, <1 cm parenchymal depth	865.02 865.12	
II.	Hematoma:	Subcapsular, 10% to 50% surface area; Intraparenchymal, <5 cm in diameter	865.01 865.11	2
	Laceration:	1–3 cm parenchymal depth that does not involve a trabecular vessel	865.02 865.12	2
III.	Hematoma:	Subcapsular, >50% surface area or expanding; Ruptured subcapsular hematoma with active bleeding; Intraparenchymal hematoma >2 cm or expanding		3
	Laceration:	>3 cm parenchymal depth or involving trabecular vessels	865.03 865.13	3
IV.	Laceration:	Laceration involving segmental or hilar vessels producing major devascularization (>25% of spleen)	865.04 865.14	4
V.	Laceration:	Completely shattered spleen	865.04 865.14	5
	Vascular:	Hilar vascular injury which devascularizes spleen		5

*Advance one grade for multiple injuries to the same organ.
†Based on most accurate assessment at autopsy, laparotomy, or radiologic study.
From Moore EE, Cogbill TH, Jurkovich GJ, et al: Organ injury scaling V: Spleen and liver. J Trauma 1995;38(3):323.

Table 18–2. Liver Injury Scale

Grade*	Type	Injury Description†	ICD-9	AIS-90
I.	Hematoma:	Subcapsular, nonexpanding, <10% surface area	864.01 864.11	2
	Laceration:	Capsular tear, <1 cm parenchymal depth	864.02 864.12	2
II.	Hematoma:	Subcapsular, 10% to 50% surface area Intraparenchymal, <10 cm in diameter	864.01 864.11	2
	Laceration:	1–3 cm parenchymal depth, <10 cm in length	864.03 864.13	2
III.	Hematoma:	Subcapsular, >50% surface area or expanding; Ruptured subcapsular hematoma; Intraparenchymal hematoma >10 cm or expanding		3
	Laceration:	>3 cm parenchymal depth	864.04 864.14	3
IV.	Hematoma:	Ruptured intraparenchymal hematoma with active bleeding		4
	Laceration:	>3 cm parenchymal disruption involving 25% to 75% of hepatic lobe or 1 to 3 Couinaud's segments within a single lobe	864.04 864.14	4
V.	Laceration:	Parenchymal disruption involving >75% of hepatic lobe or >3 Couinaud's segments within a single lobe		5
	Vascular:	Juxtahepatic venous injuries; i.e., retrohepatic vena cava/major hepatic veins		5
VI.	Vascular:	Hepatic avulsion		6

ᵃAdvance one grade for multiple injuries to the same organ.
†Based on most accurate assessment at autopsy, laparotomy, or radiologic study.
From Moore EE, Cogbill TH, Jurkovich GJ, et al: Organ injury scaling V: Spleen and liver. J Trauma 1995;38(3):323.

Table 18–3. Extrahepatic Biliary Tree Injury Scale

Grade*	Injury Description	ICD-9	AIS-90
I.	Gallbladder contusion	868.02	2
	Portal triad contusion	868.02	2
II.	Partial gallbladder avulsion from liver bed; cystic duct intact	868.02	2
	Laceration or perforation of the gallbladder	868.12	2
III.	Complete gallbladder avulsion from liver bed	868.02	3
	Cystic duct laceration/transectoin	868.12	3
IV.	Partial or complete right hepatic duct laceration	868.12	3
	Partial or complete left hepatic duct laceration	868.12	3
	Partial common hepatic duct laceration (≤ 50%)	868.12	3
	Partial common bile duct laceration (≤ 50%)	868.12	3
V.	>50% transection of common hepatic duct	868.12	3–4
	>50% transection of common bile duct	868.12	3–4
	Combined right and left hepatic duct injuries	868.12	3–4
	Intraduodenal or intrapancreatic bile duct injuries	868.12	3–4

*Advance one grade for multiple injuries up to Grade III.
From Moore EE, Jurkovich GJ, Knudson M, et al: Organ injury scaling VI: Extrahepatic biliary, esophagus, stomach, vulva, vagina, uterus (non-pregnant), uterus (pregnant), fallopian tube, and ovary. J Trauma 1995;39(6):1069.

Table 18–4. Pancreatic Organ Injury Scale

Grade*	Type	Injury Description†	ICD-9	AIS-90
I.	Hematoma:	Minor contusion without duct injury	863.81–863.84	2
	Laceration:	Superficial laceration without duct injury		2
II.	Hematoma:	Major contusion without duct injury or tissue loss	863.81–863.84	2
	Laceration:	Major laceration without duct injury or tissue loss		3
III.	Laceration:	Distal transection or parenchymal injury with duct injury	863.92–863.94	3
IV.	Laceration:	Proximal[a] transection or parenchymal injury involving ampulla	863.91	4
V.	Laceration:	Massive disruption of pancreatic head	863.91	5

.81, .91 = Head; .82, .92 = Body; .83, .93 = Tail

*Advance one grade for multiple injuries to the same organ.
†Based on most accurate assessment at autopsy, laparotomy, or radiologic study.
[a]Proximal pancreas is to the patients' right of the superior mesenteric vein.
From Moore EE, Cogbill TH, Malangoni MA, et al: Organ injury scaling II: Pancreas, duodenum, small bowel, colon and rectum. J Trauma 1990;30(11):1427.

Table 18–5. Adrenal Organ Injury Scale

Grade*	Injury Description	ICD-9	AIS-90
I.	Contusion	868.01/.11	1
II.	Laceration involving only cortex (<2 cm)	868.01/.11	1
III.	Laceration extending into medulla (≥2 cm)	868.01/.11	2
IV.	>50% parenchymal disruption	868.01/.11	2
V.	Total parenchymal destruction (including massive intraparenchymal hemorrhage) Avulsion from blood supply	868.01/.11	3

*Advance one grade for multiple injuries up to Grade V.
From Moore EE, Malangoni MA, Cogbill TA, et al: Organ injury scaling VII: Cervical vascular, peripheral vascular, adrenal, penis, testes, and scrotum. J Trauma 1996;41(3):523.

Table 18–6. Esophagus Injury Scale

Grade*	Injury Description	ICD-9	AIS-90
I.	Contusion/hematoma	862.22/.32	2
	Partial-thickness laceration	862.22/.32	3
II.	Laceration ≤50% circumference	862.22/.32	4
III.	Laceration >50% circumference	862.22/.32	4
IV.	Segmental loss or devascularization ≤2 cm	862.22/.32	5
V.	Segmental loss or devascularization >2 cm	862.22/.32	5

*Advance one grade for multiple injuries up to Grade III.
From Moore EE, Jurkovich GJ, Knudson M, et al: Organ injury scaling VI: Extrahepatic biliary, esophagus, stomach, vulva, vagina, uterus (non-pregnant), uterus (pregnant), fallopian tube, and ovary. J Trauma 1995;39(6):1069.

Table 18–7. Stomach Injury Scale

Grade*	Injury Description	ICD-9	AIS-90
I.	Contusion/hematoma	863.0/.1	2
	Partial-thickness injury	863.0/.1	2
II.	Laceration ≤ 2 cm in GE junction or pylorus	863.0/.1	3
	≤ 5 cm in proximal one third of stomach	863.0/.1	3
	≤ 10 cm in distal two thirds of stomach	863.0/.1	3
III.	Laceration > 2 cm in GE junction or pylorus	863.0/.1	3
	> 5 cm in proximal one third of stomach	863.0/.1	3
	> 10 cm in distal two thirds of stomach	863.0/.1	3
IV.	Tissue loss or devascularization ≤ two thirds of stomach	863.0/.1	4
V.	Tissue loss or devascularization > two thirds of stomach	863.0/.1	4

GE, gastroesophageal.
*Advance one grade for multiple injuries up to Grade III.
From Moore EE, Jurkovich GJ, Knudson M, et al: Organ injury scaling VI: Extrahepatic biliary, esophagus, stomach, vulva, vagina, uterus (non-pregnant), uterus (pregnant), fallopian tube, and ovary. J Trauma 1995;39(6):1069.

Table 18–8. Duodenum Organ Injury Scale

Grade*	Type	Injury Description†	ICD-9	AIS-90
I.	Hematoma:	Involving single portion of duodenum	863.21	2
	Laceration:	Partial thickness, no perforation	863.21	3
II.	Hematoma:	Involving more than one portion	863.21	2
	Laceration:	Disruption <50% of circumference	863.31	4
III.	Laceration:	Disruption 50% to 75% circumference of D2†	863.31	4
		Disruption 50% to 100% circumference of D1, D3, D4‡		4
IV.	Laceration:	Disruption >75% circumference of D2‡	863.31	5
		Involving ampulla or distal common bile duct		5
V.	Laceration:	Massive disruption of duodenopancreatic complex	863.31	5
	Vascular:	Devascularization of duodenum	863.31	5

*Advance one grade for multiple injuries to the same organ.
†Based on most accurate assessment at autopsy, laparotomy, or radiologic study.
‡D1 = first portion duodenum, D2 = second portion duodenum, D3 = third portion duodenum, D4 = fourth portion duodenum.
From Moore EE, Cogbill TH, Malangoni MA, et al: Organ injury scaling II: Pancreas, duodenum, small bowel, colon and rectum. J Trauma 1990;30(11):1427.

Table 18–9. Small Bowel Organ Injury Scale

Grade*	Type	Injury Description†	ICD-9	AIS-90
I.	Hematoma:	Contusion or hematoma without devascularization	863.20	2
	Laceration:	Partial thickness, no perforation	863.20	2
II.	Laceration:	Laceration <50% of circumference	863.30	3
III.	Laceration:	Laceration ≥50% of circumference without transection	863.30	3
IV.	Laceration:	Transection of the small bowel	863.30	4
V.	Laceration:	Transection of the small bowel with segmental tissue loss	863.30	4
	Vascular:	Devascularized segment	863.30	4

*Advance one grade for multiple injuries to the same organ.
†Based on most accurate assessment at autopsy, laparotomy, or radiologic study.
From Moore EE, Cogbill TH, Malangoni MA, et al: Organ injury scaling II: Pancreas, duodenum, small bowel, colon and rectum. J Trauma 1990;30(11):1427.

Table 18–10. Colon Organ Injury Scale

Grade*	Type	Injury Description†	ICD-9	AIS-90
I.	Hematoma:	Contusion or hematoma without devascularization	863.40–863.44	2
	Laceration:	Partial thickness, no perforation	863.40–863.44	2
II.	Laceration:	Laceration <50% of circumference	863.50–863.54	3
III.	Laceration:	Laceration ≥50% of circumference without transection	863.50–863.54	3
IV.	Laceration:	Transection of the colon	863.50–863.54	4
V.	Laceration:	Transection of the colon with segmental tissue loss	863.50–863.54	4
	Vascular:	Devascularized segment	863.50–863.54	4

.41, .51 = Ascending; .42, .52 = Transverse; .43, .53 = Descending; .44, .54 = Rectum

*Advance one grade for multiple injuries to the same organ.
†Based on most accurate assessment at autopsy, laparotomy, or radiologic study.
From Moore EE, Cogbill TH, Malangoni MA, et al: Organ injury scaling II: Pancreas, duodenum, small bowel, colon and rectum. J Trauma 1990;30(11):1427.

Table 18–11. Rectal Organ Injury Scale

Grade*	Type	Injury Description†	ICD-9	AIS-90
I.	Hematoma:	Contusion or hematoma without devascularization	863.45	2
	Laceration:	Partial thickness laceration	863.45	2
II.	Laceration:	Laceration <50% of circumference	863.55	3
III.	Laceration:	Laceration ≥50% of circumference	863.55	4
IV.	Laceration:	Full-thickness laceration with extension into the perineum	863.55	5
V.	Vascular	Devascularized segment	863.55	5

*Advance one grade for multiple injuries to the same organ.
†Based on most accurate assessment at autopsy, laparotomy, or radiologic study.
From Moore EE, Cogbill TH, Malangoni MA, et al: Organ injury scaling II: Pancreas, duodenum, small bowel, colon and rectum. J Trauma 1990;30(11):1427.

Table 18–12. Renal Injury Scale

Grade*	Type	Injury Description†	ICD-9	AIS-90
I.	Contusion:	Microscopic or gross hematuria; urologic studies normal		2
	Hematoma:	Subcapsular, nonexpanding without parenchymal laceration	866.01 866.11	2
II.	Hematoma:	Nonexpanding perirenal hematoma confined to renal retroperitoneum	866.01	2
	Laceration:	<1.0 cm parenchymal depth of renal cortex without urinary extravasation	866.02 866.12	2
III.	Laceration:	>1.0 cm parenchymal depth of renal cortex without collecting system rupture or urinary extravasation	866.02 866.12	3
IV.	Laceration:	Parenchymal laceration extending through the renal cortex, medulla, and collecting system		4
	Vascular:	Main renal artery or vein injury with contained hemorrhage		4
V.	Laceration:	Completely shattered kidney	866.03	5
	Vascular:	Avulsion of renal hilum which devascularizes kidney	866.13	5

*Advance one grade for multiple injuries to the same organ.
†Based on most accurate assessment at autopsy, laparotomy, or radiologic study.
From Moore EE, Cogbill TH, Jurkovich GJ, et al: Organ injury scaling III: Chest wall, abdominal vascular, ureter, bladder, and urethra. J Trauma 1992;33(3):337.

Table 18–13. Ureter Organ Injury Scale

Grade*	Type	Injury Description†	ICD-90	AIS-90
I.	Hematoma:	Contusion of hematoma without devascularization	867.2–867.3	2
II.	Laceration:	<50% transection	867.2–867.3	2
III.	Laceration:	>50% transection	867.2–867.3	3
IV.	Laceration:	Complete transection with 2 cm devascularization	867.2–867.3	3
V.	Laceration:	Avulsion with >2 cm of devascularization	867.2–867.3	3

*Advance one grade for multiple injuries to the same organ.
†Based on most accurate assessment at autopsy, laparotomy, or radiologic study.
From Moore EE, Cogbill TH, Jurkovich GJ, et al: Organ injury scaling III: Chest wall, abdominal vascular, ureter, bladder, and urethra. J Trauma 1992;33(3):337.

Table 18–14. Bladder Organ Injury Scale

Grade*	Type	Injury Description†	ICD-9	AIS-90
I.	Hematoma:	Contusion, intramural hematoma	867.0–867.1	2
	Laceration:	Partial thickness		3
II.	Laceration:	Extraperitoneal bladder wall laceration <2 cm	867.0–867.1	4
III.	Laceration:	Extraperitoneal (>2 cm) or intraperitoneal (<2 cm) bladder wall lacerations	867.0–867.1	4
IV.	Laceration:	Intraperitoneal bladder wall laceration >2 cm	867.0–867.1	4
V.	Laceration:	Intra- or extraperitoneal bladder wall laceration extending into the bladder neck or ureteral orifice (trigone)	867.0–867.1	4

*Advance one grade for multiple injuries to the same organ.
†Based on most accurate assessment at autopsy, laparotomy, or radiologic study.
From Moore EE, Cogbill TH, Jurkovich GJ, et al: Organ injury scaling III: Chest wall, abdominal vascular, ureter, bladder, and urethra. J Trauma 1992;33(3):337.

Table 18–15. Urethra Organ Injury Scale

Grade*	Type	Injury Description†	ICD-9	AIS-90
I.	Contusion:	Blood at urethral meatus; urethrograph normal	867.0–867.1	2
II.	Stretch injury:	Elongation of urethra without extravasation on urethrograph	867.0–867.1	2
III.	Partial disruption:	Extravasation of urethrograph contrast at injury site with contrast visualized in the bladder	867.0–867.1	2
IV.	Complete disruption:	Extravasation of urethrograph contrast at injury site without visualization in the bladder; <2 cm of urethral separation	867.0–867.1	3
V.	Complete disruption:	Complete transection with >2 cm urethral separation, or extension into the prostate or vagina	867.0–867.1	4

*Advance one grade if multiple lesions/injuries exist.
†Based on most accurate assessment at autopsy, laparotomy, or radiologic study.
From Moore EE, Cogbill TH, Jurkovich GJ, et al: Organ injury scaling III: Chest wall, abdominal vascular, ureter, bladder, and urethra. J Trauma 1992;33(3):337.

Table 18–16. Vulva Injury Scale

Grade*	Injury Description	ICD-9	AIS-90
I.	Contusion/hematoma	922.4	1
II.	Laceration—superficial (skin only)	878.4	1
III.	Laceration—deep (into fat/muscle)	878.4	2
IV.	Avulsion—skin, fat, muscle	878.5	3
V.	Injury into adjacent organs (anus/rectum/urethra/bladder)	878.5	3

*Advance one grade for multiple injuries up to Grade III.
From Moore EE, Jurkovich GJ, Knudson M, et al: Organ injury scaling VI: Extrahepatic biliary, esophagus, stomach, vulva, vagina, uterus (non-pregnant), uterus (pregnant), fallopian tube, and ovary. J Trauma 1995;39(6):1069.

Table 18–17. Vagina Injury Scale

Grade*	Injury Description	ICD-9	AIS-90
I.	Contusion/hematoma	922.4	1
II.	Laceration—superficial (mucosa only)	878.6	1
III.	Laceration—deep (into fat/muscle)	878.6	2
IV.	Laceration—complex, into cervix or peritoneum	878.7	3
V.	Injury into adjacent organs (anus/rectum/urethra/bladder)	878.7	3

*Advance one grade for multiple injuries up to Grade III.
From Moore EE, Jurkovich GJ, Knudson M, et al: Organ injury scaling VI: Extrahepatic biliary, esophagus, stomach, vulva, vagina, uterus (non-pregnant), uterus (pregnant), fallopian tube, and ovary. J Trauma 1995;39(6):1069.

Table 18–18. Uterus (Non-pregnant) Injury Scale

Grade*	Injury Description	ICD-9	AIS-90
I.	Contusion/hematoma	867.4/.5	2
II.	Superficial laceration (≤1 cm)	867.4/.5	2
III.	Deep laceration (>1 cm)	867.4/.5	3
IV.	Laceration involving uterine artery	902.55	3
V.	Avulsion/devascularized	867.4/.5	3

*Advance one grade for multiple injuries up to Grade III.
From Moore EE, Jurkovich GJ, Knudson M, et al: Organ injury scaling VI: Extrahepatic biliary, esophagus, stomach, vulva, vagina, uterus (non-pregnant), uterus (pregnant), fallopian tube, and ovary. J Trauma 1995;39(6):1069.

Table 18–19. Uterus (Pregnant) Injury Scale

Grade*	Injury Description	ICD-9	AIS-90
I.	Contusion/hematoma (without placental abruption)	867.4/.5	2
II.	Superficial laceration (≤1 cm) or partial placental abruption <25%	867.4/.5	3
III.	Deep laceration (>1 cm) occurring in second trimester or placental abruption >25% but <50%	867.4/.5	3
	Deep laceration (>1 cm) in third trimester	867.4/.5	4
IV.	Laceration involving uterine artery	902.55	4
	Deep laceration (>1 cm) with >50% placental abruption	867.4/.5	4
V.	Uterine rupture		
	-second trimester	867.4/.5	4
	-third trimester	867.4/.5	5
	Complete placental abruption	867.4/.5	4–5

*Advance one grade for multiple injuries up to Grade III.
From Moore EE, Jurkovich GJ, Knudson M, et al: Organ injury scaling VI: Extrahepatic biliary, esophagus, stomach, vulva, vagina, uterus (non-pregnant), uterus (pregnant), fallopian tube, and ovary. J Trauma 1995;39(6):1069.

Table 18–20. Fallopian Tube Injury Scale

Grade*	Injury Description	ICD-9	AIS-90
I.	Contusion/hematoma	867.6/.7	2
II.	Laceration (≤50% circumference)	867.6/.7	2
III.	Laceration (>50% circumference)	867.6/.7	2
IV.	Transection	867.6/.7	2
V.	Vascular—devascularized segment	902.89	2

*Advance one grade for multiple injuries up to Grade III.
Moore EE, Jurkovich GJ, Knudson M, et al: Organ injury scaling VI: Extrahepatic biliary, esophagus, stomach, vulva, vagina, uterus (non-pregnant), uterus (pregnant), fallopian tube, and ovary. J Trauma 1995;39(6):1069.

Table 18–21. Ovary Injury Scale

Grade*	Injury Description	ICD-9	AIS-90
I.	Contusion/hematoma	867.6/.7	1
II.	Superficial laceration (depth ≤0.5 cm)	867.6/.7	2
III.	Deep laceration (depth >0.5 cm)	867.6/.7	3
IV.	Partial disruption of blood supply	902.81	3
V.	Avulsion or complete parenchymal disruption	902.81	3

*Advance one grade for multiple injuries up to Grade III.
From Moore EE, Jurkovich GJ, Knudson M, et al: Organ injury scaling VI: Extrahepatic biliary, esophagus, stomach, vulva, vagina, uterus (non-pregnant), uterus (pregnant), fallopian tube, and ovary. J Trauma 1995;39(6):1069.

Table 18–22. Penis Injury Scale

Grade*	Injury Description	ICD-9	AIS-90
I.	Cutaneous laceration/contusion	911.0/922.4	1
II.	Buck's fascia (cavernosum) laceration without tissue loss	878.0	1
III.	Cutaneous avulsion	878.1	3
	Laceration through glans/meatus		
	Cavernosal or urethral defect < 2 cm		
IV.	Partial penectomy	878.1	3
	Cavernosal or urethral defect ≥ 2 cm		
V.	Total penectomy	878.1	3

*Advance one grade for multiple injuries up to Grade III.
From Moore EE, Malangoni MA, Cogbill TA, et al: Organ injury scaling VII: Cervical vascular, peripheral vascular, adrenal, penis, testis, and scrotum. J Trauma 1996;41(3):523.

Table 18–23. Testis Injury Scale

Grade*	Injury Description	ICD-9	AIS-90
I.	Contusion/hematoma	911.0/922.4	1
II.	Subclinical laceration of tunica albuguinea	922.4	1
III.	Laceration of tunica albuguinea with <50% parenchymal loss	878.2	2
IV.	Major laceration of tunica albuguinea with ≥50% parenchymal loss	878.3	2
V.	Total testicular destruction or avulsion	878.3	2

*Advance one grade for multiple injuries up to Grade V.
From Moore EE, Malangoni MA, Cogbill TA, et al: Organ injury scaling VII: Cervical vascular, peripheral vascular, adrenal, penis, testis, and scrotum. J Trauma 1996;41(3):523.

Table 18–24. Scrotum Injury Scale

Grade	Injury Description	ICD-9	AIS-90
I.	Contusion/hematoma	922.4	1
II.	Laceration <25% of scrotal diameter	878.2	1
III.	Laceration ≥25% of scrotal diameter or stellate	878.3	2
IV.	Avulsion < 50%	878.3	2
V.	Avulsion ≥ 50%	878.3	2

From Moore EE, Malangoni MA, Cogbill TA, et al: Organ injury scaling VII: Cervical vascular, peripheral vascular, adrenal, penis, testis, and scrotum. J Trauma 1996;41(3):523.

Table 18–25. Chest Wall Organ Injury Scale*

Grade†	Type	Injury Description	ICD-9	AIS-90
I.	Contusion:	Any size	911.0/922.1	1
	Laceration:	Skin and subcutaneous	875.0	1
	Facture:	<3 ribs, closed	807.01/807.02	1–2
		Nondisplaced clavicle, closed	810.00–810.03	2
II.	Laceration:	Skin subcutaneous and muscle	875.1	1
	Fracture:	≥3 adjacent ribs, closed	807.03–807.09	2–3
		Open or displaced clavicle	810.10–810.13	2
		Nondisplaced sternum, closed	807.2	2
		Scapular body, open or closed	811.00–811.19	2
III.	Laceration:	Full thickness including pleural penetration	862.29	2
				2
	Fracture:	Open or displaced sternum; flail sternum	807.2/807.3	3–4
		Unilateral flail segment, (<3 ribs)	807.4	
IV.	Laceration:	Avulsion of chest wall tissues with underlying rib fractures	807.10–807.19	4
	Fracture:	Unilateral flail chest, (≥3 ribs)	807.4	3–4
V.	Fracture:	Bilateral flail chest; (≥3 ribs on both sides)	807.4	5

*This scale is confined to the chest wall alone and does not reflect associated internal thoracic or abdominal injuries. Therefore, further delineation of upper versus lower or anterior versus posterior chest wall was not considered, and a grade VI was not warranted. Specifically, thoracic crush was not used as a descriptive term; instead, the geography and extent of fractures and soft tissue injury were used to define the grade.
†Upgrade by one grade for bilateral injuries.
From Moore EE, Cogbill TH, Jurkovich GJ, et al: Organ injury scaling III: Chest wall, abdominal vascular, ureter, bladder, and urethra. J Trauma 1992;33(3):337.

Table 18–26. Lung Organ Injury Scale

Grade*	Type	Injury Description†	ICD-9	AIS-90
I.	Contusion:	Unilateral, <1 lobe	861.12/861.31	3
II.	Contusion:	Unilateral, single lobe	861.20/861.30	3
	Laceration:	Simple pneumothorax	860.0/1 860.4/5	3
III.	Contusion:	Unilateral, >1 lobe	861.20/861.30	3
	Laceration:	Persistent (>72 hours), airleak from distal airway	860.0/1 860.4/5 862.0/861.30	3–4
	Hematoma:	Nonexpanding intraparenchymal		
IV.	Laceration:	Major (segmental or lobar) airway leak	862.21/861.31	4–5
	Hematoma:	Expanding intraparenchymal		
	Vascular:	Primary branch intrapulmonary vessel disruption	901.40	3–5
V.	Vascular:	Hilar vessel disruption	901.41/901.42	4
VI.	Vascular:	Total, uncontained transection of pulmonary hilum	901.41/901.42	4

*Advance one grade for bilateral injuries; hemothorax is graded according to the thoracic vascular organ injury scale (OIS) (see Table 18–30).
†Based on most accurate assessment at autopsy, laparotomy, or radiologic study.
From Moore EE, Malangoni MA, Cogbill TH, et al: Organ injury scaling IV: Thoracic vascular, lung, cardiac, and diaphragm. J Trauma 1994;36(3):299.

Table 18–27. Diaphragm Organ Injury Scale

Grade*	Injury Description	ICD-9	AIS-90
I.	Contusion	862.0	2
II.	Laceration ≤2 cm	862.1	3
III.	Laceration 2–10 cm	862.1	3
IV.	Laceration >10 cm with tissue loss ≤25 cm²	862.1	3
V.	Laceration with tissue loss >25 cm²	862.1	3

*Advance one grade for bilateral injuries.
From Moore EE, Malangoni MA, Cogbill TH, et al: Organ injury scaling IV: Thoracic vascular, lung, cardiac, and diaphragm. J Trauma 1994;36(3):299.

Table 18–28. Cardiac Injury Organ Scale

Grade*	Injury Description	ICD-9	AIS-90
I.	Blunt cardiac injury with minor ECG abnormality (nonspecific ST or T wave changes, premature atrial, ventricular contraction or persistent sinus tachycardia)	861.01	3
	Blunt or penetrating pericardial wound without cardiac injury, cardiac tamponade or cardiac herniation		
II.	Blunt cardiac injury with heart block (right or left bundle branch, left anterior fascicular, or atrioventricular) or ischemic changes (ST depression or T-wave inversion) without cardiac failure	861.01	3
	Penetrating tangential myocardial wound up to, but not extending through endocardium, without tamponade	861.12	3
III.	Blunt cardiac injury with sustained (≥5 beats/min) or multifocal ventricular contractions	861.01	3–4
	Blunt or penetrating cardiac injury with septal rupture, pulmonary or tricuspid valvular incompetence, papillary muscle dysfunction, or distal coronary arterial occlusion without cardiac failure	861.01	3–4
	Blunt pericardial laceration with cardiac herniation		
	Blunt cardiac injury with cardiac failure	861.01	3–4
	Penetrating tangential myocardial wound up to, but not extending through endocardium, with tamponade	861.12	3
IV.	Blunt or penetrating cardiac injury with septal rupture, pulmonary or tricuspid valvular incompetence, papillary muscle dysfunction or distal coronary arterial occlusion producing cardiac failure	861.12	3
	Blunt or penetrating cardiac injury with aortic or mitral valve incompetence		
	Blunt or penetrating cardiac injury of the right ventricle, right atrium, or left atrium	861.03 861.13	5
V.	Blunt or penetrating cardiac injury with proximal coronary arterial occlusion		
	Blunt or penetrating left ventricular perforation	861.03 861.13	5
	Stellate injuries <50% tissue loss of the right ventricle, right atrium or left atrium	861.03 861.13	5
VI.	Blunt avulsion of the heart; penetrating wound producing >50% tissue loss of a chamber		6

*Advance one grade for multiple penetrating wounds to a single chamber or multiple chamber involvement.
From Moore EE, Malangoni MA, Cogbill TH, et al: Organ injury scaling IV: Thoracic vascular, lung, cardiac, and diaphragm. J Trauma 1994;36(3):299.

Table 18–29. Cervical Vascular Organ Injury Scale

Grade*	Injury Description	ICD-9	AIS-90
I.	Thyroid veins	900.8	
	Common facial vein	900.8	
	External jugular vein	900.81	1–3
	Non-named arterial/venous branches	900.9	
II.	External carotid arterial branches (ascending pharyngeal, superior thyroid, lingual, facial, maxillary, occipital, posterior auricular)	900.8	
	Thyrocervical trunk or primary branches	900.8	
	Internal jugular vein	900.1	1–3
III.	External carotid artery	900.02	2–3
	Subclavian vein	901.3	3–4
	Vertebral artery	900.8	2–4
IV.	Common carotid artery	900.01	3–5
	Subclavian artery	901.1	3–4
V.	Internal carotid artery (extracranial)	900.03	3–5

*Increase one grade for multiple Grade III or IV injuries involving >50% vessel circumference. Decrease one grade for <25% vessel circumference disruption for Grades IV or V.

From Moore EE, Malangoni MA, Cogbill TH, et al: Organ injury scaling VII: Cervical vascular, peripheral vascular, adrenal, penis, testis, and scrotum. J Trauma 1996;41(3):523.

Table 18–30. Thoracic Vascular Organ Injury Scale

Grade*	Injury Description†	ICD-9	AIS-90
I.	Intercostal artery/vein	901.81	2–3
	Internal mammary artery/vein	901.82	2–3
	Bronchial artery/vein	901.89	2–3
	Esophageal artery/vein	901.9	2–3
	Hemizygous vein	901.89	2–3
	Unnamed artery/vein	901.9	2–3
II.	Azygous vein	901.89	2–3
	Internal jugular vein	900.1	2–3
	Subclavian vein	901.3	3–4
	Innominate vein	901.3	3–4
III.	Carotid artery	900.01	3–5
	Innominate artery	901.1	3–4
	Subclavian artery	901.1	3–4
IV.	Thoracic aorta, descending	901.0	4–5
	Inferior vena cava (intrathoracic)	902.10	3–4
	Pulmonary artery, primary intraparenchymal branch	901.41	3
	Pulmonary vein, primary intraparenchymal branch	901.42	3
V.	Thoracic aorta, ascending and arch	901.0	5
	Superior vena cava	901.2	3–4
	Pulmonary artery, main trunk	901.41	4
	Pulmonary vein, main trunk	901.42	4
VI.	Uncontained total transection of thoracic aorta or pulmonary hilum	901.0	5

*Increase one grade for multiple Grade III or IV injuries if >50% circumference; decrease one grade for Grade IV or V injuries if <25% circumference.

†Based on most accurate assessment at autopsy, laparotomy, or radiologic study.

From Moore EE, Malangoni MA, Cogbill TH, et al: Organ injury scaling IV: Thoracic vascular, lung, cardiac, and diaphragm. J Trauma 1994;36(3):299.

Table 18–31. Abdominal Vascular Organ Injury Scale*

Grade†	Injury Description	ICD-9	AIS-90
I.	Non-named superior mesenteric artery or superior mesenteric vein branches	902.20–902.39	NS
	Non-named inferior mesenteric artery or inferior mesenteric vein branches	902.27–902.32	NS
	Phrenic artery/vein	902.89	NS
	Lumbar artery/vein	902.89	NS
	Gonadal artery/vein	902.89	NS
	Ovarian artery/vein	902.81–902.82	NS
	Other non-named small arterial or venous structures requiring ligation	902.90	NS
II.	Right, left or common hepatic artery	902.22	3
	Splenic artery/vein	902.23–902.34	3
	Right or left gastric arteries	902.21	3
	Gastroduodenal artery	902.24	3
	Inferior mesenteric artery, trunk or inferior mesenteric vein, trunk	902.27–902.32	3
	Primary named branches of mesenteric artery (e.g., ileocolic artery or mesenteric vein)	902.26–902.31	3
	Other named abdominal vessels requiring ligation/repair	902.89	3
III.	Superior mesenteric vein, trunk	902.31	3
	Renal artery/vein	902.41–902.42	3
	Iliac artery/vein	902.53–902.54	3
	Hypogastric artery/vein	902.51–902.52	3
	Vena cava, infrarenal	902.10	3
IV.	Superior mesenteric artery, trunk	902.25	3
	Celiac axis proper	902.24	3
	Vena cava, suprarenal and infrahepatic	902.10	3
	Aorta, infrarenal	902.00	4
V.	Portal vein	902.33	3
	Extraparenchymal hepatic vein	902.11	
	Hepatic vein		3
	Liver + veins		5
	Vena cava, retrohepatic or suprahepatic	902.19	5
	Aorta, suprarenal, subdiaphragmatic	902.00	4

*This classification system is applicable for extraparenchymal vascular injuries. If the vessel injury is within 2 cm of the organ parenchyma, refer to specific organ injury scale.

†Increase one grade for multiple Grade III or IV injuries involving >50% vessel circumference. Downgrade one grade if <25% vessel circumference laceration for Grade IV or V.

From Moore EE, Cogbill TH, Jurkovich GJ, et al: Organ injury scaling III: Chest wall, abdominal vascular, ureter, bladder, and urethra. J Trauma 1992;33(3):337.

Table 18–32. Peripheral Vascular Organ Injury Scale

Grade*	Injury Description	ICD-9	AIS-90
I.	Digital artery/vein	903.5	1–3
	Palmar artery/vein	903.4	1–3
	Deep palmar artery/vein	904.6	1–3
	Dorsalis pedis artery	904.7	1–3
	Plantar artery/vein	904.6	1–3
	Non-named arterial/venous branches	903.8/904.7	1–3
II.	Basilic/cephalic vein	903.8	1–3
	Saphenous vein	904.3	1–3
	Radial artery	903.2	1–3
	Ulnar artery	903.3	1–3
III.	Axillary vein	903.02	2–3
	Superficial/deep femoral vein	903.02	2–3
	Popliteal vein	904.42	2–3
	Brachial artery	903.1	2–3
	Anterior tibial artery	904.51/904.52	1–3
	Posterior tibial artery	904.53/904.54	1–3
	Peroneal artery	904.7	1–3
	Tibioperoneal trunk	904.7	2–3
IV.	Superficial/deep femoral artery	904.1/904.7	3–4
	Popliteal artery	904.41	2–3
V.	Axillary artery	903.01	2–3
	Common femoral artery	904.0	3–4

*Increase one grade for multiple Grade III or IV injuries involving >50% vessel circumference. Decrease one grade for <25% vessel circumference disruption for Grade IV or V.

From Moore EE, Malangoni MA, Cogbill TH, et al: Organ injury scaling VII: Cervical vascular, peripheral vascular, adrenal, penis, testis, and scrotum. J Trauma 1996;41(3):523.

References

1. Moore EE, Cogbill TH, Jurkovich GJ, et al: Organ injury scaling V: Spleen and liver (1994 revision). J Trauma 1995;38(3):323.
2. Moore EE, Cogbill TH, Malangoni MA, et al: Organ injury scaling II: Pancreas, duodenum, small bowel, colon and rectum. J Trauma 1990;30(11):1427.
3. Moore EE, Cogbill TH, Jurkovich GJ, et al: Organ injury scaling III: Chest wall, abdominal vascular, ureter, bladder, and urethra. J Trauma 1992;33(3):337.
4. Moore EE, Malangoni MA, Cogbill TH, et al: Organ injury scaling IV: Thoracic vascular, lung, cardiac, and diaphragm. J Trauma 1994;36(3):299.
5. Moore EE, Jurkovich GJ, Knudson M, et al: Organ injury scaling VI: Extrahepatic biliary, esophagus, stomach, vulva, vagina, uterus (non-pregnant), uterus (pregnant), fallopian tube, and ovary. J Trauma 1995;39(6):1069.
6. Moore EE, Malangoni MA, Cogbill TH, et al: Organ injury scaling VII: Cervical vascular, peripheral vascular, adrenal, penis, testis, and scrotum. J Trauma 1996;41(3):523.

Chapter 19

Approach to the Acute Abdomen

Abdominal pain is one of the most common conditions that call for prompt diagnosis and treatment. Specifically, "the acute abdomen" encompasses a clinical syndrome whose principal manifestation occurs in the abdominal area and requires prompt diagnosis and possible early surgical intervention. It is only through a thorough history and physical examination, combined with appropriate laboratory tests and imaging studies, that a diagnosis can be confirmed.

The patient with an acute abdomen requires a systematic approach. Early surgical consultation is warranted because many of the causes of the acute abdomen require prompt surgical treatment.[1] Undue delay in diagnosis and treatment can adversely affect patient outcome. During the last several decades there has been a considerable reduction in morbidity and mortality associated with acute abdominal diseases. There may be several reasons for this, including better access to medical care, more uniform standards of health care, use of antibiotics, recognition of the importance of fluid resuscitation, and adjunctive diagnostic modalities. However, the history and physical examination remain the most important tools in the diagnosis of the acute abdomen.

CHARACTERIZATION OF PAIN

The nature, severity, periodicity, progression, location, onset, factors that aggravate or alleviate, and past episodes of pain must be fully characterized because these often elucidate the underlying cause. Pain patterns in acute abdominal disorders have specific characteristics depending on the underlying clinical disorder. Abdominal pain is divided into visceral and parietal pain. Visceral pain is mediated primarily by afferent C fibers in the walls of the hollow viscera and in the capsules of solid organs. It is perceived as dull and continuous and is poorly localized. It is elicited by distention, direct inflammation, ischemia, or infiltration of nerves (as in a malignancy).[15] For example, in the case of a small bowel obstruction, luminal distention of a hollow viscus such as the small intestine, with associated smooth muscle contraction, leads to a diffuse, vague, poorly localized, deep pain in the midabdomen. It is possible to crush, cut, or tear intestines in the fully conscious patient without causing pain, yet excruciating pain often accompanies stretching or distention of the intestines or extensive contraction against resistance (e.g., in intestinal, biliary, renal colic).

In contrast to visceral pain, afferent C and A delta fibers mediate parietal pain. This type of pain is perceived as a sharp and well-localized sensation. It

The Acute Abdomen

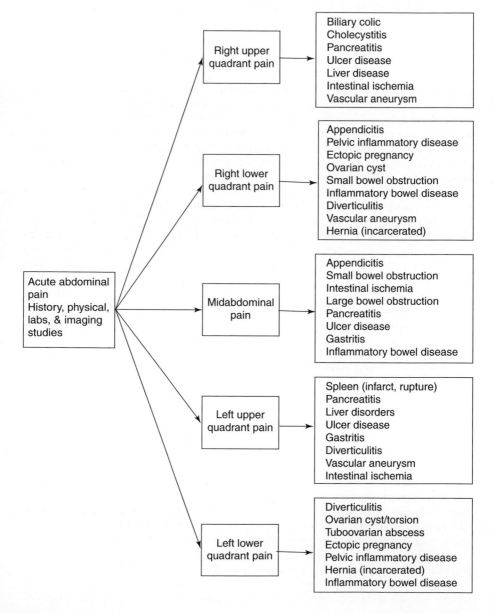

Diagnostic Pearls for the Acute Abdomen

Diagnosis	Key Pearls
Appendicitis	Emergent OR. Consider laparoscopy in females. CT scan in late presentation (>3 days of symptoms)
Pelvic inflammatory disease[2]	Antibiotics oral or IV depending on severity. OR for unresponsive cases.
Ectopic pregnancy[2]	Serial beta-human chorionic gonadotropin assays, pelvic sonography, and laparoscopy may be diagnostic. Treatment is surgical excision of implant.
Partial small bowel obstruction	Keep patient NPO and consider nasogastric tube (NGT). Follow serial exams and kidney-ureter-bladder (KUB) x-ray for evidence of progression or nonresolution that will require surgery.
Complete small bowel obstruction	Keep patient NPO or use NGT. Emergent OR may be necessary. Rule out carcinomatosis, inflammatory bowel disease, early postop bowel obstruction.
Inflammatory bowel disease[6]	Nonoperative treatment with steroids/sulfasalazine/cyclosporine in refractory cases. Flagyl for perianal Crohn's disease. Surgery reserved for obstruction/perforation/abscess/growth failure in children.
Diverticulitis	CT scan/antibiotics/(+/−) CT-guided abscess drainage. Surgery reserved for refractory cases or 4 to 6 weeks after resolution of symptoms.
Large bowel obstruction	Water-contrast enema is diagnostic. Sigmoid volvulus may be decompressed endoscopically, but it recurs in 50% of cases if surgery is not performed. Cecal volvulus may be decompressed endoscopically, but surgery is generally mandated with resection or cecopexy. Consider obstructing carcinoma.
Abdominal aortic aneurysm[12]	Emergent OR for suspected leak. Immediate vascular consultation in all suspected cases.
Mesenteric ischemia/ infarction	Emergent OR for suspected infarction. Suspected ischemia requires vascular consultation.
Strangulated/ incarcerated hernia	Emergent OR for suspected strangulation of all hernia types. Incarcerated hernias require surgical consultation with attempted reduction and elective repair.
Nephrourolithiasis	Flank pain, hematuria, costovertebral angle tenderness are prominent. Excretory urography is confirmatory.
Ulcer (perforated)	Emergent OR. KUB or upright chest x-ray usually reveals pneumoperitoneum.
Biliary colic	Cholelithiasis on right upper quadrant (RUQ) ultrasound. Fever and leukocytosis are absent. If patient is able to tolerate food PO, he may be sent home, with elective cholecystectomy scheduled.
Cholecystitis	Cholelithiasis on RUQ ultrasound. Fever and leukocytosis are present. Cholecystectomy should be performed.
Pancreatitis	Elevated amylase level. Choledocholithiasis or alcohol are usual causes. Patient is kept NPO, and endoscopic retrograde cholangiopancreatography may be performed. Elective cholecystectomy is scheduled when pancreatitis has resolved.
Liver disorder (laceration/tumor/ abscess)	Emergent surgical consultation for laceration/possible OR.
Splenic disorder (laceration/tumor/ abscess)	Emergent surgical consultation for laceration/possible OR.

is elicited by direct irritation of the parietal peritoneum, which is innervated by the somatic sensory nerves, corresponding to the cutaneous nerves. The pain may be exactly localized to a particular quadrant or to a very specific area of the abdomen. For example, a patient with a perforated appendix presents with evidence of localized peritonitis (i.e., pus in contact with the anterior visceral peritoneum with an associated inflammatory response) and demonstrates localized pain in the specific area of peritoneal irritation.

Some disorders demonstrate both visceral and parietal pain at different times in the progression of the disease. For example, in its classic presentation appendicitis begins with a poorly localized, vague, continuous, midepigastric pain associated with the obstructed appendiceal lumen. During the next several hours to days, this visceral pain may progress to a localized and sharp pain resulting from the inflamed appendix coming into direct contact with the parietal peritoneum, or from a perforated appendix and pus in contact with the peritoneum.

The character of the pain can provide useful clues to the underlying cause of the acute abdomen. Pain characterized as crescendo with intermittent intervals of relief, poorly localized, and deep-seated, is known as "colic pain," which physiologically reflects intermittent spasms of hollow smooth muscle structures. An example of this is nephrolithiasis with partial or complete obstruction of the ureter. Other examples of colicky pain include small bowel obstruction with spasmodic contraction of the proximal intestine against a fixed obstruction. Sharp, well-localized pain that is aggravated by movement best characterizes disease processes that directly involve the peritoneum, for example, by an inflammatory response such as that seen in perforated appendicitis, gangrenous bowel with perforation, or an intra-abdominal abscess in contact with the peritoneum. Other body fluids can cause inflammation of the peritoneum—for example, blood (hemoperitoneum from a ruptured abdominal aneurysm) and infected bile from a damaged bile duct. The patient with deep-seated, vaguely localized, and generalized abdominal pain who is unable to find a comfortable position that assuages the pain has pain characteristic of visceral ischemia. The deep-seated pain that is described as "boring" from the midepigastric region anteriorly to the back posteriorly is characteristic of pancreatitis but may also be seen in an eroding posterior duodenal ulcer.

The location of the pain may also provide clues to the underlying diagnosis (see Algorithm). Pain in the right and left upper quadrants may reflect a process that is thoracic in origin. A wide variety of thoracic processes such as pneumonia, exacerbation of chronic obstructive pulmonary disease, myocardial infarction, pneumothorax, and pulmonary embolus may result in an acute abdomen.[1] The history and physical examination as well as a high index of suspicion aid in separating these processes from true intra-abdominal conditions. In general, the location of the pain may give a clue to the underlying cause, such as a perforated appendicitis with focal right lower quadrant peritonitis. However, in many situations, the location does not accurately reflect the etiology. An example of this is a patient with right lower quadrant peritonitis after a perforated duodenal ulcer; the gastric contents track along the right paracolic gutter, producing focal peritonitis in the right lower quadrant. Once an inflammatory process has progressed to involve the entire peritoneum in the form of diffuse peritonitis, there are few clues to the underlying cause except from the history of onset and progression.[1] Early recognition of this particular entity is crucial because early surgical intervention is almost always warranted. The lower abdominal quadrants may be involved in females with processes involving the ovaries, oviducts, and uterus.[2] Pelvic examination is mandatory in all females of childbearing age or older.

The progression of the pain syndrome also plays an important role in evaluation of the acute abdomen. A rapidly progressive picture with associated systemic findings such as hypotension, tachycardia, and mental status change indicates a rapidly progressive intra-abdominal catastrophe that mandates immediate surgical consultation.[1] It should be stressed that initial efforts must be directed toward immediate resuscitation with no delay in performing definitive laparotomy, which may be both diagnostic and therapeutic. Abdominal pain syndromes with a more moderate presentation are more common and are characteristic of biliary disease (biliary colic or cholecystitis), pancreatitis, or such intestinal problems as appendicitis, bowel obstruction, or diverticulitis. Milder forms of abdominal pain with vague symptoms, little or no evidence of progression, and no associated symptoms may represent the earliest stage of an acute abdominal process or a nonsurgical process such as gastroenteritis. A period of observation may be warranted.

Finally, alleviating and aggravating factors in many instances may provide a clue to the underlying cause. Postprandial pain in the right upper quadrant in association with rich meals composed of high fat content or carbohydrate (dietary factor) may indicate a biliary cause. Pain that is alleviated by eating only to return in the postprandial state may indicate an ulcer diathesis. The past medical history should be explored for possible clues. An accurate drug history may reveal the cause of an acute abdominal pain syndrome, such as narcotic withdrawal or cocaine abuse. Pain coincidental with the menstrual cycle may suggest an ovarian process.

ASSOCIATED SYMPTOMS

Associated symptoms may also provide clues to the underlying cause of the acute abdomen. Vomiting is a prominent feature in most upper gastrointestinal causes but may also be a prominent feature in lower gastrointestinal processes, such as early appendicitis. In general, vomiting occurs in persons with disturbances of the small intestine. Most important of these are partial and complete small bowel obstructions, in which vomiting and acute abdominal pain are key features. In patients with small bowel obstruction, vomiting that occurs early in the development of pain may indicate a proximal obstruction, whereas vomiting that occurs later may indicate a more distally located obstruction. The nature of the vomiting may offer clues as well, such as bile staining, which indicates a process distal to the pylorus. Clear gastric vomitus is a key feature of gastric outlet obstruction as in pyloric stenosis or in advanced peptic ulcer disease, in which the pyloric channel is obstructed.[3]

Anorexia is a nonspecific associated symptom that is generally present in most patients with acute abdominal processes. Classically, anorexia that precedes the onset of midepigastric pain that later localizes to the right lower quadrant is an important component in the diagnosis of acute appendicitis.

Anorexia is also a prominent symptom when oral intake triggers acute abdominal pain or worsens preexisting pain, as in biliary processes, pancreatitis, or intestinal ischemia.

Constipation is not a prominent feature of the acute abdomen. Its presence may reflect a generalized ileus, which may be associated with any number of acute intra-abdominal processes. However, constipation in the absence of flatus is strongly associated with complete bowel obstruction, especially in the presence of accompanying abdominal pain, distention, and vomiting.

Diarrhea is generally characteristic of nonsurgical causes of the acute abdomen such as gastroenteritis. However, bloody diarrhea is characteristic of ischemic colitis, and in this setting, an acute intestinal vascular occlusion must be considered.[4] Other symptoms to be considered are jaundice (hepatobiliary disease), hematemesis (upper gastrointestinal disorders such as peptic ulcer disease), hematochezia (upper and lower gastrointestinal disorders such as peptic ulcer disease and diverticulitis), and finally, hematuria (urinary tract calculi), all of which may present with acute abdominal pain.

ADDITIONAL ELEMENTS IN THE HISTORY

Past medical and surgical histories, allergies, drugs, and time of the last meal are key elements in completing the history of the present illness. Specific attention paid to the medical history may produce clues to an underlying medical cause of the acute abdomen. However, a surgical cause for the acute abdomen must be excluded with a high degree of certainty before a nonsurgical diagnosis is considered. In this setting, early surgical consultation is warranted. A thorough medical history may alert the clinician to an underlying medical condition that may affect preoperative and postoperative care. For example, active cardiopulmonary or renal disease may require specific interventions such as placement of a right heart catheter or hemodialysis. Moreover, early medical consultation may be warranted preoperatively to maximize the patient's medical condition and minimize the risks of surgery.

PHYSICAL EXAMINATION

A complete physical examination is mandatory in all patients presenting with an acute abdomen. Special attention must be given to both the cardiopulmonary and the abdominal examinations. Initial vital signs should be observed, paying special attention to signs of shock (hypotension, tachycardia, tachypnea, and fever). Patients with an acute abdomen who are in shock require immediate surgical consultation because early surgical intervention may alter subsequent morbidity and mortality.

Cardiopulmonary examination of the patient with an acute abdomen should focus on signs that may account for the acute abdominal pain syndrome or indicate the presence of coexisting medical conditions. For example, the patient who presents with right upper quadrant pain, fever, productive sputum, and right basilar egophony, all of which suggest pulmonary consolidation, represents a variant presentation of primary bacterial pneumonia. The patient with diffuse peritonitis may demonstrate bilateral decreased breath sounds secondary to decreased diaphragmatic excursion resulting from pain. Special attention should be given to signs commonly elicited in patients with acute abdominal pain. Tachypnea may be an early sign of a compensated shock state resulting from an intra-abdominal process. Decreased respiratory excursion is commonly seen secondary to diaphragmatic irritation due to peritonitis. Tachycardia should also alert the physician to the possibility of a shock state or severe abdominal pain. Cardiac auscultatory abnormalities may be a clue to a decompensated cardiovascular status and may warrant more thorough preoperative consultation or intraoperative monitoring.

The abdominal examination should include the basic elements of inspection, auscultation, and palpation. Inspection should focus on obvious anatomic considerations such as prior surgical scars, distention, and abnormal contours that may be highly suggestive of an underlying diagnosis. For example, a tender mass in a surgical scar may suggest a bowel obstruction, or marked distention with dilated superficial veins on the anterior abdominal wall may suggest a diagnosis of cirrhosis and end-stage liver disease. Auscultation may be nonspecific; however, marked absence of bowel sounds or marked hyperactivity may be important clinical findings in the acute abdomen. The finding of tenderness on palpation is highly suggestive of an intra-abdominal process with associated peritoneal irritation. Early recognition of generalized peritonitis (diffuse tenderness on palpation and muscular rigidity) is mandatory because this condition requires early and mandatory celiotomy in most clinical circumstances.

Focal tenderness is indicative of a localized inflammatory involvement of the peritoneum, as commonly seen in acute appendicitis. Site-specific tenderness with associated peritoneal inflammation may represent a process that is anatomically discontinuous, as in a patient with perforated duodenal ulcer with spillage of duodenal contents and tracking along the pelvic gutter, which produces localized tenderness in the right lower quadrant. Thus, caution must be exercised in interpreting localized tenderness. The absence of localized tenderness in the presence of acute abdominal pain may suggest a noninflammatory process such as vascular intestinal ischemia or infarction.[4] Acute urinary calculus may also present with severe abdominal pain and a little abdominal tenderness. Eliciting tenderness may only require gentle percussion without deep palpation, sparing the patient from severe discomfort during the abdominal examination. The abdominal examination is dynamic and may reflect the natural progression of the underlying process, and this progression may be a clue to the underlying cause. Frequent examinations in certain clinical situations by the same clinician may be warranted.

Rectal examination and a bimanual pelvic examination in females is required in the evaluation of the acute abdomen. The presence of occult blood and associated tenderness may help to establish a possible pelvic cause of the acute abdomen. Lower quadrant tenderness with associated rectal tenderness may represent a primary inflammatory process in the adnexa.[2]

The presence of occult blood is nonspecific and may be present in many clinical conditions. Finally, examination of the external genitalia with close attention to both external and internal inguinal rings is most important to exclude hernias and associated bowel incarceration or strangulation.

Certain findings in the evaluation of the acute abdomen are highly indicative of a particular diagnosis. For example, Murphy's sign (an abrupt cessation of inspiratory effort during right upper quadrant palpation) is consistent with acute cholecystitis because pain impedes the ability of the patient to inspire fully.

LABORATORY EVALUATION

The selection of appropriate laboratory tests must be guided by the complete history and physical examination and should be used to confirm the suspected diagnosis. Caution must be exercised to avoid overreliance on laboratory tests that are ordered without clinical guidance. Careful selection based on clinical findings, correct interpretation, and knowledge of the limitations of each test allows optimum use of these ancillary tests. Initial laboratory tests in most patients should include determination of hemoglobin and hematocrit levels and a white blood cell count. Leukocytosis is commonly encountered in patients with many abdominal inflammatory processes, as well as a shift to the left toward more immature white cells. Abnormally low white blood cell counts may be encountered in patients at the extremes of age and in those with immunosuppression. Serum electrolytes, blood urea nitrogen (BUN), and serum creatinine should also be included in most initial laboratory screenings. Patients with profound diarrhea, vomiting, and hypovolemia may have serious electrolyte derangements that may require early treatment prior to definitive diagnosis and surgical therapy.

Clotting studies (partial thromboplastin time, prothrombin time, and platelet count or functional study) should be included if suspicion of an underlying hematologic disorder is high. Patients receiving anticoagulant therapy should have clotting studies performed early in anticipation of possible surgery. A specimen for type and screen or cross-match should be drawn initially and kept in case component transfusion therapy may be necessary.

An elevated serum amylase concentration in patients with clinical symptoms of acute pancreatitis is highly supportive of the diagnosis.[5] However, an elevated amylase level may also be seen in patients with small bowel ischemia or infarction, perforated ulcer, sialadenitis, or tubo-ovarian processes. Normal amylase levels may also be seen in patients with both acute and chronic pancreatitis.

Liver function tests (alkaline phosphatase, bilirubin, alanine aminotransferase [ALT], and aspartate aminotransferase [AST]) may be useful in patients with primary hepatobiliary disease. These tests are indicative of liver parenchymal reserve and may be valuable in differentiating medical from surgical diseases of the liver.

The urinalysis may offer valuable information. In nephrourolithiasis that presents as an acute abdomen, a urinalysis with hematuria can establish the true diagnosis. Pyuria may confirm the presence of a urinary tract infection. Additional information may be obtained from routine urinalysis. A high specific gravity may indicate hypovolemia, and ketones may suggest diabetic ketoacidosis presenting as abdominal pain.

The fecal occult blood test should be performed as part of the rectal examination in all patients with abdominal pain. The presence of occult blood may indicate an underlying carcinoma or mucosal abnormality such as inflammatory bowel disease.[6] The presence of occult blood, however, is non-specific, and further diagnostic tests may be required. Stool specimens may be submitted for culture when an infectious enteritis or colitis is suspected.

IMAGING STUDIES

Plain radiographs of the chest and abdomen are not necessary in all patients with abdominal pain.[7] Patients in whom the clinical presentation suggests an obvious diagnosis, such as appendicitis, complete small bowel obstruction, or acute cholecystitis, do not require plain radiographs. However, when the diagnosis remains in question or when the history indicates active cardiopulmonary risk, chest radiographs may be warranted.

Plain radiographs of the abdomen (flat and upright or decubitus views) are useful in corroborating a clinical diagnosis.[7] The presence of pneumoperitoneum may be indicative of a perforation of the gastrointestinal tract as in patients with a perforated ulcer or diverticulitis in those who have undergone instrumentation of the gastrointestinal tract. Free intra-abdominal air is also seen in patients in the first few days after abdominal surgery. The presence of air in the portal vein or its tributaries may indicate an inflammatory abdominal process with abscess formation. Air in the biliary tree may be seen in those with gallstone ileus. Calcifications may be seen in patients with gallstones, chronic pancreatitis, urinary stones, abdominal vascular disease, or an appendicolith. Abnormal intestinal gas patterns may suggest a generalized ileus in the presence of a variety of intra-abdominal processes or may indicate a specific underlying diagnosis.

Computed tomography (CT) is a most useful imaging modality in the investigation of abdominal pain.[8] CT can visualize solid organs, retroperitoneum, and gastrointestinal tract when oral and intravenous contrast is utilized. The usefulness of CT as a diagnostic tool and as primary therapy is demonstrated in the use of CT guided percutaneous procedures in the setting of intra-abdominal abscess. Use of CT scans should be limited to clinical situations in which the diagnosis remains in question. Ultrasonography as an imaging modality is valuable primarily in evaluating biliary tract disease, appendicitis, and pelvic causes of abdominal pain.

ENDOSCOPY

Although not usually performed in patients with acute abdominal pain, proctosigmoidoscopy or colonoscopy can be considered in patients with large bowel obstruction because it may be diagnostic in those with an obstructing carcinoma or therapeutic in those with volvulus. Endoscopic esophagogastroduodenoscopy is usually indicated in most patients with an upper gastrointestinal hemorrhage.

LAPAROSCOPY

Laparoscopy plays an important role in the evaluation of females with lower quadrant abdominal pain of questionable cause.[9] The differentiation of appendicitis or a gynecologic disorder may be possible only under direct vision. Laparoscopy may obviate the need for celiotomy in both instances. Laparoscopy may also have a diagnostic role in the small group of patients with ongoing mild abdominal pain of uncertain etiology.

EARLY LAPAROTOMY

Urgent laparotomy should be considered in patients with acute abdominal pain and tenderness, overt peritonitis, and uncertain diagnosis when these are associated with signs of progressive shock (tachycardia, oliguria, and hypotension).[1] Undue delay in diagnostic evaluation may result in an adverse outcome. Additionally, progressive physical findings of guarding, rigidity, progressive tenderness, or distention may warrant urgent laparotomy. The presence of pneumoperitoneum or extravasation of contrast medium also warrants prompt laparotomy. Early surgical consultation is important in these clinical situations.

DIFFERENTIAL DIAGNOSIS

The approach to the patient with acute abdominal pain requires synthesis of the presenting history, physical examination findings, and formulation of a differential diagnosis (Table 19–1) with corroboration through selective laboratory tests and imaging studies.[10] Examining the abdomen by quadrants will help in arriving at a site-specific differential diagnosis (see Algorithm at the beginning of this chapter).

PREOPERATIVE PREPARATION

After completing the initial evaluation of the patient with acute abdominal pain and establishing the indications for laparotomy, pain medication in moderate doses should be administered to make the patient comfortable. Resuscitation of patients with signs and symptoms of hypovolemia should be carried out prior to induction of anesthesia because these patients may show hemodynamic instability on administration of anesthetic agents. Special attention should be paid to identifying those patients with underlying intravascular depletion, and

Table 19–1. Common Nonsurgical Causes of Acute Abdominal Pain

Myocardial infarction	Uremia
Esophageal spasm	Sickle cell crisis
Pericarditis	Acute intermittent porphyria
Pneumonia	Henoch-Schönlein purpura
Pleuritis	Narcotic withdrawal
Pulmonary embolus	Herpes zoster
COPD exacerbation	Addisonian crisis
Asthma exacerbation	Radiculitis
Systemic lupus erythematosus	Lead poisoning
Polyarteritis nodosum	Psychogenic causes
Diabetic ketoacidosis	

resuscitation of these patients with warm balanced intravenous crystalloid solutions should be undertaken. Correction of electrolyte, hemoglobin, and clotting abnormalities should begin prior to surgery, and this may require close coordination with the anesthesiologist. Placement of indwelling catheters such as nasogastric tubes and Foley catheters should be done not as a routine measure but only in warranted clinical circumstances. Administration of medications preoperatively should be limited. Special attention should be paid to cardiovascular drugs such as beta blockers, digoxin, and antihypertensives. Corticosteroids should be administered prior to surgery in patients with adrenal suppression resulting from chronic corticosteroid use. Antibiotics are given at least 30 minutes prior to surgical incision to gain adequate tissue levels.[11] The antibiotics chosen should be broad-spectrum and should have coverage against gram-negative aerobes, gram-positive cocci, and anaerobes. Informed consent should be obtained prior to administration of analgesics or preoperative sedation. No substitute for the primary surgeon is acceptable in carrying out a complete discussion of all risks and benefits and in answering all pertinent questions from both the patient and the family members prior to surgery.

References

1. Martin RF, Flynn P: The acute abdomen in the critically ill patient. Surg Clin North Am 1997;77(6):1455.
2. Tarraza HM, Moore RD: Gynecologic causes of the acute abdomen and the acute abdomen in pregnancy. Surg Clin North Am 1997;77(6):1333.
3. Moir CR: Abdominal pain in infants and children. Mayo Clin Proc 1996;71(10):984.
4. Howard TJ, Plaskon LA, Wiebke EA: Nonocclusive mesenteric ischemia remains a diagnostic dilemma. Am J Surg 1996;171(4):405.
5. Chase CW, Barker DE, Russell WL: Serum amylase and lipase in the evaluation of acute abdominal pain. Am Surg 1996;62(12):1028.
6. Roy MA: Inflammatory bowel disease. Surg Clin North Am 1997;77(6):1419.
7. Mindelzun RE, McCort JJ: What radiographic views constitute acute abdominal series? AJR Am J Roentgenol 1996;166(3):716.
8. Gupta H, Dupuy DE: Advances in imaging of the acute abdomen. Surg Clin North Am 1997;77(6):1245.
9. Memon MA, Fitzgibbons RJ: The role of minimal access surgery in the acute abdomen. Surg Clin North Am 1997;77(6):1333.
10. Martin RF, Rossi RL: The acute abdomen. An overview and algorithms. Surg Clin North Am 1997;77(6):1227.
11. Farber MS, Abrams JH: Antibiotics for the acute abdomen. Surg Clin North Am 1997;77(6):1395.
12. Walker JS, Dire DJ: Vascular abdominal emergencies. Emerg Med Clin North Am 1996;14(3):571.
13. Pollack ES: Pediatric abdominal emergencies. Pediatr Ann 1996;25(8):448.
14. Gill BD, Jenkins JR: Cost effective evaluation and management of the acute abdomen. Surg Clin North Am 1996;76(1):71.
15. Boey JH: The acute abdomen. In Wag L (ed): Current Surgical Diagnosis and Treatment, 10th ed. Stamford, CT, Appleton & Lange, 1994.

Chapter 20

Acute Gastrointestinal Hemorrhage

Acute gastrointestinal (GI) hemorrhage is one of the most common causes of hospital admission in this country. Despite advances in both diagnostic and therapeutic measures, GI hemorrhage continues to result in significant morbidity and mortality. Although the majority of patients presenting with GI hemorrhage of both upper and lower sources stop bleeding spontaneously, ongoing or recurrent blood loss during hospitalization occurs in approximately 20%. It is this subset that presents a clinical challenge, which often requires the combined efforts of the emergency department physician, gastroenterologist, radiologist, and surgeon. The most common causes of upper GI hemorrhage include peptic ulcer disease, gastroesophageal varices, erosive gastritis, and the Mallory-Weiss syndrome. The most frequent causes of lower GI hemorrhage are diverticulosis, vascular ectasia, hemorrhoids, cancer, and various colitides.

The care of the patient with acute GI hemorrhage is divided into three distinct phases that may overlap temporally: initial assessment and resuscitation, localization of the bleeding source, and therapeutic intervention. Rapid accomplishment of all three steps is necessary to ensure the greatest chance of a satisfactory outcome. This chapter will outline a general approach to the patient with acute GI hemorrhage and review the techniques currently available for diagnosis and therapy.

INITIAL ASSESSMENT AND RESUSCITATION

All patients arriving in the emergency department with significant upper or lower GI hemorrhage should have two large-bore (14- to 16-gauge) peripheral intravenous lines established. Mandatory laboratory tests include complete blood count, platelet count, prothrombin and activated partial thromboplastin times, as well as blood type and cross-match. Resuscitation is begun with isotonic crystalloid (usually lactated Ringer's solution), guided by the patient's vital signs and estimated blood loss. A Foley catheter should be placed to monitor urinary output. The decision to transfuse blood products must be made on an individual basis and is based on the volume of blood loss, hemodynamic status, and underlying disease process while taking into account the risks associated with transfusion. It should be noted that GI hemorrhage may precipitate myocardial ischemia or infarction in the elderly or in patients with preexisting coronary artery disease. Supplemental oxygen is administered, and endotracheal intubation should be considered in patients with severe or recalcitrant hemodynamic decompensation. Pulmonary artery catheterization and monitoring in the intensive care unit (ICU) are appropriate measures in selected patients with ongoing hemorrhage, hemodynamic instability, or severe underlying medical illness.[1]

The history and physical examination play important roles in establishing the etiology and location of hemorrhage. The presentation of bleeding (e.g., hematemesis, hematochezia, melena) often suggests either an upper or a lower source. *Hematemesis*, the vomiting of bright red blood or "coffee grounds," points toward an upper GI source. *Melena*, the passage of black tarry stools, results from the breakdown of blood within the GI tract and is usually associated with upper GI bleeding. *Hematochezia*, the passage of bright red blood per rectum, is usually associated with colorectal lesions. A frequent pitfall, however, is the assumption that passage of bright red blood per rectum is diagnostic of a lower GI source. A brisk upper GI bleed may produce hematochezia, and the unwary surgeon may be fooled into performing a nontherapeutic subtotal colectomy for a bleeding duodenal ulcer. Additional important historical data include associated abdominal pain, previous peptic ulcer disease, liver disease, weight loss, change in bowel habits, alcohol abuse, aspirin, steroid, or nonsteroidal anti-inflammatory drug (NSAID) use, and a history of previous GI bleeding.

Physical examination is initially directed at the patient's general appearance, vital signs, and assessment of the magnitude of hemorrhage. Examination should document the presence of abdominal masses or tenderness, hepatomegaly, and the stigmata of portal hypertension or cirrhosis. A careful anorectal examination may reveal bright red blood or melena as well as the presence of masses, hemorrhoids, fistulas, or fissures.

Passage of a nasogastric tube should be the initial diagnostic maneuver to assist in the differentiation of upper and lower GI sources of hemorrhage. Initial aspiration of fresh blood or coffee-ground material is virtually diagnostic of a bleeding source located in the esophagus, stomach, or duodenum. A nonbloody, bilious aspirate is highly suggestive of bleeding distal to the ligament of Treitz. Aspiration of clear, nonbilious material is nondiagnostic. Gastric lavage with approximately 500 to 1000 ml of saline assists in the determination of the character of the aspirate. Lavage also aids in the estimation of ongoing hemorrhage if the aspirate does not clear.

UPPER GASTROINTESTINAL HEMORRHAGE: LOCALIZATION

Esophagogastroduodenoscopy (EGD) is the primary initial diagnostic modality for upper GI hemorrhage. Its sensitivity is reported to be between 70% and 85%, and it has a specificity of approximately 90%.[2] It is important to perform EGD early to increase the likelihood of visualizing the offending lesion. Therefore, EGD should be performed in all patients with suspected upper GI bleeding when hemodynamic stabilization has been achieved. In addition to its diagnostic value, flexible endoscopy also offers multiple modes of therapeutic intervention (discussed later in this section). If possible, the surgeon should be present during endoscopy to facilitate the planning of possible future operations. The presence of a nonbleeding visible vessel within an ulcer correlates with a risk of rebleeding that is as high as 50%, whereas

Acute Gastrointestinal Hemorrhage

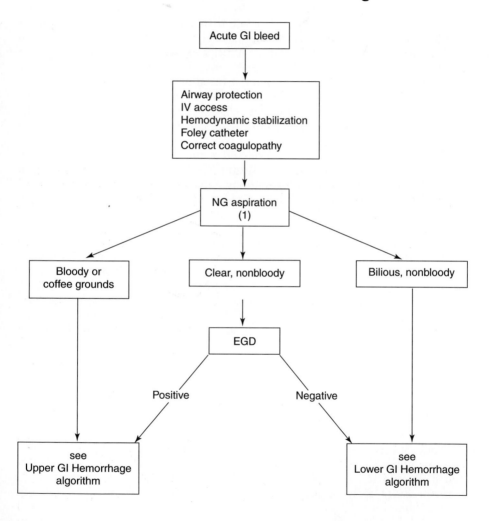

1. The upper gastrointestinal (GI) tract should be ruled out as a source of GI hemorrhage. Nonbloody drainage from a nasogastric tube (NG) will in most cases be sufficient to accomplish this. However, duodenal ulcers may bleed into the distal bowel without allowing appreciable blood to leak back through the pylorus into the stomach. A history that is suspicious for ulcer may lead to upper endoscopy even if the nasogastric aspirate is clear.

2. Variceal hemorrhage should be treated with splanchnic vasoconstrictive agents such as vasopressin (20 IU given intravenously over 20 minutes, followed by a continuous infusion at 0.2 to 0.6 IU/minute). Tamponade can be attempted with a Sengstaken-Blakemore tube. After insertion of the tube, 50 to 100 cc of air should be placed in the gastric balloon, and the intragastric position should be confirmed by abdominal radiographs. Following this, the gastric balloon should be fully inflated and the tube withdrawn to provide compression of the gastroesophageal junction. If esophageal bleeding continues, the esophageal balloon should then be inflated for up to 24 hours.

3. Portal decompression can be accomplished using portocaval or mesocaval shunts. However, the postoperative changes that occur following these surgical procedures make possible future liver transplantation a difficult challenge. A transjugular intrahepatic portosystemic shunt (TIPS), performed by an interventional radiologist, can be substituted for operative decompression for a limited time.

4. Anorectal lesions are often simply hemorrhoids, which can frequently be treated conservatively. However, rectal polyps and anorectal carcinomas can present with bleeding and require the expertise of a surgeon to correct. Colorectal surgery consultation should be considered. (See page 244.)

5. Initial localization of a GI bleeding source is usually performed with abdominal scintigraphy. Radionuclide imaging is very sensitive and can detect bleeding at a rate as low as 0.1 ml/minute. Its limiting factor is its frequent inability to pinpoint the source adequately enough to allow for a segmental resection. Although it is invasive, angiography is much better at localizing the lesion and can actually be therapeutic if selective embolization is used. Angiography does require a higher rate of blood loss (about 1 ml/minute) to detect active bleeding. (See page 244.)

Upper Gastrointestinal Hemorrhage

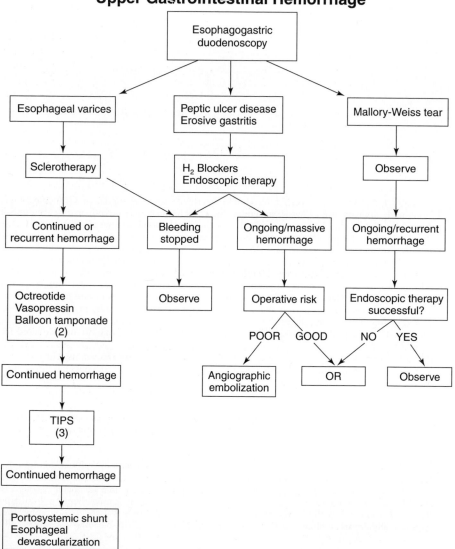

ulcers with adherent clot rebleed at a rate of 20% to 30%.[3] Although EGD is considered a very safe procedure, complications do occur rarely and include perforation, aspiration, and increased bleeding.

On occasion, however, EGD is technically not feasible or is not able to satisfactorily localize a bleeding source. In this circumstance, selective visceral angiography should be the next step in a patient with ongoing hemorrhage. The success of this procedure depends on the presence of active arterial bleeding at the time the study is performed. Hemorrhage at a rate higher than 0.5 to 1.0 ml/minute is necessary for angiographic visualization; therefore, this procedure is best performed in patients who continue to require volume resuscitation to maintain hemodynamic stability. Selective transcatheter embolization with Gelfoam or stainless steel coils is a therapeutic option in selected patients (e.g., those at increased risk for operation). The risks of selective visceral angiography include bleeding, thromboembolism, contrast reactions, and acute renal insufficiency.

Abdominal scintigraphy with ^{99m}Tc sulfur colloid or ^{99m}Tc-labeled red blood cells is a useful adjunct in patients with nondiagnostic upper GI endoscopy and bleeding that is either intermittent in nature or too slow to permit angiographic visualization. Scintigraphy with ^{99m}Tc-labeled red blood cells is particularly appealing because it allows repeat scanning up to 12 hours after administration of the labeled erythrocytes.

UPPER GASTROINTESTINAL HEMORRHAGE: ETIOLOGY AND THERAPY

Peptic Ulcer Disease

Peptic ulcer disease accounts for approximately half of all cases of upper GI hemorrhage. Spontaneous cessation of bleeding occurs in the majority of patients. In the remainder, endoscopic or surgical therapy is necessary to achieve hemostasis. Options for endoscopic therapy include the application of heater probes, multipolar electrocoagulation (Bicap), neodymium:yttrium aluminum garnet (Nd:YAG) laser photocoagulation, and injection therapy with epinephrine, ethanol, or 1% polidocanol. Patients who respond to endoscopic management should be given H_2-receptor antagonists or omeprazole and observed closely for signs of rebleeding.

The increasing use of endoscopic therapy for bleeding ulcers has resulted in a dramatic decrease in the need for emergency surgery. The decision to operate is complex and must take into account the patient's age and general condition, hemodynamic status, volume of blood loss, and chance of recurrent hemorrhage. In general, elderly patients with a lower physiologic reserve should be considered candidates for early operation. Indications for operation include failure of endoscopic or angiographic modes of hemostasis, recurrent bleeding, or massive hemorrhage that is unresponsive to resuscitation. In general, a transfusion requirement of six units of packed red blood cells within 24 hours should prompt operative intervention. The surgical procedure of choice varies with the operative findings. Bleeding duodenal ulcers may be treated by truncal vagotomy, pyloroplasty, and oversewing of the bleeding vessel. Highly selective vagotomy with oversewing of the bleeding vessel is an appropriate alternative. Bleeding gastric ulcers are best treated with gastric resection tailored to include the ulcer. The use of vagotomy is dependent on the specific type of ulcer.

Gastroesophageal Varices

Variceal hemorrhage is a relatively common manifestation of hepatic cirrhosis and is associated with significant mortality. The initial management of these patients is similar to that of patients with bleeding ulcers, with several important caveats. Maintenance intravenous fluids should be hypotonic because of the tendency toward sodium and water retention in these patients. Coagulopathy and thrombocytopenia are quite common and should be aggressively corrected. A lower threshold for pulmonary artery catheterization is advisable in hemodynamically unstable patients.

The first therapeutic maneuver in patients with active variceal hemorrhage is an attempt to decrease portal venous pressure medically. This can be accomplished by administering 20 IU of vasopressin over 20 minutes followed by continuous infusion of 0.2 to 0.6 IU/minute. Vasopressin causes systemic vasoconstriction and decreased portal flow but can result in severe hypertension or myocardial ischemia. Because of this, it is often administered concomitantly with intravenous nitroglycerin. An alternative regimen is octreotide, a synthetic somatostatin analogue that appears to be as effective as vasopressin but has fewer deleterious side effects.[4] Endoscopy for both diagnostic and therapeutic reasons should be performed when the patient's condition permits. Even in patients with known esophageal varices, the acute bleeding episode may not necessarily be due to a bleeding varix but may result from erosive gastritis or peptic ulcer disease. Once confirmed, bleeding varices are addressed with sclerotherapy or rubber band ligation, which results in hemostasis in more than 90% of patients. Patients who continue to bleed despite these measures should undergo placement of a Sengstaken-Blakemore tube. After insertion of the tube, an abdominal x-ray is obtained to confirm intragastric placement. The gastric balloon is inflated first and placed on traction; if this fails to control hemorrhage, the esophageal balloon is then inflated. The duration of balloon tamponade should not exceed 24 to 48 hours because of the risk of pressure necrosis of the esophageal wall. All patients requiring balloon tamponade should undergo endotracheal intubation to decrease the risk of aspiration. Although the majority of patients respond to balloon tamponade, it should be considered a temporizing measure because 25% to 50% of patients rebleed after the balloons are deflated.

Transjugular intrahepatic portosystemic shunting (TIPS) has recently played an increasingly prominent role in the management of patients with acute variceal hemorrhage that is refractory to other modalities.[5] This procedure involves the percutaneous placement of an expandable metallic stent between a hepatic vein and the portal vein, thereby decreasing portal venous pressure. TIPS is of particular value in patients who are poor surgical candidates and those being considered for hepatic transplantation because the procedure does not induce any scarring or anatomic distortion of the right upper quadrant. Recurrent variceal hemorrhage secondary to shunt thrombosis has been reported several months following TIPS. Surgical options for emergent control of variceal hemorrhage include portocaval and mesocaval shunting as well as esophageal transection and devascularization (Sugiura procedure). Distal splenorenal shunting should not be used in the emergent setting.

Mallory-Weiss Syndrome

The Mallory-Weiss syndrome involves upper GI hemorrhage from a mucosal tear at the gastroesophageal junction. In the typical scenario, the patient gives a history of antecedent vomiting or retching, often after an alcoholic binge. Hematemesis with or without melena may follow. Most cases of bleeding secondary to Mallory-Weiss tears stop spontaneously; those that do not are best approached with endoscopic coagulation or injection therapy.[6] Recurrent bleeding after these measures is unusual. In the rare case requiring surgical management, the bleeding tear may be oversewn through an anterior gastrotomy.

Erosive Gastritis

Erosive gastritis refers to the presence of gastric mucosal erosions, which are most commonly noted in critically ill patients. The pathogenesis of stress gastritis is believed to be impaired function of the gastric mucosal barrier that occurs in this patient population. The overall incidence of the disease appears to be declining, presumably secondary to routine prophylaxis with sucralfate, H_2-receptor antagonists, and antacids in most intensive care units, as well as improvements in resuscitation and nutritional support. Endoscopically, multiple superficial ulcers or erosions are noted within the stomach. Treatment of acute hemorrhage includes alkalinization of gastric pH with H_2-receptor antagonists or antacids, resuscitation with crystalloid or blood products, correction of coagulopathy, and treatment of the underlying disease process. Endoscopic treatment has shown some promise in selected cases.[7] Angiographic transcatheter embolization or selective intra-arterial infusion of vasopressin may be attempted in refractory cases. Surgical options include vagotomy and hemigastrectomy, vagotomy with pyloroplasty and oversewing of bleeding sites, subtotal or total gastrectomy, and gastric devascularization. The mortality rate in patients requiring operation is high.

LOWER GI HEMORRHAGE: LOCALIZATION

Lower GI hemorrhage is defined as hemorrhage arising distal to the ligament of Treitz. The first objective in the localization of a lower GI bleed is the exclusion of an upper GI source. As mentioned earlier, both melena and hematochezia may occur in patients with upper GI hemorrhage. Liberal use of nasogastric aspiration and upper GI endoscopy is encouraged in an effort to reduce the rate of missed upper GI lesions. Early rigid proctoscopy plays a critical role in ruling out anorectal disorders and diffuse proctocolitis. Patients who stop bleeding in the emergency department or who bleed intermittently

Lower Gastrointestinal Hemorrhage

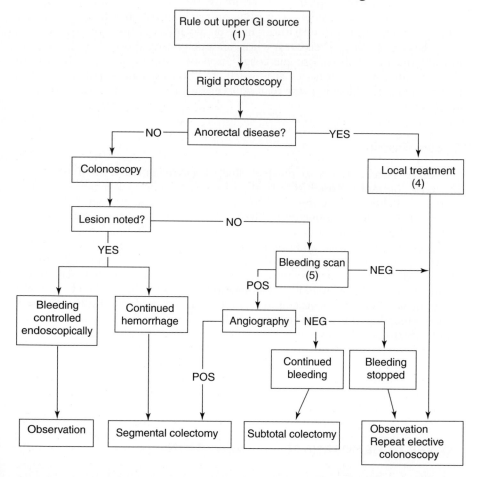

should be admitted for observation and undergo semielective total colonoscopy after adequate mechanical bowel preparation has been performed. Although it may be technically difficult, colonoscopy performed during an episode of acute hemorrhage is not only cost effective,[8] it may also be the diagnostic procedure of choice when it is performed by a highly skilled endoscopist.[9]

Ongoing hemorrhage in the presence of nondiagnostic colonoscopy should prompt further attempts at localization with selective visceral angiography or abdominal scintigraphy with ^{99m}Tc-labeled red blood cells or ^{99m}Tc-sulfur colloid. The choice of test depends on availability and the patient's status. In many institutions, the preference is to obtain a bleeding scan first and then proceed with angiography if the scan is positive. Radionuclide imaging has the advantage of being exceedingly sensitive, since it can detect hemorrhage at a rate of 0.1 ml/minute. As mentioned previously, tagged RBC scans may be repeated within 12 hours if intermittent hemorrhage is suspected. However, it is sometimes difficult to pinpoint the exact location of hemorrhage or to exclude an underlying duodenal or small bowel source. Selective visceral angiography is less sensitive but allows definitive localization when the rate of hemorrhage exceeds 0.5 to 1.0 ml/minute. Selective transcatheter embolization or vasopressin infusion may be considered in the poor-risk patient, although embolization carries a finite risk of transmural necrosis and bowel perforation. Barium enema has no role in the management of patients with acute lower GI hemorrhage because the contrast serves only to impede subsequent attempts at colonoscopic or angiographic visualization.

LOWER GI HEMORRHAGE: ETIOLOGY AND THERAPY

Colonic Diverticulosis

Most lower GI bleeds arise from colonic diverticulosis or colonic vascular ectasia. Colonic diverticula are common in Western society and appear to be related to dietary factors. The incidence of colonic diverticulosis increases with age, although hemorrhage occurs in less than 5% of all patients with diverticulosis. Acquired colonic diverticula occur most frequently in the sigmoid and descending colon. Diverticular bleeding is characteristically massive but usually stops spontaneously. Hemorrhage in the presence of acute diverticulitis is unusual. A second hemorrhage is often a harbinger of future recurrent bleeding and should be considered an indication for definitive therapy. Ongoing or massive blood loss also signals the need for intervention. Colonoscopic methods of arresting diverticular hemorrhage are often unsuccessful, and surgery is the mainstay of therapy. Lesions located in the right colon are treated with right hemicolectomy and ileotransverse colostomy. Bleeding diverticula in the transverse, descending, and sigmoid colon are resected segmentally. Emergent subtotal colectomy should be considered a salvage procedure in patients with massive blood loss when all attempts at preoperative localization have failed.

Colonic Vascular Ectasia

Colonic vascular ectasia or angiodysplasia occurs most commonly in the cecum and right colon, although lesions may be found throughout the colon and rectum. Bleeding may be either occult or overt and is often intermittent. Although colonoscopy may be helpful, selective mesenteric angiography is usually diagnostic. Angiographic findings of vascular ectasia include a tortuous vein that empties slowly, an early-filling vein, and vascular tufts. Bleeding angiodysplasias may be treated with colonoscopic electrocoagulation or sclerotherapy, as well as with selective transcatheter embolization.[10] Continued or massive bleeding should be treated by segmental colon resection when the lesion has been localized preoperatively. Inability to localize the source of massive hemorrhage mandates subtotal colectomy.

UNCOMMON CAUSES OF GASTROINTESTINAL HEMORRHAGE

Dieulafoy's Lesion

Dieulafoy's lesion is an abnormally large submucosal vessel protruding through a small mucosal defect. Generally, the lesion is located in the cardia or fundus of the stomach within 6 cm of the gastroesophageal junction, although it may be found throughout the GI tract.[11] It is the causative lesion in less than 2% of patients with GI bleeds, but hemorrhage from these lesions may be massive or intermittent and results in painless hematemesis or melena. Treatment options include endoscopic coagulation or surgical wedge resection of the involved stomach wall.

Hemobilia

Hemobilia is a rare complication of hepatic parenchymal injury characterized by an abnormal communication between the hepatic vascular system and the biliary tree. The classic presentation of gastrointestinal hemorrhage, jaundice, and right upper quadrant pain occurs in only approximately one third of patients. Iatrogenesis has overtaken trauma as the leading cause of hemobilia, which is manifest as a complication of percutaneous liver biopsy and transhepatic stent placement.[12] The diagnosis is often elusive because upper GI endoscopy and small bowel series are usually unrevealing. CT scan may demonstrate a pseudoaneurysm, and angiography provides a definitive diagnosis. Angiographic embolization with stainless steel coils or Gelfoam is the treatment of choice. In the rare cases that require surgical intervention, ligation of the offending vessel is usually adequate.

Small Bowel Hemorrhage

Hemorrhage from the small bowel is unusual but may arise from a number of sources. These include jejunoileal diverticula, Meckel's diverticula, polyps, tumors, and inflammatory bowel disease. Localization can be difficult because these lesions are beyond the reach of standard endoscopic equipment. Small bowel series, enteroclysis, or selective visceral angiography may be diagnostic. In patients with a Meckel's diverticulum, abdominal scintigraphy after administration of ^{99m}Tc-pertechnetate confirms the diagnosis in most cases. Occasionally, intraoperative enteroscopy may be required if bleeding continues and attempts at preoperative localization have been unsuccessful.

Aortoenteric Fistula

Fistulas between the aorta and small intestine usually occur at the level of the distal duodenum in patients with prosthetic aortic grafts. The presumed cause is erosion of the vascular graft into the adjacent duodenum, which results in a smoldering inflammatory process at the level of the proximal anastomosis. Less often, abdominal aortic aneurysms or infectious aortitis may be complicated by aortoenteric fistula formation. Not infrequently, exsanguinating hemorrhage may follow a minor herald bleed. For this reason, any patient with an aortic vascular prosthesis and GI hemorrhage should be considered to have an aortoduodenal fistula until proved otherwise. Upper GI endoscopy may demonstrate the fistula as well as other potential sources of hemorrhage. Contrast-enhanced CT scan may reveal graft infection or extravasation of intravenous contrast agent into the bowel lumen. This complication is difficult to manage and is usually treated by excision of the graft, duodenal repair, and extra-anatomic vascular bypass.

Inflammatory Bowel Disease

Ulcerative colitis commonly results in bloody diarrhea; this finding is much less common in Crohn's disease. Most bleeding secondary to inflammatory bowel disease stops spontaneously, and massive hemorrhage occurs in only 2% to 3% of patients. Patients with fulminant ulcerative colitis associated with hemorrhage may be treated surgically by subtotal colectomy with ileostomy. Continence may be restored at a later date by elective completion proctectomy and ileal pouch–anal anastomosis.

References

1. Kollef MH, OBrien JD, Zuckerman GR, et al: BLEED: A classification tool to predict outcomes in patients with acute upper and lower gastrointestinal hemorrhage. Crit Care Med 1997;25(7):1125.
2. Lieberman D: Gastrointestinal bleeding: Initial management. Gastroenterol Clin North Am 1993;22(4):723.
3. Gupta PK, Fleischer DE: Nonvariceal upper gastrointestinal bleeding. Med Clin North Am 1993;77(5):973.
4. Avgerinos A, Armonis A, Raptis S: Somatostatin and octreotide in the management of acute variceal hemorrhage. Hepatogastroenterology 1995;42(2):145.
5. Sahagun G, Benner KG, Saxon R, et al: Outcome of 100 patients after transjugular intrahepatic portosystemic shunt for variceal hemorrhage. Am J Gastroenterol 1997;92(9):1444.

6. Harris JM, DiPalma JA: Clinical significance of Mallory-Weiss tears. Am J Gastroenterol 1993;88(12):2056.
7. Keifhaber P, Keifhaber D, Huber F, et al: Endoscopic neodymium:YAG laser coagulation in GI hemorrhage. Endoscopy 1986;18:46.
8. Richter JM, Christensen MR, Kaplan LM, et al: Effectiveness of current technology in the diagnosis and management of lower gastrointestinal hemorrhage. Gastrointest Endosc 1995;41(2):93.
9. Vernava AM, Moore BA, Longo WE, et al: Lower gastrointestinal bleeding. Dis Colon Rectum 1997;40(7):846.
10. Foutch PG: Angiodysplasia of the GI tract. Am J Gastroenterol 1993;88:807.
11. Fockens P, Tytgat GN: Dieulafoy's disease. Gastrointest Endosc Clin N Am 1996;6(4):739.
12. Cerrniak A, Thompson JN, Hemingway AP, et al: Hemobilia: A disease in evolution. Arch Surg 1988;123(6):718.

Chapter 21

Intestinal Obstruction

By definition, an intestinal obstruction refers to a mechanical occlusion of the bowel lumen that retards passage of intraluminal contents. This is in contrast to an ileus or psuedo-obstruction, which is a result of dysfunction of intestinal muscular motility. This distinction is crucial: Treatment of ileus, of functional obstruction, focuses on treating the primary cause, often through medical modalities; mechanical occlusion can be relieved only by physical resolution of the cause of obstruction.

Both mechanical and functional obstruction can occur in the small or large bowel. The distinction between small bowel and large bowel obstruction is an important one, because each has different causes, different presentations, and different forms of management. The degree of obstruction, whether complete or partial, and, if partial, whether it is high or low grade, also affects diagnosis and management decisions.

Adhesive bands, incarcerated or strangulated hernias, and neoplasms account for the great majority of cases of mechanical bowel obstruction.[1] The incidence of these lesions differs by age. Incarcerated hernias account for far more cases of bowel obstruction in the pediatric population than neoplasms. Conversely, in geriatric patients, bowel obstruction is as likely to result from malignancy as from an incarcerated hernia.[2] Obstruction in any patient with a history of previous abdominal or pelvic surgery is most likely to result from an adhesive band. Hysterectomy and surgery for pelvic malignancy have an especially high association with adhesive band formation. Patients who have undergone emergency laparotomy for trauma also have a high incidence of adhesive obstruction.

PATHOPHYSIOLOGY

Regardless of the cause (Table 21–1), untreated intestinal obstruction behaves in a characteristic manner and results in accumulation of enteric contents, gas, and fluid proximal to the point of obstruction. Fluid is sequestered within the lumen and the wall of intestine proximal to the obstruction. This leads to proximal distention of the bowel and is a characteristic finding in patients with bowel obstruction. As the obstruction progresses, the bowel wall itself becomes increasingly edematous. Both the luminal distention and bowel wall edema further exacerbate the degree of obstruction.

Strangulation occurs when bowel edema and distention progress to the point of impedance of mesenteric venous outflow, which, if untreated, will lead eventually to frank necrosis of the bowel. Gangrene of the bowel can occur especially quickly in closed loop obstructions, in which fluid sequestration occurs rapidly within the lumen of the closed loop.

Table 21-1. Causes of Intestinal Obstruction

Obturation of the lumen	Neoplastic
Meconium	Miscellaneous
Intussusception	K^+-induced stricture
Gallstones	Radiation stricture
Impactions—fecal, barium, bezoar, worms	Endometriosis
Lesions of the bowel	Lesions extrinsic to the bowel
Congenital	Adhesive constriction or angulation
Atresia and stenosis	Hernia and wound dehiscence
Imperforate anus	Extrinsic masses
Duplications	Annular pancreas
Meckel's diverticulum	Anomalous vessels
Traumatic	Abscesses and hematomas
Inflammatory	Neoplasms
Regional enteritis	Volvulus
Diverticulitis	
Chronic ulcerative colitis	

Conversely, because of the resorptive abilities of the large bowel, even though most large bowel obstructions are theoretically closed loop obstructions (in patients with a competent ileocecal valve), they are less likely to strangulate. They are more likely to perforate owing to the high tension on the relatively thin-walled cecum.

DIAGNOSIS

History

Patients with mechanical bowel obstruction present with complaints of abdominal pain. Pain is typically described as intermittent and poorly localized. Pain that started as colicky in nature but then progressed to severe, steady, and localized pain is extremely worrisome for strangulation. Nausea and vomiting is another classic complaint. Patients with more proximal obstructions have more frequent and copious emesis, whereas patients with more distal small bowel or large bowel obstruction may not have emesis as a significant complaint at all. Obstipation is an important symptom, possibly indicating a complete obstruction; the presence of flatus is indicative of a partial, or early complete, obstruction. Patients with a closed loop obstruction may complain of pain that is out of proportion to the physical findings; rapid onset and progression of symptoms is characteristic in these patients.

Patients with ileus or colonic pseudo-obstruction frequently do not have significant pain. Typically, they complain more of abdominal distention and bloating. Nausea and vomiting and complaints of obstipation are variable.

Physical Examination

Physical findings are also variable, depending on the type, timing, and severity of the obstruction. There is a variable degree of dehydration resulting from both fluid sequestration and emesis. Vital signs may range from normal to those found in severe hypovolemic shock. Elevated temperature may be an ominous finding because it is associated with gengrenous or perforated bowel.

The entire torso must be inspected anterior and posterior from the costal margin to below the inguinal ligaments to detect potential hernias. On inspection, the classic description of a mechanical small bowel obstruction is a "soft, doughy" abdomen. Abdominal distention is usually a late finding. Conversely, patients with ileus or psuedo-obstruction may have significant abdominal distention. Careful inspection may reveal an incarcerated hernia as a cause of mechanical obstruction. If a hernia is present and is not especially tender, gentle attempts at reduction may relieve the bowel obstruction. An erythematous, tender mass may represent cellulitis overlying a strangulated hernia and should never be reduced. Digital rectal examination is mandatory in all patients.

Auscultation during periods of peristalsis may reveal classic high-pitched rushes or tinkling sounds. Gangrenous bowel is silent. Bowel sounds are usually hypoactive in patients with ileus or colonic pseudo-obstruction.

Palpation of the abdomen, except in cases of gangrenous bowel, is usually noncontributory. Tenderness may be associated with periods of hyperperistalsis. The presence of any peritoneal signs (persistent tenderness, involuntary guarding and rebound) is consistent with gangrenous bowel.

Laboratory Test

Complete blood count with differential, electrolyte series, arterial blood gas determination, and serum amylase levels are useful laboratory tests. The presence of an elevated white blood count and metabolic acidosis are worrisome for strangulation. The classic finding of hypokalemic, hypochloremic metabolic alkalosis secondary to prolonged emesis may be associated with a superimposed metabolic acidosis resulting from severe dehydration. An elevated serum amylase level may suggest pancreatitis with associated ileus.

Radiologic Test

The flat and upright abdominal plain film is an extremely useful screening tool. The plain film alone may yield a diagnosis of mechanical small bowel obstruction, ileus, large bowel obstruction, or colonic pseudo-obstruction. Conversely, other radiologic studies may be necessary to arrive at a diagnosis. The findings may be different with the various clinical entities and are discussed separately later with each entity.

PRINCIPLE OF DIAGNOSIS AND MANAGEMENT

When treating a patient with a possible bowel obstruction, the first step is to identify the surgical emergency: gangrenous bowel. As stated above, severe, unrelenting pain, peritoneal signs, a silent abdomen, and an elevated white blood count with a left shift are all ominous signs consistent with gangrenous bowel or perforation; these patients should undergo immediate laparotomy. The main goal of diagnosis is to identify the patient who is at risk for imminent strangulation or perforation *prior* to its development. All diagnostic tools and therapy are directed to this end.

MANAGEMENT

Resuscitation

Resuscitation begins as soon as the patient presents. Intravenous fluids are administered immediately. Fluid resuscitation should be accomplished with an isotonic solution such as lactated Ringer's solution. Gastric fluid losses should be replaced with either normal saline or a hypotonic solution supplemented with additional chloride. An indwelling urinary catheter should be placed to monitor the adequacy of resuscitation.

Decompression

A nasogastric tube is placed for gastric decompression. The presence of feculent material in the gastric aspirate is virtually diagnostic of a significant unrelieved small bowel obstruction. Decompression is a key component in the management of both mechanical bowel obstruction and ileus. Given the pathophysiology of mechanical obstruction, there is little chance of nonoperative resolution of the obstruction without some form of proximal decompression. Several studies have failed to show any difference between nasogastric and long intestinal tubes in the efficacy of relief of obstruction.[3, 4] Nasogastric tubes are used primarily because of their ease of placement.

For patients with a functional obstruction, nasogastric decompression decreases gastric distention and prevents progressive distal distention while the primary cause of the dysmotility is addressed. Colonic pseudo-obstruction may also be treated by distal decompression, using endoscopy or a rectal tube.

MECHANICAL SMALL BOWEL OBSTRUCTION

Diagnosis

The classic history of complete small bowel obstruction is colicky abdominal pain, nausea and vomiting, and obstipation. If the patient is still passing flatus, this may represent either an early complete obstruction or a partial small bowel obstruction.

Findings on an upright plain film of the abdomen of gas-filled, distended loops of small bowel with differential air-fluid levels (the "stairstep" pattern) and a paucity of distal colonic gas are virtually diagnostic of a complete small bowel obstruction. The presence of gas in the colon with these findings is suggestive of a partial small bowel obstruction. As fluid becomes sequestered in the small bowel, subsequent abdominal films may show a "string of pearls" sign. In cases of equivocal plain film findings, contrast media may be of use in diagnosis, either with a small bowel series or with enteroclysis.[5]

Closed loop obstructions, in which both proximal and distal ends of the bowel are obstructed, can be difficult to diagnose. The symptoms can progress rapidly without producing the characteristic radiographic findings; these patients often require resection of the strangulated loop of bowel.

CT scan has been used to diagnose equivocal cases of small bowel obstruction and may be more sensitive for closed loop or partial obstructions than plain films. It may also localize the transition zone between dilated and collapsed loops of small bowel.[6] Ultrasonography has also been used to establish a diagnosis of mechanical small bowel obstruction.[7, 8]

Management

All management decisions are made with the goal of avoiding progression of obstruction to strangulation and gangrenous bowel. However, a significant number of small bowel obstructions may resolve without the need for surgery. The choice between operative and nonoperative management is made by balancing these two conflicting facts. Currently, there are no good laboratory or radiographic markers that can confirm in timely fashion the presence or absence of gangrenous bowel. Therefore, this decision is a clinical one. For many patients, the old rule of "never let the sun rise or set on a bowel obstruction" still applies.

Any patient with signs and symptoms of strangulation should be taken to the operating room. In general, patients with complete bowel obstructions are taken to the operating room after allowing a variable amount of time for resuscitation and observation. Observation includes serial abdominal examinations, serial abdominal radiographs, and close monitoring of intake and output, complete blood count, and serum electrolytes.

Patients with a partial small bowel obstruction, or complete obstruction in the early postoperative period, inflammatory bowel disease, or known abdominal carcinomatosis are special cases that may warrant a longer trial of nonoperative management, on the order of days rather than hours.[9]

The main principles of surgical management are relief of obstruction, resection of nonviable bowel, maintenance of residual bowel function, and prevention of recurrent bowel obstruction. Laparotomy often reveals proximally dilated loops of bowel as well as collapse of loops of bowel distal to the area of obstruction. Once the transition point is found, relief of the obstruction in many cases is accomplished by simple incision of the offending adhesive band. In these cases, there is no value in further dissection to lyse every intraabdominal adhesion; they will recur. Patients with chronic small bowel obstructions or "socked-in" abdomens may require careful and tedious dissection to relieve the obstruction.

Obstructions due to metastatic carcinoma may require bypass or ostomy to relieve the obstruction. Obstructions due to a Meckel's diverticulum are best treated with resection of the small bowel rather than simple diverticulectomy. Conversely, obstructions due to Crohn's disease are best treated with stricturo-

Small Bowel Obstruction

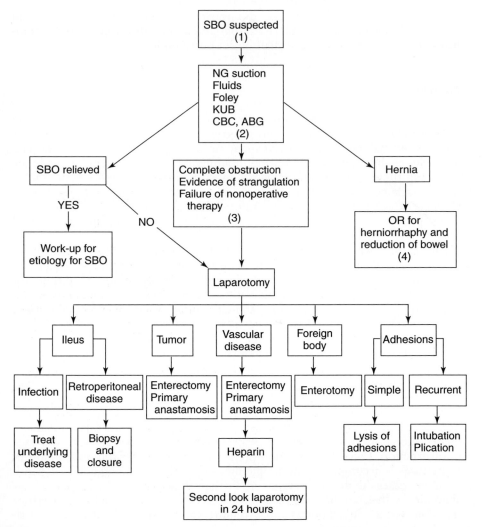

1. A history of nausea, vomiting, constipation, obstipation, and pain are all suggestive of acute small bowel obstruction (SBO). Previous abdominal surgery and subsequent adhesions may be a cause of the current problem, and it is therefore important to elicit these facts in the history. Abdominal distention, tympany, and/or a nonreducible hernia are some of the more common physical findings.
2. The work-up for patients with a suspected small bowel obstruction should include a (CBC) arterial blood gases (with specific attention paid to pH and base deficit as an indication of severity of hypoperfusion), amylase level (small bowel contains amylase, but a markedly elevated value may suggest pancreatitis as the initiating event), and determination of electrolytes. An abdominal x-ray will show dilated loops of bowel and may or may not show evidence of a closed loop obstruction. Volume resuscitation should proceed expeditiously with isotonic intravenous fluids. Urinary output should be monitored closely as the patient is resuscitated; this is best done with an indwelling bladder catheter and frequent reassessment. Intestinal decompression is accomplished with a nasogastric tube.
3. Complete obstruction, evidence of strangulation (e.g., closed loop obstruction), and failure of nonoperative management are all indications for operative intervention. In addition, patients without previous abdominal surgery are unlikely to have bowel obstruction due to adhesions; the cause is more likely to be a lesion or event not amenable to intestinal decompression and hydration alone. These patients should be explored in an urgent or semi-elective fashion.
4. Bowel obstruction due to an incarcerated hernia can be relieved with reduction of the hernia. However, unless the reduction is very easy, it is risky to reduce a segment of herniated bowel because of the possibility that the segment may be nonviable. It is much safer to reduce the bowel in the operating room under direct visualization and to resect ischemic bowel as needed. The hernia defect should be repaired at the same time.
5. Nonoperative management of a large bowel obstruction is a bit of a misnomer, since most such obstructions are due to tumors. Initial therapy may involve intestinal decompression and volume resuscitation; subsequently, a search for the cause is undertaken, and laparotomy is performed as indicated. (See page 257.)

plasty, if possible, rather than resection. Incarcerated hernias causing obstruction may be approached at the site of the hernia and do not necessarily require laparotomy.

Any frankly gangrenous bowel must be resected. Bowel of questionable viability must be carefully examined. Resection of questionable bowel is always safest; however, for patients with inadequate length of residual bowel (e.g., complete midgut volvulus), maximal conservation of bowel should be of prime importance. Assessment of intestinal viability can be a challenging problem in the operating room. Simple palpation of pulses or Doppler ultrasound examination of mesenteric arterial flow may be sufficient. In other cases intravenous fluorescein injection with Wood's lamp inspection of the bowel may be required.[10] In patients for whom maximal conservation of bowel is crucial, planned reoperation to examine segments of questionable bowel may be necessary.

In cases of strangulated hernia, bowel can be resected and reapproximated through the hernia incision as long as good margins of viable bowel can be attained.

Patients with obstruction due to Crohn's disease who fail to respond to medical management can pose a difficult problem. Given the natural history of the disease, conservation of bowel is a major concern. Resection should be reserved for severely diseases or perforated segments of bowel.

Prevention of Recurrent Bowel Obstruction

Adhesive small bowel obstructions can recur because lysis of adhesions often leads to more extensive adhesion formation in the future. Talc on surgical gloves, careless handling of tissues, inadequate hemostasis, and use of certain suture materials have all been implicated in the formation of adhesions.[11] A variety of substances intended to reduce adhesion formation have been investigated.[12, 13] To date, none have been conclusively shown to decrease the frequency of bowel obstruction. Mechanical plication and stenting of the intestine has been performed as well in an attempt to position the bowel to avoid future volvulus or obstruction.

Hernias should be repaired, electively, if possible, prior to incarceration. Attempts to reduce an incarcerated hernia, if successful, may avoid laparotomy and allow elective hernia repair at a later time. However, any hernia showing potential signs of strangulation should be operated on immediately with no attempt made at reduction, and the hernia defect should be repaired at the time of surgery.

MECHANICAL LARGE BOWEL OBSTRUCTION

Diagnosis

Large bowel obstruction is a different clinical entity than small bowel obstruction. Primary colon cancer, volvulus, and diverticulitis are the most frequent causes of large bowel obstruction; adhesions and hernias do not cause

Large Bowel Obstruction

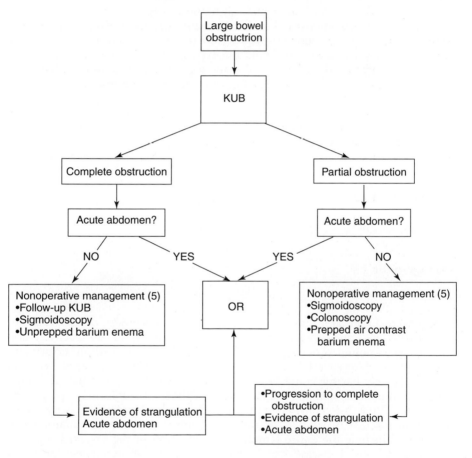

large bowel obstruction. Patients with large bowel obstruction typically present with crampy abdominal pain and a variable history of obstipation and/or abdominal distention. A history of hematochezia or heme-positive stools may be indicative of strangulation of a volvulus, diverticulitis, or cancer. As with small bowel obstruction, the signs and symptoms of diffuse peritonitis, fever, and leukocytosis are indications for laparotomy.

Digital rectal examination and plain abdominal radiographs are important early screening diagnostic tests. However, large bowel obstruction can be difficult to evaluate by plain radiograph (pneumoperitoneum would indicate an intestinal perforation).

Sigmoidoscopy and barium enema can be both diagnostic and therapeutic.[14] Both sigmoidoscopy and barium enema may differentiate true mechanical large bowel obstruction from pseudo-obstruction (Ogilvie's syndrome). A contrast enema can localize and often define the type of obstruction (e.g., neoplasm, sigmoid volvulus). Endoscopy may also allow reduction of sigmoid volvulus or decompression of the cecum in cases of imminent perforation (cecal diameter >12 cm).

CT scan has also been shown to be beneficial in cases of large bowel obstruction in patients in whom neoplasm or diverticulitis may be more likely. CT may also be helpful in demonstrating signs of intestinal ischemia.[5]

Unless there is an incompetent ileocecal valve, large bowel obstructions are closed loop obstructions. Perforation is a greater risk in large bowel obstruction due to the greater wall tension on the large, thin-walled cecum (law of LaPlace). Clinical progression may be rapid, if sigmoid volvulus is the cause, or slow, if the obstruction is due to a tumor. Once cecal diameter exceeds 10 to 14 cm, perforation becomes a significant risk.

Management

Cancer

Management of large bowel obstruction differs depending on the cause of the obstruction. Patients who undergo emergency surgery for obstructive colon cancer have a poorer prognosis, stage for stage, than those with other primary colon cancers. However, left-sided colon cancers cause progressive obstruction of the relatively narrow colon lumen and may present earlier than right-sided lesions; the patients complain of decreasing caliber of stools, constipation, or tenesmus. These lesions may demonstrate the classic "apple core" appearance on barium enema. If possible, optimal resection should proceed anatomically and should include the entire lymphatic distribution of the involved segment of colon. Advanced disease may require temporary or permanent proximal diversion.

Volvulus

Sigmoid volvulus often presents in geriatric patients with a redundant "floppy" sigmoid colon that is prone to twist on its mesentery. The symptoms of abdominal pain and obstipation are usually acute in onset, although there may be a long history of chronic intermittent abdominal pain that is self-limited, presumably as the sigmoid colon twists and then returns to its normal position. A plain radiograph may reveal a dilated "omega" closed loop of sigmoid colon. A barium enema demonstrating the classic "bird's beak" sign is pathognomonic.

Patients with sigmoid volvulus may benefit from a trial of sigmoidoscopic reduction. However, signs of strangulation, such as blood per rectum, an elevated white blood count, and peritonitis are contraindications to endoscopic decompression; similarly, if mucosal ulceration or intraluminal blood is seen on sigmoidoscopy, these patients should undergo laparotomy. In any case, because of its tendency to recur, sigmoid volvulus should eventually be treated with elective resection.

Cecal volvulus is a relatively rare cause of large bowel obstruction in the United States; however, when it does occur, it frequently progresses rapidly and will cause perforation and peritonitis if not recognized quickly. Treatment varies from right hemicolectomy to simple reduction and pexy of the cecum.

Diverticulitis

Obstruction is a relatively rare complication of diverticulitis, and operative management depends on the severity of the diverticulitis itself. Obstruction may be acute, secondary to inflammation of abscess formation, or it may be due to a chronic stricture secondary to scarring, which may be difficult to differentiate from neoplasm. Endoscopy is contraindicated in patients with acute diverticulitis because insufflation of air into the acutely diseased colon may cause perforation.

ILEUS AND COLONIC PSEUDO-OBSTRUCTION

Ileus

Diagnosis

Ileus and colonic pseudo-obstruction are functional disorders of the bowel; there is no mechanical obstruction. Small bowel dysmotility, or ileus, is characterized by abdominal distention and a variable degree of anorexia, obstipation, nausea and vomiting. Any systemic intra- or extra-abdominal infection, systemic inflammatory states such as pancreatitis or post-trauma or post-burn states, postoperative periods, metabolic abnormalities, neurologic disorders, and medications all can cause ileus. Physical examination demonstrates a distended, tympanitic, nontender abdomen with hypoactive or absent bowel sounds.

Frequently, ileus can be distinguished from mechanical small bowel obstruction by plain abdominal radiographs. Characteristically, ileus appears as diffuse, gas-filled dilated loops of both small and large bowel. In other cases, contrast studies such as an upper GI series or enteroclycis may be necessary to confidently distinguish between ileus and mechanical obstruction.

Management

Ileus is treated by decompression with a nasogastric tube and treatment of the primary cause of the ileus. Nasogastric decompression prevents ongoing dilation of the bowel while the primary problem is being treated.

Colonic Pseudo-obstruction (Ogilvie's Syndrome)

Diagnosis

Colonic pseudo-obstruction occurs when a functional obstruction is confined to the large bowel (as opposed to an ileus, which affects both the small and large bowel). Abdominal distention is the main presenting complaint, which typically occurs in a debilitated, geriatric patient, who is often taking multiple medications. Abdominal pain, nausea and vomiting usually are not significant features of the presentation. Abdominal radiographs demonstrate a massively dilated colon. On the patient's initial presentation, a barium enema should be performed to rule out mechanical obstruction. Medication, metabolic, and neurologic derangements are often implicated as causes of colonic pseudo-obstruction.

Management

Treatment, as for ileus, should be directed toward the primary cause. However, colonic pseudo-obstruction often represents a chronic relapsing condition, unlike ileus, and can be difficult to treat definitively. Also, unlike ileus, colonic pseudo-obstruction, left untreated, can result in cecal perforation, especially when the cecal diameter exceeds 12 cm. A patient with a massively distended cecum may require distal decompression with a colonoscope; often a large-bore rectal tube is left in place as a stent to prevent reaccumulation of gas within the colonic lumen. Serial abdominal films are performed to monitor the resolution of cecal distention. Promotility agents such as neostigmine[15] as well as erythromycin[16] have also been used to treat the colonic dysmotility.

References

1. Mucha P: Small intestinal obstruction. Surg Clin North Am 1987;67(3):598.
2. McEntee G, Pender D, Mulvin D, et al: Current spectrum of intestinal obstruction. Br J Surg 1987;74(11):977.
3. Gallick HL, Weaver DW, Sachs RJ, Bouwan DL: Intestinal obstruction in cancer patients. An assessment of risk factors and outcome. Am Surg 1986;8:434–437.
4. Brolin RE: The role of GI tube decompression in the treatment of mechanical intestinal obstruction. Am Surg 1983;49:131–137.
5. Ericksen AS, Krasna MJ, Mast BA, Nosher JL, Brolin RE: Use of gastrointestinal contrast studies in obstruction of the large and small bowel. Dis Colon Rectum 1990;33(1):56–64.
6. Megibow AJ: Bowel obstruction. Evaluation with CT. Radiol Clin North Am 1994;32(5):861–870.

7. Ogata M, Mateer JR, Condon RE: Prospective evaluation of abdominal sonography for the diagnosis of bowel obstruction. Ann Surg 1996;223(3):237–241.
8. Schmutz GR, Benko A, Fournier L, Peron JM, Morel E, Chiche L: Small bowel obstruction: Role and contribution of sonography. Eur Radiol 1997;7(7):1054–1058.
9. Richards WO, Williams LF: Obstruction of the large and small intestine. Surg Clin North Am 1988;68(2):360–363.
10. Horgan PG, Gorey TF: Operative assessment of intestinal viability. Surg Clin North Am 1992;72(1):143–155.
11. Fabri PJ, Rosemurgh A: Reoperation for small intestinal obstruction. Surg Clin North Am 1991;71(1):132–133.
12. Fabri PJ, Rosemurgh A: Reoperation for small intestinal obstruction. Surg Clin North Am 1991;71(1):141–143.
13. Becker JM, Dayton MT, Fazio VW, et al: Prevention of postoperative abdominal adhesions by a sodium hyaluronate-based bioresorable membrane: A prospective, randomized, double-blind multicenter study. J Am Coll Surg 1996;183(4):297–306.
14. Twist MH, Vipond MN, Veitch PS: Flexible sigmoidoscopy in addition to contrast enema in the diagnosis of left-sided large bowel obstruction. Br J Surg 1994;81(11):1670–1671.
15. Turegano-Fuentes F, Munoz-Jimenez F, Del Valle-Hernandez E, et al: Early resolution of Ogilvie's syndrome with intravenous neostigmine: A simple, effective treatment. Dis Colon Rectum 1997;40(11):1353–1357.
16. Rovira A, Lopez A, Cambray C, Gimeno C: Acute colonic pseudo-obstruction (Ogilvie's syndrome) treated with erythromycin. Intensive Care Med 1997;23(7):798.

Chapter 22

Abdominal Vascular Emergencies

ACUTE MESENTERIC ISCHEMIA

Under resting conditions, the splanchnic vascular bed receives up to 30% of cardiac output; this capacity represents the largest potential reservoir of blood. This system is composed of three vascular beds—celiac, superior mesenteric, and inferior mesenteric. Collateral flow does exist between the celiac and superior mesenteric circulation through the pancreatoduodenal arteries, and between the superior mesenteric and inferior mesenteric circulation through the marginal artery of Drummond and the arc of Riolan. These collateral sources are rarely sufficient to maintain bowel viability in the presence of occlusion of the superior mesenteric artery.

Mesenteric ischemia is a rare event. It can occur in an acute or chronic manner, the most frequently involved vessel being the superior mesenteric artery. Causes of acute mesenteric ischemia include embolus, arterial thrombosis, venous thrombosis, and nonocclusive, low-flow states. Embolus accounts for 40% of cases; it is usually of cardiac origin and occurs in patients with atrial arrhythmias, mural thrombi, valvular disease, or postmyocardial infarction. One third of the patients have had an antecedent embolic episode. Thrombosis occurs in 40% of cases, the thrombus being superimposed on a preexisting atherosclerotic plaque at the arterial orifice. Complaints of chronic mesenteric ischemia often precede the acute episode. Mesenteric venous thrombosis can occur with oral contraceptive use, intra-abdominal infection (acute appendicitis, acute diverticulitis), postsplenectomy states, myeloproliferative diseases, hematologic conditions, external compression by a cyst or tumor, venous injury, acute portal vein thrombosis, and hypercoagulable states. Nonocclusive, intense splanchnic vasoconstriction is seen in 20% of cases secondary to low-flow states in patients in shock, or who are taking vasopressors or digoxin, or who have aortic stenosis or insufficiency. Complete occlusion of the superior mesenteric artery results in a midgut infarction from the ligament of Treitz to the splenic flexure of the colon. Fortunately, the proximal jejunum and transverse colon are often spared owing to patent collateral vessels and the distal location of the embolus beyond the pancreatoduodenal and middle colic arteries.

Clinically, the hallmark of mesenteric vascular occlusion is rapidly progressive, severe midabdominal pain that is out of proportion to the relatively "benign" physical findings. The common signs are nonspecific, and a high level of suspicion is mandatory. Early symptoms include diffuse abdominal pain, nausea, vomiting, diarrhea, and hyperactive bowel sounds, but there is no distention or peritoneal signs on physical examination. Late findings reflect the presence of transmural intestinal infarction, with hypotension, fever, obvious peritonitis, and bloody diarrhea. The mortality at this clinical stage approaches 80% to 85% despite appropriate intervention. Therefore, early suspicion, rapid diagnostic evaluation, and emergent operation are essential to improve survival.

Aggressive fluid and electrolyte resuscitation, correction of the metabolic acidosis, and broad-spectrum antibiotics should be started immediately. A high neutrophil count, refractory metabolic acidosis, elevated lactic dehydrogenose (LDH) enzymes, and hyperamylasemia may contribute to the diagnosis. In the absence of peritoneal signs, mesenteric angiography with lateral views of the aorta is the definitive diagnostic test. Radiologic signs include the "meniscus sign" of an embolus, complete occlusion of the orifice with thrombosis, and "pruning" of the distal vessels with no major vascular compromise in nonocclusive mesenteric ischemia. In the case of nonocclusive mesenteric ischemia, the angiography catheter should be left in place to allow direct papaverine infusion.

Survival is determined not only by early diagnosis and restoration of effective perfusion but also by the amount of intestine that has undergone necrosis. Most surgeons agree that full systemic anticoagulation is indicated as soon as the diagnosis is suspected on clinical grounds or is confirmed by angiography.

Treatment consists of immediate abdominal exploration. Before and during laparotomy the operating room is kept as warm as possible to minimize hypothermia and vasoconstriction. At least one leg is prepped into the field to allow for harvest of saphenous vein, which is used for arterial bypass or patch. On exploration, bowel viability and vessel patency are assessed. In the case of an embolus, transverse or longitudinal arteriotomy and embolectomy are performed, followed by anticoagulation. If this is unsuccessful, or if residual clots are still blocking the small intestinal branches, fibrinolytic agents may be infused.

In patients with an ostial plaque with a thrombus, an endarterectomy or an aorto–superior mesenteric artery bypass with a saphenous vein or prosthetic graft is performed. Most surgeons prefer an antegrade or retrograde bypass technique because endarterectomy is more demanding and time consuming.

In patients with nonocclusive mesenteric ischemia with distal spasm, treatment should be nonoperative and should be aimed at optimization of hypovolemia, cardiac output, and tissue perfusion as long as there are no signs of peritonitis. Ideally, the angiographic catheter should be left in place and papaverine infusion should be started at 30 to 60 mg/hour. Bowel viability can be assessed using visual inspection, pulse palpation, continuous wave Doppler measurements, and fluorescein injection with Wood's lamp transillumination, which gives a fairly accurate estimation of blood perfusion to the bowel. Black, thin, foul-smelling, blood-filled, or distended loops of bowel are considered necrotic and should be resected. Bowel that has any degree of peristalsis is viable. Bowel that is not completely necrotic, (i.e., dusky in appearance, and with no peristalsis or audible Doppler signal) should be wrapped in warm moist towels and reevaluated at the end of the case. If uncertainty exists about bowel viability, vessel patency or anastomotic performance, a "second look" operation in 24 hours should be scheduled without hesitation.

At laparotomy in patients with mesenteric venous thrombosis, the arteries are patent but the bowel wall is cyanotic, edematous, and rigid with a discol-

Mesenteric Vascular Ischemia

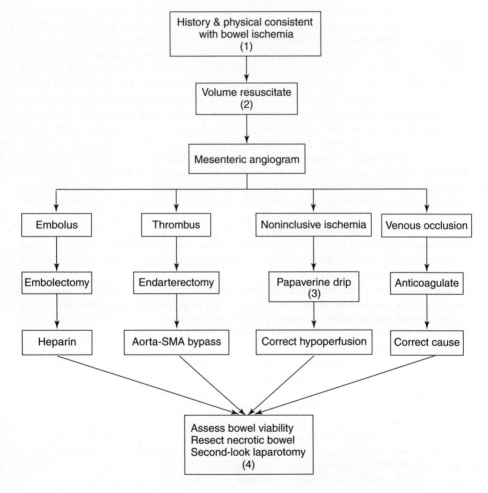

1. The diagnosis of mesenteric ischemia is a difficult one to make clinically and requires a high degree of suspicion, a very careful history, and a careful physical examination. The most common description provided by the patient is a sudden onset of severe abdominal pain, with or without nausea and vomiting. Significant risk factors include (1) arrhythmia, (2) old age, (3) cardiac disease, (4) atherosclerotic vascular disease, and (5) a hypercoagulable state. The classic description of "pain out of proportion to the physical exam" refers to the presence of significant subjective pain despite an essentially normal, soft, nondistended abdomen.
2. Mesenteric ischemia results in significant pooling of fluid in the interstitial spaces and lumen of the bowel. Intravascular hypovolemia leads to intravascular hypotension and a subsequent decrease in perfusion. Hypotension in addition to an already ischemic state further worsens the area of ischemia. Proper and aggressive volume resuscitation is therefore crucial. Close monitoring of urine output, base deficits, and serum lactate levels, as well as central pressure monitoring with pulmonary artery catheters will help to guide volume resuscitation to the proper endpoints.
3. Papaverine is given intravenously in the form of a 60-mg bolus followed by a 30–60 mg/hour drip.
4. Patients undergoing laparotomy for mesenteric ischemia must undergo a second-look procedure in 24 hours regardless of how well they appear. At this point, the patient should be adequately resuscitated, and any areas marked by questionable ischemia should be resected before they perforate.
5. The patient with a symptomatic abdominal aortic aneurysm usually presents with abdominal, flank, or back pain. Risk factors include (1) atherosclerotic vascular disease, (2) other aneurysms, and (3) older age. Seventy percent of abdominal aortic aneurysms can be diagnosed by palpation of an abdominal mass. (See page 267.)

ored, thick mesentery resulting from extravasated venous blood. The thrombus can be palpated at the level of the superior mesenteric vein extending distally to the bowel wall, or proximally if the condition is secondary to portal or splenic thrombosis. Thrombectomy is not recommended, since completeness of the procedure is impossible and rethrombosis is likely. The most commonly affected area of the bowel is the mid portion between the jejunum and ileum. A wide, fan-shaped resection that incorporates all visible thrombosed mesenteric veins is mandatory. The margins of demarcation are less clear, and resection should be performed at a safe distance to ensure a reliable anastomosis. The primary cause is evaluated, and anticoagulation is started. Second-look laparotomies should be routine in patients with mesenteric vein thrombosis.

Survival is primarily dependent on the time elapsed between onset of symptoms and restoration of intestinal perfusion. Mortality is high; for patients with embolic mesenteric occlusion, mortality is in the range of 20% to 40%, and for those with thrombotic occlusion, it is between 70% and 100%. The best results are achieved with early diagnosis of mesenteric venous thrombosis, which has a mortality of 20%. The quality of life in patients who survive depends mainly on whether enough small bowel remains to allow sufficient food absorption. Patients with 30 cm of small bowel and an intact ileocecal valve, or with 40 cm of small bowel without an ileocecal valve, probably will not be dependent on parenteral nutrition. Usually 100 cm of small bowel is required to resume a normal nutritional status.

Improvement in the outcome lies in prevention. This includes full anticoagulation of all cardiac patients with associated thrombus formation, effective treatment of arrhythmias, and appropriate evaluation and treatment of chronic mesenteric ischemia as a cause of abdominal symptoms. The best results can be expected in patients in whom there is high clinical suspicion for mesenteric ischemia and early diagnosis and operative treatment.

ABDOMINAL AORTIC ANEURYSM

Local expansion of the aorta to more than 50% of its normal size (more than 3 cm) is defined as an aneurysm. The most common cause (90% of cases) is atherosclerotic disease, whereas inflammatory and infectious causes (mycotic aneurysms) account for 5% of cases. Pseudoaneurysms and traumatic aneurysms are common in the thoracic aorta. Genetic defects in patients with connective tissue disorders such as tuberous sclerosis, Turner's syndrome, Marfan's syndrome, and Ehlers-Danlos syndrome, are also associated with aneurysmal disease.

The most common location of abdominal aortic aneurysms (AAA) is the infrarenal aorta (95% of the cases). Size varies from 3 to 15 cm; the larger the aneurysm, the greater the risk of rupture. The law of LaPlace states that wall tension is directly proportional to the diameter of the vessel. The incidence of rupture of the aneurysm increases significantly when the size doubles (>5 cm) or when the annual increase in size is more than 0.5 cm per year (<5 cm = 4% incidence of rupture; 5 to 7 cm = 6.5%; >7 cm = 20%).[4]

Most patients (up to 75%) are asymptomatic at the time of diagnosis. Discovery is usually incidental and is made during an ultrasound examination

Abdominal Aortic Aneurysm

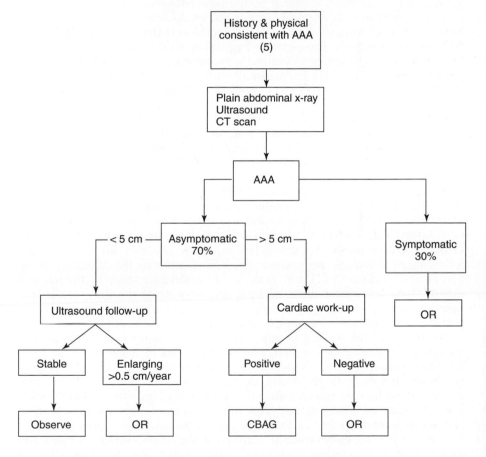

or CT scan done for unrelated reasons, or occasionally during a physical examination when a pulsatile epigastric mass is palpated. When symptoms occur they are usually due to leakage, pressure on adjacent structures, distal embolism, or a free intraperitoneal rupture. Symptoms may be mild but require a high index of suspicion because they often precede frank rupture and exsanguination. Sudden severe back and/or midabdominal pain followed by hypotension, shock, and signs of peritonitis are symptoms of a ruptured AAA. A palpable, tender, pulsatile mass in the epigastrium in this scenario precludes any further evaluation and should prompt an immediate trip to the operating room for an emergency life-saving operation.

Success is determined primarily by the time between presentation and control of hemorrhage. If diagnosis of a ruptured AAA is suspected, two large-bore intravenous lines should be started, and blood samples should be sent for type and cross-match. Preoperative aggressive fluid resuscitation should be limited to avoid converting a confined, retroperitoneal leak to a free intraperitoneal hemorrhage. Mild hypotension with a mean blood pressure of 50 mmHg is acceptable for vital organ perfusion. There is no reason to perform uncomfortable procedures preoperatively, such as Foley catheter insertion, nasogastric tube insertion, or central venous access. These maneuvers can raise the blood pressure and potentially lead to exacerbation of intra-abdominal bleeding. Rapid infusers, Cell Savers, and warming devices should be available intraoperatively to minimize blood loss, transfusion requirements, and hypothermia.

If diagnosis of a ruptured AAA is unlikely and the patient is hemodynamically stable, diagnostic tests can be obtained for further evaluation. Plain abdominal films may reveal intramural calcifications in two thirds of patients and blunting of the psoas muscle shadow, which is suggestive of retroperitoneal hematoma. Ultrasound is a simple, repeatable, less expensive modality for detection and follow-up of abdominal aortic aneurysms and is currently the screening test of first choice. Abdominal CT scan is the gold standard for studying the size and extent of the aneurysm, aortic patency, involvement of the iliac vessels, and renal perfusion. Aortography is indicated if lower extremity ischemia is suspected or if hypertension exists (to rule out a renovascular cause).

Treatment of the leaking or ruptured aneurysm is operative. Patients are prepared and draped before induction of anesthesia in order to be ready to intervene in case of sudden hypotension. The operative field includes the chest, abdomen, and both thighs. Foley catheter, nasogastric tube, and a central venous access line are inserted after the induction of anesthesia. The incision used depends on the surgeon. The most frequent approach is a midline abdominal incision extending from the xiphoid to the pubis. Intraoperatively, first priority is to gain proximal control of the aorta, which is frequently achieved by performing supraceliac clamping below the diaphragm. In the event of an intraperitoneal rupture, rapid control can be established by using an intraluminal Foley catheter placed proximally. Distal control in emergency situations is also obtained with intraluminal catheters. The aneurysmal sac is then dissected carefully, avoiding injury to the inferior vena cava and the renal vessels. The sac is opened longitudinally and all thrombotic material is evacuated. A tube or bifurcated woven Dacron graft is sutured in place with 2–0 polypropylene sutures, and the suture line is buttressed with the aneurysm flaps. The anesthesia team should be alert for possible hypotension and cardiac dysrrhythmias, which are due to reperfusion and wash-out of acidotic and hyperkalemic blood, following restoration of distal blood flow. Intra- and postoperative correction of hypovolemia, hypothermia, and coagulopathy is crucial for patient survival and prevents complications of renal insufficiency and myocardial infarction.

Early postoperative complications include acute tubular necrosis, thromboembolic paraplegia, impotence, colonic ischemia, prolonged ileus, cardiac ischemia, and pulmonary insufficiency. Colonic ischemia can be prevented by judicious assessment of the patency and collateral flow of the inferior mesenteric artery and determination of the need for reimplantation. If hematochezia develops postoperatively, immediate sigmoidoscopy should be performed. Mucosal ischemia may resolve spontaneously; transmural involvement requires reexploration and colonic resection. Lower extremity pulses should be monitored postoperatively for possible emboli from the aneurysmal debris or thrombosis of the graft and distal vessels. Spinal cord ischemia is unusual in patients with infrarenal aortic aneurysms (0.2%).[5]

Mortality ranges from 15% to 88%. The preoperative level of hemodynamic instability clearly correlates with outcome. Decreased urinary output is a poor prognostic sign, and renal failure is almost universally fatal.

Asymptomatic patients with detected aneurysms of 5 cm in diameter or more, or with an annual increase in size of more than 0.4 cm, are candidates for surgical repair unless other concomitant medical problems increase the operative risk beyond the risk of rupture. Elective surgery candidates should undergo evaluation of the cardiovascular system and, if indicated, of the carotid and renal vessels because of their frequent involvement in atherosclerotic disease and compromised flow. If the patient becomes symptomatic, the operation becomes imperative regardless of aneurysm size because rupture is imminent. Optimal cardiovascular preparation, bowel preparation, and controlled circumstances in the operating room contribute to the low mortality in elective cases (1% to 2%). Postoperatively, selective invasive monitoring is valuable in the management of fluids and vasoactive drugs.

Complications after elective surgery include pulmonary atelectasis and infections, deep venous thrombosis, embolism, and ventral hernias. Prevention starts with early ambulation, pain management, and close follow-up care.

VISCERAL VASCULAR ANEURYSMS

Aneurysms affecting the visceral arteries are uncommon. Causes include atherosclerosis, arterial dysplasia, infectious arteritis, and periarterial inflammatory processes (e.g., pancreatitis).

Visceral aneurysms rarely rupture, and most patients are asymptomatic. The most common symptoms include epigastric, midabdominal, or flank pain that is not associated with food. The diagnosis should be suspected if the patient presents with the "double rupture" sign—nonspecific abdominal complaints followed by hemorrhagic shock and peritoneal signs. At this point, the rupture is no longer contained, and there is imminent danger of exsanguination. This is a life-threatening state, and the patient belongs in the operating room.

The highest incidence of rupture occurs in patients with splenic aneurysms, which rupture in close to 20% of cases. Pregnant women with splenic aneurysms are of special concern. Because of the anatomic and physiologic changes of pregnancy, these aneurysms are most likely to rupture, and the incidence of rupture approaches 90%.

Aneurysms as small as 2 cm may be seen on plain abdominal radiographs as calcified vessel dilatations. Diagnosis is confirmed with celiac, superior mesenteric artery, renal, and inferior mesenteric artery angiography.

Asymptomatic aneurysms less than 2 cm in diameter may be observed. Symptomatic aneurysms or aneurysms larger than 2 cm should be repaired, usually with resection and reanastomosis or with graft interposition. In addition, splenic artery aneurysms must be repaired in all women of childbearing potential. Splenic artery aneurysms may be embolized in patients who have a high operative risk.

References

1. Boley SJ, Brandt J: Intestinal ischemia. Surg Clin North Am 1992;72(1):1.
2. Crawford ES: Ruptured abdominal aortic aneurysm. An editorial. J Vasc Surg 1991;18:348.
3. Mannick JA, Whittemore AD: Management of ruptured symptomatic abdominal aneurysms. Surg Clin North Am 1988;68:377.
4. Nevitt MP, Ballard DJ, Hallet JW: Prognosis of abdominal aortic aneurysm; a population based study. N Engl J Med 1989;321:1009.
5. Szilagyi DE, Hageman JH, Smith RF, Elliott JP: Spinal cord damage in surgery of the abdominal aorta. Surgery 1978;83:38.

Chapter 23
Antibiotics

Peritonitis is broadly defined as inflammation of the peritoneal cavity. Bacterial peritonitis is the most clinically relevant form of this condition and results from violation of the integrity of a hollow viscus with ensuing contamination. Although the chemical peritonitis that occurs in such situations as bile peritonitis is not initially infectious, it may quickly become so as inflammation of the peritoneal cavity, the systemic inflammatory response syndrome (SIRS), and bacterial translocation occur. The mainstays of treatment are surgical intervention, hemodynamic support, and antibiotic therapy.

The principle of prophylactic antibiotic usage in surgical patients has been fairly well elucidated. Over 30 years ago it was demonstrated that after contamination has occurred there is a brief time period during which tissue is infection free.[1] Studies have proved that initiation of antibiotic therapy during this period dramatically decreases the incidence of infection and results in a 7% rate of infection when started preoperatively versus approximately a 30% rate when given postoperatively.[2] These data have been confirmed by various laboratory investigations, and the efficacy of antibiotics in reducing infection is no longer a subject of debate.

Animal models[3, 4] have demonstrated the existence of two stages in abdominal sepsis. Initially, acute peritonitis ensues secondary to gram-negative aerobes; this is associated with a nearly 40% mortality rate. Animals surviving this initial insult develop intra-abdominal abscesses by the seventh postoperative day due to anaerobic organisms. The synergy between anaerobes and facultative bacteria has been demonstrated to be the mechanism of intra-abdominal abscess formation. Clinical studies have shown that patients who lack antibiotic anaerobic coverage have an increased incidence of postoperative intra-abdominal abscesses, with *Bacteroides fragilis* being cultured in approximately half of patients.

An understanding of the bacterial flora of the gastrointestinal tract leads to an educated choice of antibiotic coverage. The concentration of bacteria in the stomach is very low because of the acidic gastric pH (pH 2 to 3); the flora are composed mainly of *Streptococcus*, yeast, and some swallowed oral bacteria. There are no obligate anaerobes. The small bowel contains 10^6 to 10^8 colonies/ml, the ileum being more heavily populated. Aerobic bacteria, mainly *Streptococcus*, dominate the proximal small bowel, while the microflora in the distal ileum, for the most part, mimic that of the colon. The concentration of bacteria increases dramatically beyond the ileocecal valve, and in fact, two thirds of dry fecal matter consist of bacteria. The ratio of anaerobic to aerobic organisms is 3000 to 10,000:1, with *Bacteroides* species predominating. Many other bacteria are part of the normal colonic flora (e.g., *Klebsiella, Enterobacter, Pseudomonas*), and thus, perforation results in leakage of mixed flora into the peritoneal cavity.

The intestines are therefore the predominant source of pathogens that cause intra-abdominal infections. Knowledge of the type and frequency of bacteria residing in the different portions of the gastrointestinal (GI) tract allows appropriate antibiotic coverage prior to culture availability. Gram-positive organisms predominate after perforations of the esophagus or stomach, whereas more distal perforations lead to an increased proportion of gram-negative and anaerobic organisms. The gastrointestinal flora can, however, change depending on a multitude of conditions: age, race, diet, previous operations, nutritional status, gastric acidity, bile salt excretion, gut motility, immune mechanisms, and prior antibiotic administration.

Only those bacteria that can withstand host defenses can survive long enough to establish an infectious process. Therefore, the pathogenicity of individual bacterial species is important in the mixed infections seen in patients with intra-abdominal infections. *Escherichia coli*, the most commonly isolated aerobe, occurs with a frequency in abdominal infections that exceeds its intraluminal frequency by greater than 300 times, indicating an enhanced ability to survive host defenses. Gram-negative anaerobes also possess this ability and are frequently responsible for abscess formation. Other bacteria such as enterococci are frequently isolated, but their pathogenicity is still in question; they may act as cofactors rather than as sources of abscess formation.

Antibiotic therapy must be started as soon as an intra-abdominal infection is considered. This initial therapy may then be modified when sensitivity data are available. Several agents or combinations of agents can treat peritonitis effectively (Table 23–1). Efficacy studies of various antibiotic regimens have not proved the superiority of single agent therapy over combination therapy. Therefore, other factors must be considered when choosing antibiotics. Drug allergies must be known. In the elderly and patients with renal insufficiency, doses of aminoglycosides may have to be adjusted due to the associated renal toxicity. Though single agent therapy is usually slightly higher in cost, the laboratory evaluation of the antibiotic levels necessary to prescribe the proper dosage of antibiotics such as gentamicin or tobramycin may negate the cost differences. Both metronidazole and clindamycin are effective, safe, and inexpensive choices for anaerobic bacterial coverage, and patients receiving metronidazole have even shown a decreased incidence of *Clostridium difficile* colitis.

Table 23–1. Parenteral Antibiotic Agents Used for Coverage of Colonic Microflora and Peritonitis

Single Agent Therapy	Ceftriaxone
Ampicillin–sulbactam	Cefoperazone
Cefotetan	Cefotaxime
Cefoxitin	Ciprofloxacin
Ceftizoxime	Gentamicin
Imipenem–cilastatin	Levofloxacin
Piperacillin	Ofloxacin
Ticarcillin–clavulanic acid	Tobramycin
Combination Therapy	*Anaerobic Coverage*
Aerobic Coverage	Metronidazole
Amikacin	Clindamycin
Aztreonam	Chloramphenicol

TRAUMA

Victims of penetrating abdominal injury are at increased risk of infection due to both introduction of a contaminated missile or knife into the peritoneal cavity and, more importantly, injury to the gastrointestinal tract. The importance of surgical technique cannot be overstressed: irrigation, debridement of all devitalized tissue, and removal of all debris, including clots, are imperative. Antibiotic therapy in these patients must be considered an adjunct to prompt surgical intervention and control of gastrointestinal spillage.

Antibiotics used in patients with penetrating abdominal trauma must cover a wide variety of potential contaminants. Broad-spectrum antibiotic coverage has classically included a penicillin or ampicillin-type antibiotic for gram-positive coverage, an aminoglycoside for aerobic gram-negative coverage, and clindamycin or metronidazole for anaerobic coverage. The evolution of broad-spectrum cephalosporins has forced a reevaluation of this regimen in favor of a single agent with fewer potential side effects, decreased costs, and ease of administration. Many studies have compared single drug to multiple drug therapy and have shown no statistical differences in wound infection or intra-abdominal abscess formation, confirming the adequacy of single agent, broad-spectrum coverage for most cases of peritoneal contamination and infection.

Several studies have addressed the question of duration of therapy. A review of the literature shows little consistency in the duration of treatment after penetrating abdominal trauma. A retrospective evaluation of only those regimens with adequate anaerobic and aerobic coverage showed no statistical advantage to prolonged therapy (greater than 24 hours).[5] This finding was confirmed by a prospective study that showed that regardless of contamination and degree of injury, 24 hours of antibiotic therapy was satisfactory for all patients with penetrating abdominal trauma.[8] Unfortunately, although most surgeons believe this on paper, when confronted with a high-risk patient, many revert to the "more is better" theory and continue antibiotic therapy for more than 24 hours.

Penetrating abdominal trauma has an infection rate of 7% to 16% and the following associated risk factors: number of organs injured, injury to the colon, shock, age, and gunshot wounds.[6] Lengthening the course of antibiotic therapy does nothing to decrease the risk of infection, but further investigation is needed for these high-risk patients. Prolonged antibiotic administration also alters endogenous flora, promotes the emergence of resistant organisms, increases the risk of side effects, increases costs, and may even mask coexisting intra-abdominal infections.

APPENDICITIS

Appendectomy is the treatment of choice for patients presenting with signs and symptoms consistent with acute appendicitis. Antibiotics are an adjunct to prompt surgical intervention. The optimal duration of antibiotic therapy is unclear; it is clear that preoperative dosing is important in decreasing wound infection rates. Prior to the use of antibiotics, mortality rates associated with acute appendicitis ranged from 8% to 15%. The current practice of prophylactic antibiotic therapy has decreased this rate to less than 1%. And while morbidity (specifically wound infection) increases with the severity of appendicitis, studies have demonstrated that antibiotics decrease the incidence of infectious complications at all stages of the disease.

The most common pathogens encountered in the acutely inflamed appendix are *Escherichia coli* (aerobe) and *Bacteroides fragilis* (anaerobe); therefore, antibiotic therapy must be directed against these bacteria. Regardless of the degree of contamination, single agent therapy with a broad-spectrum cephalosporin or penicillin should suffice. Therapy should be initiated preoperatively, with intraoperative findings determining the total course of antibiotic treatment required. If a normal appendix is identified, no postoperative antibiotic therapy is indicated unless another source of infection that requires treatment is identified. For patients with uncomplicated appendicitis, only perioperative (24 hours) antibiotics are needed. When perforation or abscess is encountered, a longer duration of treatment is required. Intravenous antibiotic therapy should be continued for 5 postoperative days, or until the patient is tolerating oral intake and has been afebrile for 24 hours. At that point, the antibiotics regimen may be changed to an appropriate oral agent given over a course of 7 to 10 days. The patient need not remain in the hospital to complete the antibiotic course. If the patient remains febrile or if ileus persists beyond 7 days, an intra-abdominal abscess or wound infection should be suspected and investigated by means of physical examination and further studies.

DIVERTICULITIS

Treatment of diverticulitis centers on treatment of the acute infection and its complications—hemorrhage, abscess, fistula, and peritonitis. Approximately 80% of patients admitted with an acute episode of diverticulitis can be managed with antibiotics and a low-residue diet. Antibiotic therapy is directed against those bacteria commonly cultured from stool; therefore, antimicrobial coverage must include both aerobes and anaerobes, especially *E. coli, Bacteroides*, and *Klebsiella*. Mild episodes (low-grade fever and crampy abdominal pain) may be treated with a 10-day regimen of oral antibiotics that provide broad aerobic and anaerobic coverage, such as a fluoroquinolone in combination with clindamycin or metronidazole. An alternative regimen could be an oral broad-spectrum penicillin, such as amoxicillin trihydrate/clavulanate potassium. More severe episodes require hospitalization and possibly surgical intervention. Intravenous antibiotics are used to achieve adequate tissue levels rapidly. Depending on the severity of infection, single agent, broad-spectrum therapy may be adequate, although triple agent therapy (e.g., ampicillin, an aminoglycoside, and metronidazole/clindamycin) may be necessary. Intravenous therapy is continued until the patient has been afebrile for greater than 48 hours and is able to tolerate oral intake. At this point, an oral agent may be substituted and the patient discharged. If fevers or ileus continue for more than 7 to 10 days despite adequate antibiotic therapy, further diagnostic work-up should be pursued in search of an abscess.

INTRA-ABDOMINAL ABSCESS

There are a multitude of causes of intra-abdominal abscesses, but most, if not all, are treated with a combination of antibiotic therapy and drainage. Antibiotic therapy alone rarely effects a cure because the bacterial inoculum is usually large, antibiotics penetrate poorly into the abscess center, and the acidic hypoxic micro-environment of the abscess inhibits efficacy. Drainage of the abscess reverses some of these conditions and increases the efficacy of antibiotic therapy.

The presumptive choice of antibiotic is directed against the microorganisms most likely to be recovered from the abscess and is adjusted when culture and sensitivity results are available. The most common pathogens are a combination of aerobic and anaerobic bacteria, and single or combination antibiotic therapy is chosen as previously discussed.

PERFORATED PEPTIC ULCERS

Bacteria counts in the stomach tend to be low owing to the acidic environment. Therefore, patients who present early with a perforated ulcer usually do not require long-term antibiotic therapy postoperatively because the peritonitis is typically a chemical condition rather than a bacterial one. There are exceptions, however. Patients who are already being treated for peptic ulcer disease with H_2 blockers or proton pump blockers have a medically altered gastric pH that allows bacteria to proliferate. In these patients, antibiotic therapy should be continued as empiric coverage (3 days). Patients with purulent peritonitis—typically those with a delayed presentation—require a full course (7 to 10 days) of antibiotic administration. Once the patient can tolerate oral intake, antibiotics can be changed to an oral agent to complete the antibiotic course.

PANCREATITIS

Based on retrospective and prospective studies, antibiotics are not indicated for the treatment of mild to moderate pancreatitis.[7] Prospective studies that evaluated the role of prophylactic antibiotics in severe pancreatitis (three or more of Ranson's criteria) showed promising results; antibiotics reduced abscess formation and increased survival. Pancreatic infection is thought to result from bacterial translocation from the gut, allowing colonization of the necrotic material. The most common pathogens, as expected, include gram-negative aerobes such as *Escherichia coli*, *Proteus*, *Pseudomonas*, and *Enterococcus*. Studies have been convincing in demonstrating differences in antibiotic penetration of the necrotic tissue. Ceftazidime, imipenem, and metronidazole all have an acceptable penetration rate and achieve therapeutic concentrations in the necrotic pancreatic area. It must be stressed that once infection occurs, antibiotics alone are not enough to cure the condition, and surgical debridement should be considered.

CHOLECYSTITIS

Patients with biliary colic require no antibiotic therapy. However, once bacterial invasion is present, as evidenced by increased temperature or an elevated white blood cell count, antibiotic therapy is indicated. Since biliary excretion of some drugs may be impaired because of acute biliary disease, therapeutic *tissue* levels rather than biliary levels should be sought. Second-generation cephalosporins or antimicrobials with a similar spectrum of activity will suffice. For patients with acute cholecystitis, perioperative (24 hours) therapy has been shown to decrease rates of infection. A full course (5 to 7 days) of antibiotics is necessary if a gangrenous gallbladder is found intraoperatively or if cholangitis is present.

The need for routine anaerobic coverage has not been clearly established, but in the high-risk patient, it may offer some benefit. The one exception is emphysematous cholecystitis. This is a particularly virulent form of acute cholecystitis produced by bacterial invasion rather than gallstones. *Clostridium welchii* is the most common organism cultured, but other clostridia as well as gram-negative aerobes may also be the cause. In this case, anaerobic coverage is necessary. Antibiotics, however, are only an adjunct to surgical removal of the gallbladder.

CHEST TUBES

Victims of either blunt or penetrating trauma may develop a hemothorax or pneumothorax that requires the emergent insertion of a chest tube. The urgency with which thoracostomy is performed may be associated with an increased infection rate of the pleural space. The literature is inconclusive about the need for antibiotics; improving sterile technique is probably the best method of avoiding this complication. However, a single dose of a first-generation cephalosporin or oxacillin may be effective in lowering the infection rate. Short- or long-term antibiotic therapy is not recommended and may, in fact, lead to the emergence of resistant organisms.

BURNS

At the time of injury, burn wounds are rarely infected, and no prophylactic therapy is indicated. However, more than 50% of patients who die as a consequence of burn wounds do so because of uncontrolled infection. Sources include indigenous flora and nosocomial bacteria. Systemic antibiotic therapy should be directed toward specific infections. *Pseudomonas* has great invasive potential, can spread quickly through eschar to infect viable tissue, and may lead to disseminated sepsis. *Staphylococcus*, in contrast, usually only causes a local infection. *Candida* is rapidly and often covertly disseminated, resulting in a 60% mortality rate.

Since gram-positive coverage is lacking in topical antimicrobial agents (Table 23–2), cellulitis is often due to one of these organisms, which are effectively covered with oxacillin or vancomycin. Doses may have to be maximized because burn patients metabolize and excrete drugs more rapidly. If wounds do not

Table 23–2. Topical Antimicrobial Agents Used for Thermally Injured Patients

Silver Sulfadiazine (Silvadene)
Topical agent of first choice
Effective against gram-negative and yeast organisms
Moderate penetration of eschar
Resistant organisms: *Pseudomonas, Enterobacter*
Complication: leukopenia
Mafenide Acetate (Sulfamylon)
Effective against gram-positive and gram-negative organisms and some yeast
Deep penetration of eschar; levels attained in 8 hours
Painful on application
Complication: carbonic anhydrase inhibition (metabolic acidosis results; usually noted after
   3 to 5 days of use)
Silver Nitrate
Effective against gram-positive and gram-negative organisms and yeast
Poor to no eschar penetration
Complications: electrolyte imbalances (especially Na$^+$)

improve with oxacillin alone, an aminoglycoside may be added for synergism. Drug blood levels are followed so that adequate tissue levels can be maintained. If the wound remains cellulitic or if the patient's condition worsens despite broad-spectrum antibiotic coverage, quantitative cultures of the wounds should be performed and antibiotic therapy adjusted accordingly.

References

1. Burke JF: The effective period of preventive antibiotic action in experimental incisions and dermal lesions. Surgery 1961;50:161.
2. Stone HH, Haney BB, Kolb LD, et al: Prophylactic and preventative antibiotic therapy: Timing, duration, and economics. Ann Surg 1979;189:691.
3. Weinstein WM, Onderdonk AB, Bartlett JG, et al: Experimental intraabdominal abscesses in rats: Development of an experimental model. Infect Immunol 1974;10:1250.
4. Onderdonk AB, Bartlett JG, Louie T, et al: Microbial synergy in experimental intraabdominal abscess. Infect Immunol 1976;13:22.
5. Dellinger ER: Antibiotic prophylaxis in trauma: Penetrating abdominal injuries and open fractures. Rev Infect Dis 1991;13:S847.
6. Nichols RL, Smith JW, Klein DB, et al: Risk of infection after penetrating abdominal trauma. N Engl J Med 1984;311:1065.
7. Bradley EL: Antibiotics in acute pancreatitis. Am J Surg 1989;158:472.
8. Kirton OC, O'Neill P, Kestner M, Tortella B: Antibiotic prophylaxis in high risk penetrating hollow viscus injury: A prospective randomized double-blinded, placebo-controlled multicenter trial. J Trauma 1999;45:1107.

Chapter 24

Resuscitative and Emergent Diagnostic Procedures

Emergent injuries (i.e., immediately or soon-to-be life-threatening injuries) in trauma patients are rapidly detected and corrected in the primary survey and resuscitation phases of care, with the focus on the Airway (with cervical spine control), Breathing, and Circulation. The goal is to maintain the flow of oxygenated blood to the brain. Further assessment occurs in the secondary survey, which most commonly involves diagnostic peritoneal tap and lavage. Therapeutic procedures temporize for the underlying pathophysiology. Knowledge of the anatomy is essential for rapid performance of these procedures.

This chapter reviews the common procedures used for resuscitation, rapid diagnosis, and therapy in the trauma patient. Indications, contraindications, techniques, and complications are reviewed, and salient features are then discussed. Depending on the urgency of the condition and the status of the patient, local anesthesia may or may not be needed. For expedient skin preparation, an iodine or chlorhexidene solution may be used.

RESUSCITATIVE PROCEDURES

Surgical Airway

Indications. Inability to obtain an airway with chin lift/jaw thrust maneuvers, suctioning, or endotracheal intubation.

Contraindications. Crushed larynx; ability to obtain an airway nonsurgically.

Technique
1. Maintain neck with in-line traction.
2. Perform quick preparation of skin.
3. Identify the cricothyroid membrane. If the membrane is difficult to identify, a 12-gauge intravenous catheter can be placed through the membrane, directed at a 45-degree angle inferiorly, to provide temporary "jet" ventilation with an oxygen source delivering at least 50 psi.[1]
4. Make a 4-cm incision over the membrane and through the skin, fascia, and membrane. Do not remove any portion of the membrane.
5. Insert the knife handle parallel through the wound and turn the handle 90 degrees (Fig. 24–1).
6. Place a No. 6 Shiley tracheostomy tube (or a 7-Fr endotracheal tube)

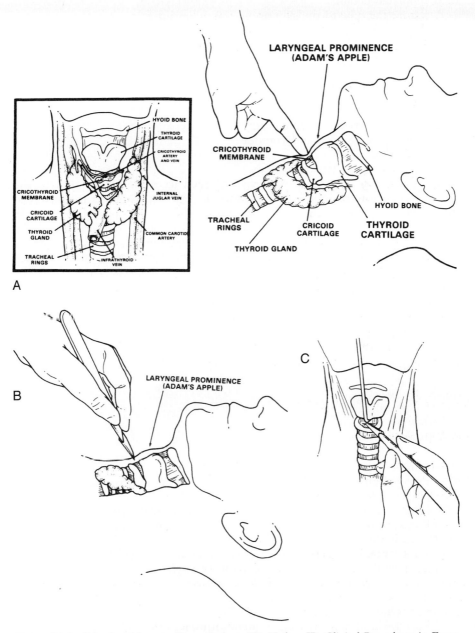

Figure 24–1. Cricothyroidotomy. (From Roberts JR, Hedges JR: Clinical Procedures in Emergency Medicine, 4th ed. Philadelphia, WB Saunders, 1998, p. 63.)

through the opening in the airway and inflate the cuff. Verify breath sounds with ventilated breaths.

7. Suture the tube to the skin using 2–0 nylon suture.

8. Apply dressing.

Complications. Complications are usually related to difficulty in identifying the surface anatomy overlying the cricothyroid membrane.

1. Bleeding.
2. False subcutaneous or subfascial passage.
3. Infection.
4. Recurrent laryngeal nerve injury.
5. Tracheal or esophageal laceration.
6. Aspiration.
7. Subglottic or laryngeal stenosis.

Discussion. Cricothyroidotomy provides rapid access for airway control; the airway can be secured in less than 20 seconds. Inability to obtain the airway at this point leads to asphyxia. Needle cricothyroidotomy can provide temporary access when surgical cricothyroidotomy is difficult due to thickness of the neck or the surgeon's unfamiliarity with the technique. Oxygenation can be maintained indefinitely, but inadequate ventilation for over 45 minutes leads to hypercarbia. Tracheostomy is difficult in trauma patients owing to the mechanism of neck injury and the patient's inability to extend the neck. Resuscitation tracheostomy is indicated only for patients with a crushed larynx. A cricothyroidotomy should be converted to a tracheostomy after 36 hours to avoid subglottic stenosis.

Breathing

Needle Thoracostomy

Indication. Tension pneumothorax.
Contraindication. Simple pneumothorax.

Technique

1. Perform quick preparation of skin overlying the upper anterior chest on the side of the tension pneumothorax.

2. Identify second intercostal space in the midclavicular line.

3. Puncture the chest wall with 12-gauge intravenous (IV) catheter at this site (Fig. 24–2).

4. If a tension pneumothorax is present, a gush of air will be audible.

5. Remove the needle, leaving the catheter in place.

6. Insert a chest tube (see Discussion, below).

Complication

1. Laceration of lung, causing a pneumothorax.

2. Inadequate release of tension pneumothorax in individuals with a thick chest wall (i.e., the IV catheter is too short to traverse the chest wall).

3. Soft tissue infection or hematoma.

Discussion. A tension pneumothorax is air in the chest cavity under pressure,

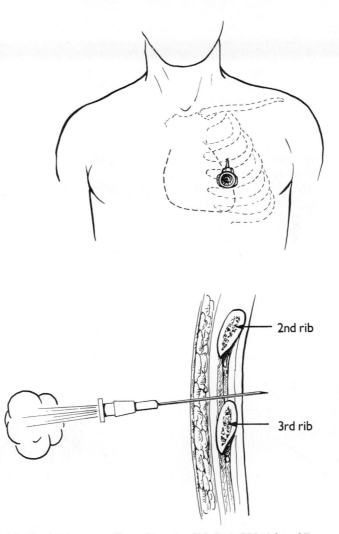

2nd rib

3rd rib

Figure 24–2. Needle thoracostomy. (From Dunmire SM, Paris PM: Atlas of Emergency Procedures. Philadelphia, WB Saunders, 1994, p. 56.)

which causes a mediastinal shift with subsequent hemodynamic compromise (hypotension, jugular venous distention) due to inadequate venous return to the heart. This is a clinical diagnosis, and therefore it should not be made radiographically. Needle thoracostomy rapidly converts a tension pneumothorax to an open pneumothorax, which requires placement of a chest tube, removal of the needle thoracostomy catheter, and placement of a Vaseline gauze dressing over the catheter site.

Tube Thoracostomy (Chest Tube)

Indications. Simple pneumothorax; open pneumothorax; hemothorax.
Contraindications. Initial treatment of tension pneumothorax.

Technique

1. Prepare the skin of the ipsilateral chest anteriorly and laterally.

2. Identify the fourth intercostal space, found most easily at the level of the nipple. For a pneumothorax, identify the anterior axillary line; for a hemothorax, identify the middle or posterior axillary line. The skin incision should be made over the upper fifth intercostal space, with entry into the thorax at the fourth; this creates a skin flap that seals the entrance of the tube, preventing a mechanical air leak.

3. In the awake patient, infiltrate the planned incision and area of entry with a generous amount of local anesthetic. The pleura is particularly sensitive, so depth of local infiltration is important.

4. Incise the skin over the upper fifth intercostal space at the anterior axillary line for a pneumothorax; at the middle or posterior axillary line for a hemothorax (Fig. 24–3).

5. With a Kelly clamp, spread the tissues overlying the fifth rib, then

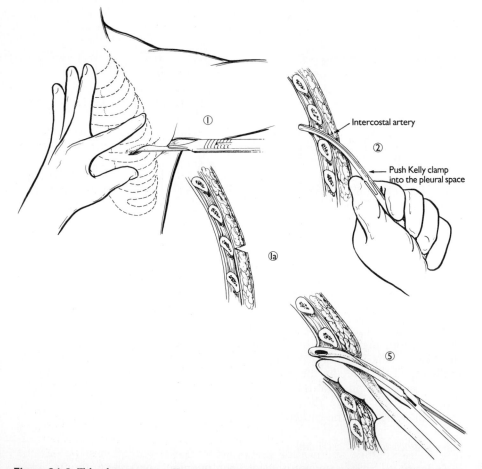

Figure 24–3. Tube thoracostomy. (From Dunmire SM, Paris PM: Atlas of Emergency Procedures. Philadelphia, WB Saunders, 1994, p. 61.)

spread through the muscles of the fourth intercostal space *over* the rib (the neurovascular bundle runs on the inferior margin of the rib). The clamp should "pop" through the pleura. Be careful to maintain total control of the clamp to avoid injuring structures deep in the chest.

6. Place the index finger through the opening and feel around the parietal pleural surface to ensure that adhesions are absent and to determine the direction of tube placement.

7. Use a Kelly clamp on the tip of the chest tube to guide placement through the opening, directing the tube to the posterior apex. A size 36-Fr chest tube is standard in the trauma patient; however, for a patient with a spontaneous or iatrogenic pneumothorax, a smaller size, such as a 24- or 28-Fr, is acceptable.

8. Ensure that all of the holes in the chest tube are positioned within the pleural cavity, generally at the 10-cm mark beyond the most proximal hole.

9. Have an assistant connect the tube to the drainage or suction system.

10. Suture the tube to the margins of the wound using 0 silk suture, one on each side of the tube, with each suture then wrapped around the tube.

11. Place a Vaseline gauze dressing over the tube entrance. In a patient with an open pneumothorax, place a similar dressing over the open wound.

Complications
1. Inadequate local anesthesia in the awake patient.
2. Subcutaneous tunnel with tube outside the chest wall.
3. Incorrect intrathoracic tube position (e.g., anterior position for a hemo-thorax).
4. Subdiaphragmatic and/or transdiaphragmatic placement, causing injury to the liver or spleen (this can be avoided with proper surface anatomy orientation).
5. Injury to the intrathoracic structures (which can be avoided by placing a finger through the opening before positioning the tube to ensure absence of pleural adhesions): the lung, heart, diaphragm, great vessels, esophagus, or herniated abdominal contents may be injured.
6. Bleeding (particularly if the intercostal artery or vein is injured by placing the tube *under* the rib rather than *over*).
7. Infection, both cutaneous and intrathoracic (empyema).
8. Mechanical leak resulting from (a) tube placement directly through the chest wall rather than indirectly with an overlying skin flap, (b) positioning the tube with a hole outside the pleural or chest cavity, or (c) loose tube connections.
9. Clogged or kinked tube or tubing.

Discussion. A simple pneumothorax is air within the chest cavity between the visceral and parietal pleura; it represents an alveolar or bronchial leak. An open pneumothorax results from a defect in the musculoskeletal chest wall, such that air enters the pleural space through this defect; there may be a pulmonary leak as well. Placement of a chest tube is a rapid procedure, which is summed up by the sequence, "cut, spread, spread, in, finger, tube." The goal is to evacuate the air and/or blood from within the pleural space, thus permitting expansion of the lung for breathing. Negative intrapleural pressure is then recreated, using a water seal/suction/drainage apparatus. Since the great majority of pneumothoraces represent alveolar leaks, the air leak stops when the parietal and visceral pleura are apposed, thus sealing the alveolar leak. Persistent air leak is determined by disconnecting the suction from the apparatus, thus putting the apparatus at atmospheric pressure. The apparatus then merely represents an extension of the chest wall. If air bubbles are present during this water seal, an air leak exists. It is important to ensure that this does not represent a mechanical leak (No. 8 in complications listed above). Hemothorax output is monitored closely after chest tube placement. Output of more than 1 liter during the first hour is an indication for exploratory thoracotomy.

Circulation

Vascular Access

Central Venous Access. Options include subclavian, internal jugular, and femoral venous lines.

Indications. Inability to obtain peripheral venous access; placement of monitoring devices, such as a pulmonary artery catheter; infusion of solutions that cannot be given peripherally.

Contraindications. None of the above indications; venous thrombosis at, or injury proximal to, the proposed location.

Technique

1. Position the patient.
   a. For insertion of a subclavian or internal jugular line in an *elective* procedure, turning the head to the contralateral side and placing a roll between the shoulder blades provide excellent exposure. Often during urgent or emergent placement this is not possible because cervical spine protection is needed. The patient is then positioned in the Trendelenburg position to facilitate venous distention and to prevent air embolus.
   b. For insertion of a femoral line, externally rotating and slightly abducting the thigh provides good exposure.
2. Prepare and drape the area. Emphasis is placed on performing the procedure in sterile fashion.
3. Identify the surface anatomy.
   a. Subclavian: The subclavian vein lies posterior to the medial clavicle and is separated from the subclavian artery by the anterior scalene muscle. The clavicular head of the sternocleidomastoid muscle overlies this area and serves as a direction mark for venipuncture.
   b. Internal jugular: The internal jugular vein lies posterior to the belly of the sternocleidomastoid muscle and anterolateral to the carotid artery. Venipuncture can be accomplished using an anterior, middle (between the sternal and clavicular heads of the sternocleidomastoid muscle), or posterior approach, all of which are based on the vertical relationship of the vein to the muscle.
   c. Femoral: The femoral vein lies inferior to the inguinal ligament in the groin and medial to the femoral artery.
4. In the awake patient, infiltrate a generous amount of local anesthetic.

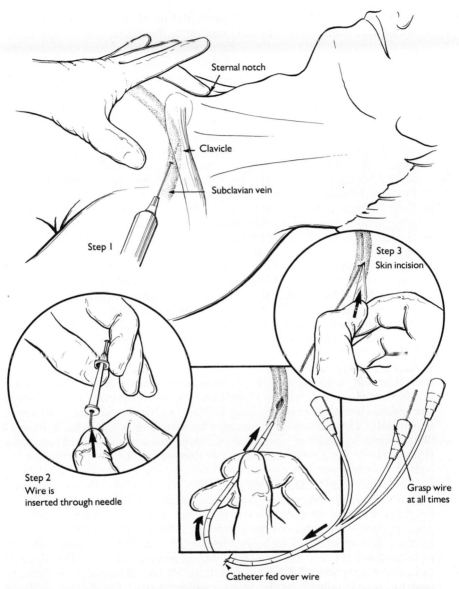

Sternal notch

Clavicle

Subclavian vein

Step 1

Step 3
Skin incision

Step 2
Wire is
inserted through needle

Grasp wire
at all times

Catheter fed over wire

Figure 24–4. Subclavian central line placement. (From Dunmire SM, Paris PM: Atlas of Emergency Procedures. Philadelphia, WB Saunders, 1994, p. 199.)

5. Venipuncture (Fig. 24–4). The 14-gauge needle is attached to a 10-cc syringe with the bevel aligned with the numbers on the syringe. One cubic centimeter of air is drawn into the syringe and then expelled after the needle has punctured the skin; this removes any skin "plug" from the hollow of the needle.

   a. Subclavian: The skin is pierced (with the bevel of the needle directed anteriorly) 2 cm inferior to the junction of the lateral and middle thirds of the clavicle. The needle is then directed toward the origin of the clavicular head of the sternocleidomastoid muscle by "walking" it along the clavicle in a series of in and out motions in the frontal plane, redirecting the needle shaft with the thumb of the opposite hand and keeping the plane of the needle as close to the frontal plane as possible. The needle is directed posterior to the clavicle with the thumb. Constant syringe back pressure is maintained as the needle is passed under the clavicle and into the vein. Backflow of venous blood, usually vigorous, signals that the subclavian vein has been punctured. The syringe is turned 90 degrees, using the numbers as a guide, to position the bevel of the needle tip inferiorly.

   b. Internal jugular: The skin is pierced (with the bevel of the needle directed anteriorly) at the apex of the triangle of the junction of the sternal and clavicular heads of the sternocleidomastoid muscle. Using the anterior approach, the needle is directed inferolaterally; in the middle approach, inferiorly; and in the posterior approach, inferomedially. The carotid artery may be retracted medially with the opposite hand. Backflow of venous blood signals that the internal jugular vein has been punctured.

   c. Femoral: The skin is pierced (with the bevel of the needle directed anteriorly) medial to the femoral artery pulse and directed superiorly. Backflow of venous blood indicates that the femoral vein has been punctured.

6. Guidewire and dilator placement. The syringe is disconnected, and a guidewire is passed. Resistance to the guidewire indicates that the needle tip is not in the vein and should be repositioned with the syringe. **Do not force the guidewire**: Guidewire kinking at best, and vessel puncture at worst, may result. The skin over the guidewire entrance is cut with a No. 11 scalpel blade to facilitate placement of the dilator and catheter. The dilator is passed over the guidewire, using a twisting motion through the soft tissues.

7. Catheter placement. After removing the dilator, the catheter is passed similarly, and the guidewire is removed. For internal jugular and subclavian lines, the catheter tip should be at the junction of the superior vena cava and the right atrium. Approximate measured distances from the catheter tip to the skin exit site are: right subclavian, 15 cm; left subclavian, 18 cm; right internal jugular, 10 cm; left internal jugular, 12 cm. The femoral catheter may be placed to the hub (20 to 30 cm, depending on catheter length). An introducer is placed by passing it over the dilator, and the dilator and guidewire are then removed. Easy return of blood from all catheter ports should be matched by easy flushing with saline. All hubs are secured. The catheter is sutured to the skin in several places with 3–0 nylon suture. Povidone-iodine ointment and a sterile dressing are applied.

Complications[2]
1. Placement
   a. Pneumothorax.
   b. Hemothorax.

   c. Mediastinal hematoma.

   d. Arterial puncture or placement.

   e. Thoracic duct laceration (left neck).

   f. Cardiac dysrhythmias.

   g. Superficial hematoma.

   h. Nerve puncture.

2. Catheter

   a. Tip improperly positioned intravascularly (e.g., either not at the superior vena cava–right atrium junction or in the right atrium.

   b. Tip positioned extraluminally.

   c. Occlusion of catheter.

   d. Leak in catheter.

3. Long term

   a. Infection

   b. Venous thrombosis

Discussion

The choice of site depends on the technical skill and preference of the physician as well as the long-term use of the line. The line that is easiest to care for is the subclavian; femoral lines have fewer complications associated with placement but have a greater risk of deep venous thrombosis. The most direct route to the right atrium is through the right internal jugular vein. According to Poiselle's law, rapid infusion requires a short, large-diameter catheter. Introducer catheters fit this description, but standard triple-lumen catheters do not and thus must not be used for initial resuscitation.

Venous Cut-down

Indication. Inability to obtain peripheral or introducer central venous access, usually because of severe hypovolemia and venous collapse.

Contraindications. Percutaneous central access obtainable; previous vein stripping or harvest.

Technique

1. Site: The most common location is the saphenous vein at the ankle because of its constant anatomy and superficial location. Other sites include the saphenous vein in the groin (just distal to the saphenofemoral junction), and the antecubital fossa in the upper extremity.

2. Prepare the skin.

3. Administer local anesthesia (in the awake patient).

4. Make a transverse incision through the skin 2 cm anterior and 2 cm superior to the medial malleolus (Fig. 24–5).

5. Spread the subcutaneous tissues with a hemostat; the vein, usually collapsed, "pops out" from the surrounding tissue, and the clamp is spread beneath the vein.

6. Obtain distal venous control with a 3–0 silk suture tie; proximal control is obtained with a proximal suture, *untied.*

7. Perform a transverse venotomy between the sutures with a No. 11 scalpel blade by approaching the vein from the side and cutting up.

8. Insert a large-gauge catheter or even the intravenous tubing through the

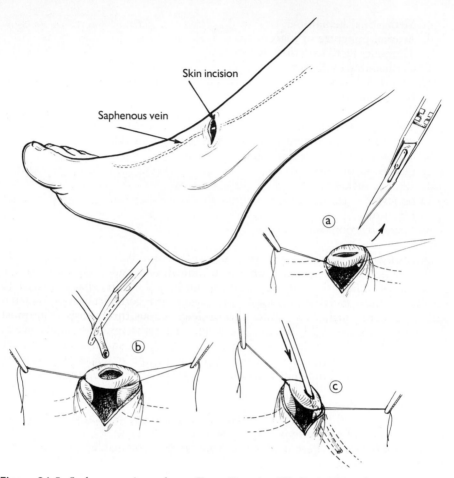

Figure 24–5. Saphenous vein cutdown. (From Dunmire SM, Paris PM: Atlas of Emergency Procedures. Philadelphia, WB Saunders, 1994, p. 205.)

venotomy and advance it proximally, tying the proximal suture. The venous lumen can be visualized by using a "vein pic," either a commercially available device or one made by bending the tip of an 18-gauge needle.

9. Close the skin with 3–0 silk suture and apply a dressing.

Complications
1. Infection.
2. Superficial hematoma.
3. Injury to the saphenous nerve, which often lies adherent to the vein. This results in a variety of paresthesias and dysthesias over the medial foot and distal leg, depending on the nature of the injury.
4. Phlebitis.

Discussion. A cut-down is usually performed in a patient in extremis. Vascular access is achieved within 30 seconds. The sequence is "cut, spread, isolate and incise (the vein), in (with the catheter or tubing)."

Intraosseous Puncture[1]
Indications. Inability to obtain emergent venous access in children less than 7 years of age.

Contraindications. Ability to obtain venous access with another route; injury proximal to the tibia on the side of the proposed puncture.

Technique
1. Positioning: The patient should be supine, with the knee flexed to 30 degrees.
2. Site: Two centimeters inferior to the tibial tuberosity on the anteromedial surface of the proximal tibia.
3. Prepare and drape the skin.
4. Infiltrate local anesthetic in the awake patient.
5. Puncture the skin at a 90-degree angle to the ground (45 to 60 degrees to the skin—the knee is bent), with the bevel of the needle directed toward the foot, using a short, large-bore bone-marrow-aspiration needle or a short 18-gauge spinal needle with a stylet (Fig. 24–6). Advance the needle using a gentle twisting motion through the cortex of the bone and into the marrow.
6. Remove the stylet and aspirate the marrow with a 10-ml syringe filled with 5 ml of saline. Aspiration of marrow indicates appropriate entrance. Saline can be used to expel clot that may occlude the needle. Proper placement is further verified when the needle remains upright without support and the intravenous solution flows freely without subcutaneous infiltration. Infuse the saline solution.
7. Screw the needle in further until the hub rests on the skin. Stabilize the apparatus with a generous dressing preceded by an application of antibiotic ointment.

Complications
1. Infection.
2. Hematoma.
3. Osteomyelitis.
4. Incorrect placement, resulting in subcutaneous or subperiosteal infusion or through-and-through puncture of the bone.
5. Physeal plate injury (hence the reason for bending the knee so that the needle is directed toward the foot).

Discussion. Intraosseous puncture requires frequent reassessment to ensure continued placement within the marrow cavity. It must be discontinued as soon as other routes of venous access can be obtained to prevent long-term complications such as osteomyelitis and transient bone marrow hypocellularity.

Cardiac Access

Pericardiocentesis
Indication. Suspected pericardial tamponade (most commonly in patients

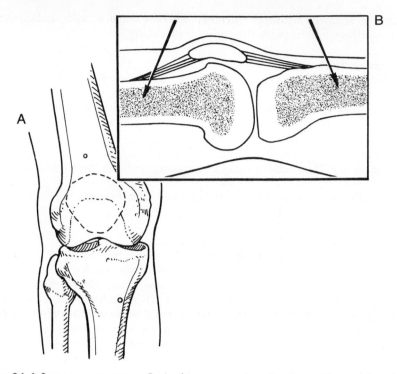

Figure 24–6. Intraosseous puncture. Optimal intraosseous insertion sites are those with a relatively flat surface, such as the anterior medial surface of the tibia, about 2 cm below the tibial tuberosity. (From Walsh-Sukys M, Krug S [eds]: Procedures in Infants and Children. Philadelphia, WB Saunders, 1997, p. 135.)

with penetrating trauma located within the "precordial box"); temporizing release of tamponade when this has been diagnosed by echocardiogram or ultrasound while awaiting the resources to correct the source of the tamponade.

Contraindications. In the stable patient, other means of diagnosing pericardial tamponade, such as echocardiography, trauma ultrasound, or pericardial window (see next section); in the unstable patient, resources to perform an emergent thoracotomy or sternotomy.

Technique

1. Establish electrocardiographic (ECG) monitoring.
2. Perform surgical preparation. Local anesthesia is rarely indicated given patient instability.
3. Site: Left of the xyphoid process, just inferior to the xyphochondral junction.
4. Puncture: Using an 18-gauge, 15-cm long catheter over a needle attached to a syringe, puncture the skin at a 45-degree angle to the skin, aiming cephalad toward the tip of the left scapula, applying constant back pressure on the syringe.
5. Aspiration of blood with improvement in blood pressure indicates release

of tamponade; if hypotension worsens, ventricular puncture should be suspected.

6. After the initial aspiration of blood, remove the needle, leaving the catheter within the pericardial sac; a three-way stopcock is attached to the catheter to allow further aspiration if tamponade recurs (while the patient progresses to the operating room).

7. Suture the catheter in place, and apply a sterile cover dressing.

Complications
1. Puncture of ventricle.
2. Laceration of coronary vessels.
3. Partial thickness laceration of myocardium.
4. Iatrogenic hemopericardium with tamponade, secondary to the complications 1 to 3.
5. Ventricular dysrhythmias.
6. Injury to other intrathoracic structures.
   a. Lung, leading to pneumothorax.
   b. Aorta, leading to hemothorax or mediastinal hematoma.
   c. Esophagus, leading to mediastinitis.
   d. Inferior vena cava, leading to hemopericardium.
7. Injury to peritoneal structures, with consequent hemoperitoneum or peritonitis.
8. Pericarditis.
9. Superficial bleeding.
10. Superficial infection.

Discussion. Pericardiocentesis is a blind tap of the pericardial sac that relies on a knowledge of anatomy. The pericardial base lies on the superior surface of the mid-diaphragm, which is at the level of the xyphoid base. Mediastinal shift changes the anatomy and requires redirection of the needle. The needle is directed to the left scapular tip because most of the pericardial sac lies to the left.

Pericardiocentesis is both diagnostic and therapeutic for cardiac tamponade but is not therapeutic for correction of the injury that caused the tamponade. The quality of the aspirated blood is not helpful for diagnosis; nonclotting blood, the classic teaching, is present in only 50% of patients with tamponade, no better than a coin toss. Thus, pericardiocentesis is a temporizing measure for nonsurgeon physicians; diagnosis is better made with ultrasound or the pericardial window and, in the unstable patient, emergent thoracotomy.

Pericardial Window[3]
Indication. Suspected pericardial tamponade.

Contraindication. Stable patient in an institution that has ultrasound capability.

Technique
1. Perform surgical preparation and draping.
2. Administer general anesthesia.
3. Site: Xiphoid process.
4. Incision (Fig. 24–7): Center the incision on the xiphoid process, cutting

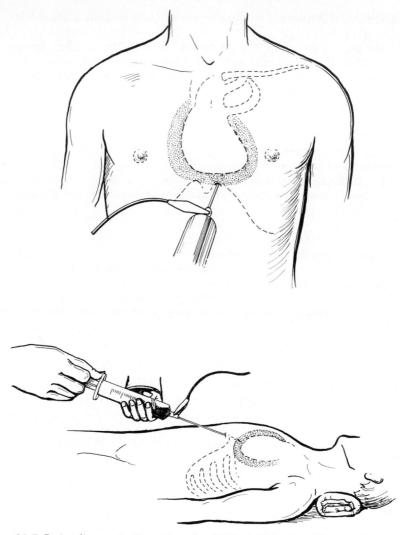

Figure 24–7. Pericardiocentesis. (From Dunmire SM, Paris PM: Atlas of Emergency Procedures. Philadelphia, WB Saunders, 1994, p. 64.) [Do not use alligator clips in the trauma patient—only in a stable, medical patient.]

through skin and subcutaneous fat. The midline fascia is incised, allowing further exposure along the lateral borders of the xiphoid. The xiphoid is removed by grasping it with a Kocher clamp and dividing its base. The peritoneum must not be entered.

5. Expose the pericardium by lifting up on the sternum and bluntly dissecting away the anterior mediastinal fat.

6. If the pericardium is obviously bulging with blood and tamponade is not immediately life-threatening, do not open the pericardium but perform a median sternotomy instead. Otherwise, the pericardium is grasped with an

Allis clamp, and a small incision is made. Hemopericardium also leads to median sternotomy. Irrigation of the pericardial sac with saline may be useful to rule out a clotted hemopericardium.

7. If no blood is present (in the normal situation, a small amount of serous fluid is seen), close the fascia with a 0 Vicryl suture and the skin with suture or staples.

Complications
1. False-negative result due to clotted blood in the pericardial sac.
2. False-positive result due to pooling of superficial bleeding.
3. Bleeding, superficial and mediastinal.
4. Infection, superficial and mediastinal.
5. Peritoneal entry, with extension of intraperitoneal contamination into pericardium and consequent pericarditis or mediastinitis.
6. Pneumothorax.

Discussion. A subxiphoid, or pericardial, window is an operative procedure using an anterior mediastinal approach to the pericardium that allows a direct diagnosis and treatment of hemopericardium. Complications are minimal, and conversion to median sternotomy for a positive result is readily accomplished.

Emergent (Left Anterolateral) Thoracotomy[3, 4]
Indications. Penetrating thoracic trauma with uncontrolled hemorrhage, deterioration in condition, or cardiac arrest; uncontrolled massive hemothorax; penetrating abdominal trauma with cardiopulmonary arrest in the treatment facility.

Contraindications. Blunt abdominal or thoracic trauma with cardiac arrest; prehospital arrest for more than 10 minutes regardless of mechanism; stable patient with penetrating thoracic or abdominal trauma; surgeon unavailable.

Technique
1. Perform rapid skin preparation and draping.
2. Site: Left fourth intercostal space (level of the inframammary line) from the sternum to the anterior axillary line.
3. Incision: Incise through the skin, intercostal muscles, and pleura; insert chest wall retractor with the handle toward the left axilla. Further exposure can be gained by extending the incision across the sternum into the right fourth intercostal space (Fig. 24–8).
4. Retract the left lung posteriorly or anteriorly, depending on the priority of exposure of the pericardium or the descending aorta.
5. For apparent pericardial tamponade, incise the pericardium longitudinally, parallel with but anterior to the left phrenic nerve. Grasping the distended pericardium can be difficult, and the pericardiotomy can be initiated with the scalpel, followed by scissors.
6. After evacuating blood and clots, mobilize the heart out of the pericardial sac, identify the injury, and control it with direct finger pressure. Alternative control measures include placement of temporary sutures (two 2–0 Ethibond sutures placed parallel to the wound on each side vs. running 3–0 Prolene sutures), application of a vascular clamp for atrial injuries, or insertion of a

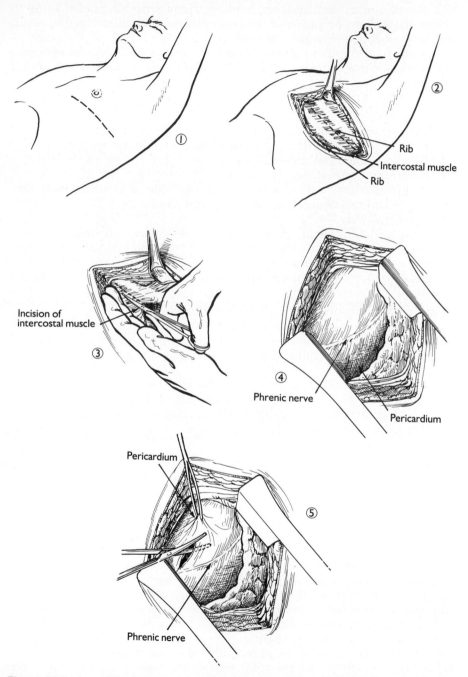

Figure 24–8. Anterolateral thoracotomy. (From Dunmire SM, Paris PM: Atlas of Emergency Procedures. Philadelphia, WB Saunders, 1994, p. 71.)

Foley catheter through the wound and then inflating it (this may cause further tearing, however).

7. Once control of the cardiac wound has been obtained, perform open cardiac massage in the nonbeating heart by placing one hand posterior to the heart and the other anterior, moving compressions from the cardiac apex to the outflow tracts.

8. Aortic cross-clamping is performed by identifying the collapsed aorta anterior to the midthoracic vertebral column, identifying any aortic injury, spreading (with a DeBakey vascular clamp) through the left mediastinal pleura both anterior and posterior to the aorta above the level of injury, and applying the vascular clamp across the aorta, taking care not to injure or include in the clamp the anteriorly located esophagus and vagus nerves.

9. Following further repair in the operating room, the pericardium is closed, chest tubes are placed (or maintained), and the chest is closed by reapproximating the ribs with multiple interrupted figure-of-eight 0-Vicryl sutures and placing subcutaneous and cutaneous running sutures.

Complications
1. Thoracotomy
   a. Pulmonary laceration.
   b. Untied internal mammary artery division.
   c. Intercostal neurovascular injury.
   d. Infection.
2. Pericardiotomy.
   a. Division of phrenic nerve(s).
   b. Laceration of heart or coronary vessel.
3. Aortic cross-clamping.
   a. Injury to descending aorta, esophagus, or vagus nerves.
   b. Clamp position distal to the site of aortic injury.

Discussion. Emergent thoracotomy is a heroic measure performed in patients who are in extremis from penetrating torso trauma. Patients with stab wounds have the best survival rate (to patient hospital discharge) at 38%, whereas those with gunshot wounds fare less well, with only a 4.5% survival rate. This surgical procedure has serious complications and should not be undertaken by nonsurgically trained physicians.

DIAGNOSTIC PROCEDURES

Diagnostic Peritoneal Tap and Lavage

Indications
1. Equivocal abdominal examination.
2. Altered mental status resulting from head injury, drugs or alcohol, or spinal injury, which precludes an adequate abdominal examination.
3. Inaccessibility of patient for further evaluation or serial examinations, such as a patient requiring emergent nonabdominal operations.
4. In penetrating trauma, assessment of transperitoneal penetration, which is rare.

Contraindications

1. Indication for operation (peritonitis, unstable patient with abdominal source of problem).
2. Coagulopathy, cirrhosis.
3. Relative (distorted anatomy): pregnancy, obesity, previous operations (adhesions).

Technique

1. Perform periumbilical and infraumbilical midline surgical preparation, which is rare.
2. Administer local anesthetic.
3. Insert nasogastric tube and decompress the bladder.
4. Site of incision: Junction of upper third with lower two thirds of distance in the midline between the umbilicus and the pubic symphysis. In patients with a pelvic fracture or pregnancy of more than 20 weeks, the site is midline supraumbilical.
5. Make a 3-cm incision through skin, subcutaneous fat, and Scarpa's fascia to the linea alba (Fig. 24–9).
6. Grasp and elevate the linea alba with Kocher or Allis clamps, then incise it.
7. Identify the peritoneum through preperitoneal fat and incise it.
8. Insert a peritoneal dialysis catheter toward the right or left pelvis.
9. Connect a syringe to the catheter and aspirate.
10. If nothing is aspirated, perform lavage: instill 1 liter (or 10 ml/kg) of warmed normal saline or lactated Ringer's solution into the peritoneal cavity through intravenous tubing attached to the catheter. Gently shake the abdomen to assist in the even distribution of the fluid throughout the cavity.
11. After 5 minutes, drain the lavage fluid by putting the (vented) IV bag on the floor, permitting drainage by gravity. Ideally, two thirds of the infused volume should be returned for analysis, but one half is acceptable. Send the entire IV bag to the laboratory for unspun analysis.
12. Remove the catheter and close the linea alba with 2–0 Vicryl suture. Close the skin with suture or staples, and place a sterile dressing.

Complications

1. Abdominal wall bleeding (may cause a false-positive study).
2. Injury to intraperitoneal structures (bowel, distended bladder).
3. Wound infection.

Discussion. Diagnostic peritoneal lavage (DPL) is best considered a diagnostic peritoneal *tap* and lavage. If the tap is revealing, the lavage does not have to be performed, thus saving time. Criteria[5] for a positive test, necessitating operative exploration, include:

Tap: 5 to 10 ml of gross blood, enteric contents, or bile.
Lavage: more than 10^5 red blood cells (RBCs)/ml (with blunt trauma) or 5000 RBCs/ml (with penetrating trauma); more than 500 white blood cells (WBCs)/ml; bacteria; enteric contents; bile; more than 2000 IU/L amylase; lavage fluid draining through chest tube or bladder drainage catheter.

DPL provides an indirect evaluation of injury by determining the presence

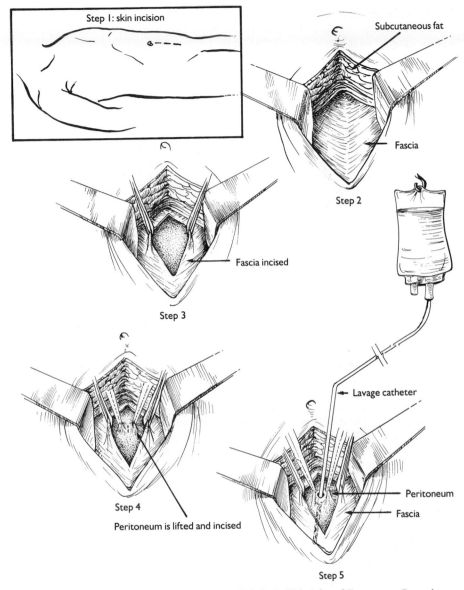

Figure 24–9. Peritoneal lavage. (From Dunmire SM, Paris PM: Atlas of Emergency Procedures. Philadelphia, WB Saunders, 1994, p. 7.)

and the character of the intraperitoneal fluid. From this assessment, a decision is made about the need for operative intervention. When describing the results, it is best to quantitate the findings to avoid misleading conclusions. A truly negative lavage shows no RBCs or WBCs, and so on, yet the term negative lavage is often used to describe the operative decision (i.e., the findings were less than the criteria listed above for operation). The presence of 50,000 RBCs/ml in the lavage fluid is still abnormal, but it does not necessitate operative exploration at that time; observation is still required for any evolving injury.

DPL is very good at finding intraperitoneal injury; it has a 98% sensitivity for detecting intraperitoneal bleeding. However, not all intraperitoneal bleeding (e.g., liver) requires operative intervention, and thus, for the decision to operate, DPL is overly sensitive. It does not find retroperitoneal injuries (pancreas, duodenum) and is less helpful in finding diaphragmatic tears.

Before DPL is performed in a setting that requires patient transfer, a surgeon should be consulted. Often, the delay introduced in the transfer is not justified by the need for the procedure.

Operating Table Angiography

Indications. Exclusion of arterial injury following extremity trauma in a patient with equivocal signs of injury; delineation of the character, exact location, extent, and nature of a known arterial injury (i.e., creation of a "roadmap"); follow-up of an arterial repair (completion angiogram).

Contraindications. In the preoperative phase, a hemodynamically stable patient who can undergo a formal arteriogram in the radiology department.

Technique

1. Perform surgical preparation and draping of the entire extremity of interest.

2. Infiltrate local anesthetic.

3. Obtain arterial access proximal to the level of suspected injury using a 20-gauge needle arterial puncture either transcutaneously or via a cut-down. For the lower extremity, the common or superficial femoral artery is a good choice.

4. Place a radiograph cassette (in its sterile cover) under the area of interest. This is a uniplanar study.

5. Inject 20 to 30 ml of contrast agent (60% Renografin); without inflow occlusion, injection is rapid, and film exposure occurs at the conclusion of the injection. With inflow occlusion, injection is slower (5 to 10 seconds), and is followed by film exposure.

6. Remove catheter and apply direct pressure, or close the arterial puncture site with a single 6–0 Prolene suture.

Complications

1. Missed injury (not typically a biplanar study).
2. Arterial dissection.
3. Contrast reaction.
4. Contrast nephropathy.

Discussion. To exclude arterial injury to an extremity, the clinical examination coupled with ankle/brachial indices and/or a Doppler ultrasound examination is quite useful. The operating table angiogram is most useful when there is simply not enough time to obtain an angiogram, given logistical constraints, the extent of patient injuries, or a compromised extremity.

One-Shot Intravenous Pyelogram

Indications. Gross hematuria resulting from blunt or penetrating injury, or injury promixity; to ensure contralateral renal function and identify renal injuries.

Contraindications. Hemodynamically stable blunt trauma patient who can undergo CT scan.

Technique
1. Establish intravenous access.
2. Inject 1.5 ml/kg of Renografin intravenously.
3. Place abdominal radiograph cassette in position and expose film 5 to 10 minutes after injection.

Complications
1. Contrast reaction.
2. Contrast nephropathy.
3. Inadequate study due to underexposure, delay in obtaining film, or low-volume contrast injection.
4. Missed injury.

Discussion. The role of the one-shot intravenous pyelogram has shrunk within the past decade, largely because of the ability of the CT scan to image better the upper urinary tract and the bladder.[6] Its role is now mostly confined to defining the presence and function of the contralateral kidney—information that is useful in decisions regarding salvage of the injured kidney.

THERAPEUTIC PROCEDURES

Fasciotomy[7]

Indications. Compartment syndrome (intracompartmental pressures >30 torr); vascular compromise to extremity of longer than 4 to 6 hours.

Contraindications. Nonviable extremity.

Technique
1. Perform surgical preparation and anesthesia of the extremity or extremities.
2. Make the incisions and perform compartment decompression (Fig. 24–10).
    a. Leg
       (1) Anterolateral longitudinal incision midway between the fibular shaft and the tibial crest, extending from the level of the tibial plateau to just proximal to the lateral malleolus: The incision is made through the underlying anterolateral fascia, decompressing the anterior compartment, as well as through the anterior intermuscular septum, decompressing the lateral compartment and avoiding the superficial peroneal nerve.
       (2) Posteromedial longitudinal incision, 2 cm posterior to the posterior border of the tibia, extending from the level of the proximal tibia to the medial malleolus: The longitudinal incision is made through the

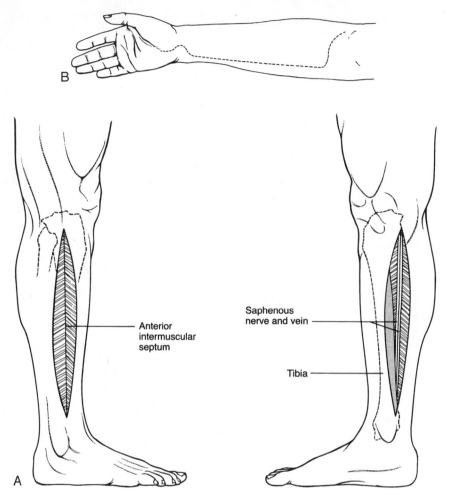

Figure 24–10. *A* and *B*, Fasciotomy. (*A*, from American Academy of Orthopaedic Surgery (AAOS) Instructional Course Lectures, Vol. 32. St. Louis, Mosby, 1983, pp. 519–520. *B*, from Whitesides T Jr, Haney TC, Morimoto K, Hirada H: Clin Orthop 1975; 113:46.)

underlying fascia covering the superficial posterior compartment (gastrocnemius, soleus), avoiding the anteriorly positioned saphenous vein and nerve. The deep posterior compartment is released by elevating the soleus muscle and incising the fascia covering the tibialis posterior and flexor digitorum longus longitudinally.

  b. Forearm

    (1) Volar incision, beginning just superior and medial to the lateral epicondyle of the humerus, extending medially and obliquely across the antecubital fossa and then distally along the ulnar border, turning to the middle finger axis at the wrist and ending at the level of the midthenar eminence. The superficial flexor compartment is released

by incising the fascia longitudinally between the flexor digitorum superficialis and the flexor carpi ulnaris muscles. The deep fascia is exposed by retracting the ulnar neurovascular bundle medially and then incised to the level of the midthenar eminence, ensuring release of the deep flexor compartment and carpal tunnel.

(2) Dorsal incision, starting just distal to the lateral epicondyle and extending longitudinally toward the midline of the wrist at the junction of the middle and distal forearm. The underlying fascia is incised longitudinally, thus releasing the extensor compartment.

3. Apply wet-to-dry saline gauze dressings.
4. Closure is considered at 7 to 10 days, once the process inciting the compartment syndrome as well as the compartment syndrome itself has resolved and all devitalized tissue has been removed. Split-thickness skin grafting and gradual primary closure with skin stretching devices are options.

Complications

1. Inadequate decompression, particularly of the deep posterior compartment of the leg and the deep flexor compartment of the forearm.

2. Injury to the superficial peroneal nerve during the lateral leg fasciotomy or to the saphenous nerve during the posteromedial leg incision.

3. Bleeding.

4. Infection.

Discussion. Compartment syndrome must be considered in patients with crush injuries, fractures, and vascular injuries of the extremity. Pulses are often intact and thus should not be used as criteria to end further investigation. The earliest signs in the awake patient are pain and neurosensory deficits. Compartment pressures can be easily measured using an 18-gauge catheter with fluid-filled tubing transduced to a pressure monitor, or using a variety of other syringe or manometer techniques. The principle behind fasciotomy is simple: release the tight wrap surrounding the muscle compartments.

Percutaneous Suprapubic Cystostomy Tube Placement[8]

Indications. Acute urinary retention with inability to catheterize the bladder through the urethra; urethral disruption.

Contraindications. Ability to place Foley catheter through urethra into bladder; nonpalpable bladder; previous lower abdominal operations; coagulopathy; clot retention; known bladder tumor.

Technique (using Stamey or Cook Urological Suprapubic Cystostomy Trochar Set)

1. Perform surgical preparation and draping.
2. Site of incision: Midline, over the distended bladder, 4 cm superior to the pubis (Fig. 24–11).
3. Infiltrate local anesthetic.
4. Localize bladder with a 22-gauge spinal needle inserted at 60 to 90

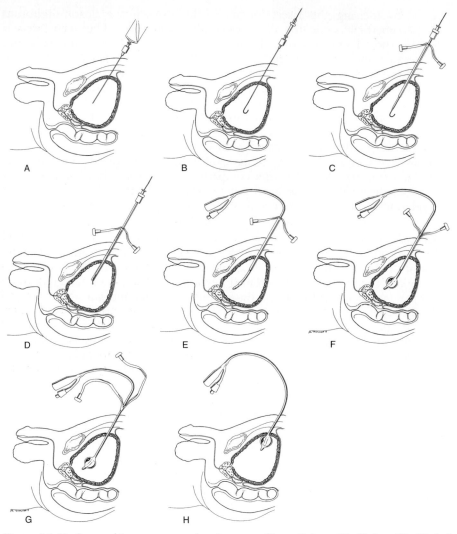

Figure 24–11. Suprapubic cystostomy tube placement. (From Roberts JR, Hedges JR: Clinical Procedures in Emergency Medicine, 4th ed. Philadelphia, WB Saunders, 1998, p. 975.)

degrees, depending on the degree of bladder distention; placement in bladder is confirmed by aspiration of urine.

5. Note the angle and depth of bladder puncture, and remove the spinal needle.

6. Make a stab wound of several millimeters through the skin at the site of the spinal needle puncture.

7. Insert the suprapubic tube (Malecot catheter)/trocar through the skin and into the bladder, again verifying puncture with aspiration of urine. The trocar is then removed, leaving the suprapubic tube in the bladder. The tube is connected to a collection bag.

8. Pull back the Malecot catheter to the anterior bladder wall and then advance it 2 cm to allow for catheter movement and prevent catheter positioning at the trigone.

9. Suture the catheter to the skin, and apply a sterile dressing.

Complications
1. Injury to bowel.
2. Through-and-through bladder perforation.
3. Intraperitoneal catheter placement with urine leak.
4. Retained catheter.
5. Hypotension (vasovagal response).
6. Hematuria.
7. Bladder spasms.
8. Postobstructive diuresis.

Discussion. In patients with nontraumatic bladder outlet obstruction, efforts should be made to catheterize the bladder through the urethra. A history of prostate or urethral surgery as well as urethral infections may indicate a bladder neck or urethral stricture. Adequate lubrication, correct catheter size (in patients with benign prostatic hypertrophy a 20- or 22-Fr catheter may be needed to push through the area), and use of a Coudé-tip catheter are all elements of success. In patients with previous surgery, ultrasound may be used to localize the bladder and direct the catheter away from potentially adhesed loops of bowel. Finally, open surgical cystostomy is always an option; it is performed through a small midline incision, with the cystostomy placed through two 2–0 chromic pursestring sutures. A separate lower quadrant exit site is used.

Tracheostomy[9]

Indications. Provision of secure airway for management of upper airway obstruction, long-term bronchopulmonary toilet, and long-term ventilatory support; emergently, crushed larynx; pediatric surgical airway.

Contraindications. Coagulopathy, infection.

Technique
1. In patients without cervical spine injuries, position the neck in hyperextension using a shoulder roll.
2. Perform surgical preparation and drape.
3. Incision: There is a choice between vertical and horizontal incisions. The vertical incision, directly over the trachea, extends from the cricoid cartilage to above the sternal notch; the horizontal transverse incision is made 2 cm above the sternal notch (Fig. 24–12).
4. Separate the strap muscles in the midline (dividing the investing layer of the deep cervical fascia).
5. Retract the thyroid isthmus superiorly (dividing the pretracheal layer of the deep cervical fascia).
6. Make a 1.5-cm incision vertically through the second and third tracheal

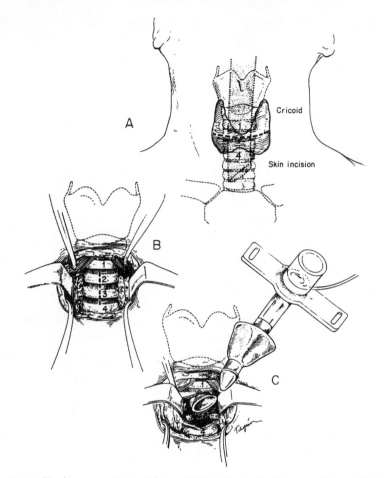

Figure 24–12. Tracheostomy. (From Sabiston DC Jr: Textbook of Surgery, 15th ed. Philadelphia, WB Saunders, 1997, p. 1816.)

rings. This incision is opened with a tracheal spreader when the tracheostomy tube is ready for insertion.

7. Place tracheal stay sutures (2–0 Prolene) at each corner of the tracheotomy (these are helpful in replacing the tube if it is dislodged).

8. Place the tracheostomy tube as the endotracheal tube is removed. Placement is confirmed by bag ventilation.

9. Secure the tracheostomy to the neck with cloth tape through the flange margins and with silk sutures at the flange margins.

Complications
1. Placement
   a. Bleeding.
   b. False subfascial passage.
   c. Injury to recurrent laryngeal nerve or esophagus.

    d. Pneumothorax.
2. Mechanical
    a. Tube obstruction.
    b. Dislodgement.
3. Long-term
    a. Stomal infection.
    b. Subglottic stenosis.
    c. Granulation tissue bleeding.
    d. Tracheoinnominate fistula.
    e. Dysphagia.

Discussion. Emergent tracheostomy is a difficult procedure, particularly when the anatomy is distorted and the neck cannot be extended. Thus, its indications are limited. Elective tracheostomy, on the other hand, is more readily accomplished, largely owing to the stability of the patient and the environment in which it is performed. Tracheostomy can be accomplished percutaneously, using a Seldinger guidewire technique and sequential dilators. It is imperative to confirm guidewire placement endoscopically before initiating the dilator sequence to ensure that posterior tracheal wall perforation has not occurred.

References

1. American College of Surgeons, Committee on Trauma: Advanced Trauma Life Support—Program for Physicians. Chicago, American College of Surgeons, 1993.
2. Mansfield PF, Hohn DC, Fornage BD, Gregurich MA, Ota DM: Complications and failures of subclavian vein catheterization. N Engl J Med 1994;331:1735–1738.
3. Stain SC, Stiles GM: Initial procedures—Resuscitation. *In* Donovan AJ (ed): Trauma Surgery: Techniques in Thoracic, Abdominal, and Vascular Surgery. St. Louis, Mosby-Year Book, 1994, p. 37.
4. Feliciano DV, Mattox KL: Indications, technique, and pitfalls of emergency center thoracotomy. Surg Rounds, Dec 1991;12:26.
5. Lucas CE: Percutaneous diagnostic puncture of the peritoneal cavity. Surgical Residents' Newsletter (Ann Surg) 1993;3(8):3.
6. Stevenson J, Battistella FD: The "one-shot" intravenous pyelogram: Is it indicated in unstable trauma patients before celiotomy? J Trauma 1994;36(6):828.
7. Rorabeck CH: A practical approach to compartment syndromes. *In* American Academy of Orthopaedic Surgeons: Instructional Course Lectures, Vol. 32. St. Louis, CV Mosby, 1983.
8. Quimby GF, Menon M: Percutaneous cystostomy. *In* Rippe JM, Irwin RS, Fink MP, Cerra FB (eds): Procedures and Techniques in Intensive Care Medicine. Boston, Little, Brown & Co, 1995, p. 257.
9. Silva WE, Harris J: Tracheostomy. *In* Rippe JM, Irwin RS, Fink MP, Cerra FB (eds): Procedures and Techniques in Intensive Care Medicine. Boston, Little, Brown & Co, 1995, p. 168.

Index

Note: Page numbers in *italics* refer to illustrations; page numbers followed by t refer to tables.